CLAUDE TIHON, Ph.D.

MITOMYCIN C

CURRENT STATUS AND NEW DEVELOPMENTS

MITOMYCIN C

CURRENT STATUS AND NEW DEVELOPMENTS

Edited by

Stephen K. Carter
Northern California Cancer Program
Palo Alto, California

Stanford University Medical Center
Stanford, California

University of California
San Francisco, California

Stanley T. Crooke
Bristol Laboratories
Syracuse, New York

Baylor College of Medicine
Houston, Texas

Upstate Medical Center
Syracuse, New York

Assisted by
Nancy A. Alder
Syracuse, New York

ACADEMIC PRESS   New York   San Francisco   London   1979
A Subsidiary of Harcourt Brace Jovanovich, Publishers

ACADEMIC PRESS, INC.
111 Fifth Avenue, New York, New York 10003

United Kingdom Edition published by
ACADEMIC PRESS, INC. (LONDON) LTD.
24/28 Oval Road, London NW1 7DX

Library of Congress Cataloging in Publication Data
Main entry under title:

Mitomycin C : current status and new developments.

    1.   Cancer—Chemotherapy.   2.   Mitomycin C—
Testing   I. Carter, Stephen K.   II. Crooke,
Stanley T.   III. Alder, Nancy A.   [DNLM:
1. Mitomycin—Therapeutic use.   2. Neoplasms—
Drug Therapy.   QV269 M684]
RC271.M53M57   616.9'94'061   79-14574
ISBN 0-12-161560-X

PRINTED IN THE UNITED STATES OF AMERICA

79 80 81 82   9 8 7 6 5 4 3 2 1

CONTENTS

CONTRIBUTORS

Numbers in parentheses indicate the pages on which authors' contributions begin.

BERTIE F. ARGYRIS (61), *Department of Microbiology, College of Medicine, State University of New York Upstate Medical Center, Syracuse, New York 13210*

LAURENCE H. BAKER (77, 121, 159, 219, 231), *Department of Oncology, Wayne State University School of Medicine, Detroit, Michigan 48201*

R. BRUCE BRACKEN (205), *Department of Urology, The University of Texas System Cancer Center, M.D. Anderson Hospital and Tumor Institute, Houston, Texas 77025*

WILLIAM T. BRADNER (33), *Antitumor Biology, Bristol Laboratories, P.O. Box 657, Syracuse, New York 13201*

DARRELL Q. BROWN (69), *Department of Radiation Therapy, American Oncologic Hospital, Philadelphia, Pennsylvania 19111*

*THOMAS BUROKER (183), *Department of Oncology, Wayne State University School of Medicine, Detroit, Michigan 48201*

PRAVIT CADNAPAPHORNCHAI (219), *Department of Medicine, Wayne State University School of Medicine, Detroit, Michigan 48201*

STEPHEN K. CARTER (251), *Northern California Cancer Program, 1801 Page Mill Road, Palo Alto, California 94304; Department of Medicine, Stanford University, Stanford, California; Department of Medicine, University of California, San Francisco, California*

ROBERT B. CATALANO (189), *Department of Medicine, American Oncologic Hospital, Philadelphia, Pennsylvania 19111*

ROBERT L. COMIS (83, 129), *Section of Hematology/Oncology, State University Hospital of New York Upstate Medical Center, Syracuse, New York 13210*

BASIL CONSIDINE (183), *Department of Radiology, Wayne State University Medical School, Detroit, Michigan 48201*

JUAN J. CORREA (231), *Department of Oncology, Wayne State University School of Medicine, Detroit, Michigan 48201*

STANLEY T. CROOKE (1, 41, 83), *Bristol Laboratories, P.O. Box 657, Syracuse, New York 13201; Department of Pharmacology, Baylor College of Medicine, Houston, Texas 77025; Department of Pharmacology, Upstate Medical Center, Syracuse, New York 13210*

*Currently at The Iowa Research Oncology Association, 1603 22nd Street, West Des Moines, Iowa 50265

YERACH DASKAL (41), *Electronmicroscopy Unit, Department of Pharmacology, Baylor College of Medicine, Houston, Texas 77030*

MICHAEL D. DeMATTIA (231), *Department of Oncology, Michigan State University, East Lansing, Michigan 48824*

ROBERT J. FRAILE (121), *Department of Oncology, Wayne State University School of Medicine, Detroit, Michigan 48201*

MICHAEL A. FRIEDMAN (113), *Cancer Research Institute, University of California School of Medicine, San Francisco, California 94143*

SANDRA J. GINSBERG (83), *Section of Hematology/Oncology, State University Hospital of the Upstate Medical Center, Syracuse, New York 13210*

THOMAS E. GODFREY (91), *Department of Medicine, Loma Linda University Medical Center, Loma Linda, California 92354*

MANUEL L. GUTIERREZ (213), *Department of Clinical Cancer Research, Bristol Laboratories, P.O. Box 657, Syracuse, New York 13201*

DAVID T. HARRIS (69, 189), *Department of Medicine, American Oncologic Hospital, Philadelphia, Pennsylvania 19111*

LANCE HEILBRUN (145), *Southwest Oncology Group, Biostatistical Office, 6723 Bertner Drive, Houston, Texas 77030*

DANIEL F. HOTH (133), *Division of Medical Oncology, Vincent T. Lombardi Cancer Research Center, Georgetown University Medical Center, Washington, D.C. 20007*

YUKIO INUYAMA (173), *Department of Otorhinolaryngology, School of Medicine, Keio University, 35 Shinano machi, Shinyu-ku-ku, Tokyo, Japan*

DOUGLAS JOHNSON (205), *Department of Urology, The University of Texas System Cancer Center, M. D. Anderson Hospital and Tumor Institute, Houston, Texas 77025*

LAWRENCE S. KOONS (69, 189), *Hematology–Oncology Associates, P.A., 1314 Park Avenue, Plainfield, New Jersey 07060*

LAWRENCE P. LEICHMAN (121), *Department of Oncology, Wayne State University School of Medicine, Detroit, Michigan 48201*

J. WILLIAM LOWN (5), *Department of Chemistry, University of Alberta, Edmonton T6G 2G2, Alberta, Canada*

JACK S. MACDONALD (133), *Division of Medical Oncology, Vincent T. Lombardi Cancer Research Center, Georgetown University Medical Center, Washington, D.C. 20007*

SILVANA MARTINO (231), *Department of Oncology, Wayne State University School of Medicine, Detroit, Michigan 48201*

TERUO MISHINA (193), *Department of Urology, Kyoto Prefectural University of Medicine, Kawaramachi-Hirokoji, Kamigyo-ku, Kyoto, Japan*

TADAAKI MIYAMOTO (163), *Hospital, National Institute of Radiological Sciences, Anagawa-4, Chiba City, Chiba Prefecture, Japan*

LEE ROY MORGAN (101), *Department of Pharmacology and Medicine, Louisiana State University Medical Center, New Orleans, Louisiana 70012*

NORMAN NIGRO (183), *Department of Surgery, Wayne State University School of Medicine, Detroit, Michigan 48201*

FRANK J. PANETTIERE (145), *Department of Medicine, Division of Hematology–Oncology, University of Texas Medical Branch, Galveston, Texas 77550*

RICHARD J. POLLARD (231), *Department of Pathology, Harper-Grace Hospital, Detroit, Michigan 48201*

VORAVIT RATANATHARATHORN (219), *Department of Oncology, Wayne State University School of Medicine, Detroit, Michigan 48201*

STEVEN D. REICH (243), *Clinical Cancer Research, Bristol Laboratories, P.O. Box 657, Syracuse, New York 13201*

WILLIAM A. REMERS (27), *College of Pharmacy, University of Arizona, Tuscon, Arizona 85721*

BARBARA F. ROSENBERG (219), *Department of Pathology, William Beaumont Hospital, Royal Oak, Michigan 48072*

JUDITH S. RUBINSTEIN (69), *Department of Radiation Therapy, American Oncologic Hospital, Philadelphia, Pennsylvania 19111*

MICHAEL K. SAMSON (121), *Department of Oncology, Wayne State University School of Medicine, Detroit, Michigan 48201*

PHILIP S. SCHEIN (133), *Division of Medical Oncology, Vincent T. Lombardi Cancer Research Center, Georgetown University Medical Center, Washington, D.C. 20007*

FREDERICK P. SMITH (133), *Division of Medical Oncology, Vincent T. Lombardi Cancer Research Center, Georgetown University Medical Center, Washington, D.C. 20007*

VAINUTIS K. VAITKEVICIUS (77, 183, 219), *Department of Oncology, Wayne State University School of Medicine, Detroit, Michigan 48201*

HIROKI WATANABE (193), *Department of Urology, Kyoto Prefectural University of Medicine, Kawaramachi-Hirokoji, Kamigyo-ku, Kyoto, Japan*

PAUL V. WOOLLEY (133), *Division of Medical Oncology, Vincent T. Lombardi Cancer Research Center, Georgetown University Medical Center, Washington, D.C. 20007*

PREFACE

Mitomycin C is an antitumor antibiotic that has demonstrated activity against a number of human neoplasms. Two problems have impeded its utilization, however: significant delayed cumulative myelosuppression and rapid emergence of resistance. With the development of the high-dose intermittent schedule, the myelosuppression has become manageable, and mitomycin C has undergone a renaissance of interest. Consequently, significant new information has evolved both in the clinic and in preclinical studies.

The purposes, then, of this volume are to provide a historical perspective on the development of mitomycin C, to summarize the recent developments, including studies on analogs, and perhaps to suggest new directions for future research. Thus, chapters such as those on the molecular mechanisms of mitomycin C (Lown) or on the morphological effects of mitomycin C (Daskal and Crooke) will be of interest to molecular biologists and pharmacologists. Chapters discussing clinical studies such as the FAM regimen (Schein, MacDonald, Smith, Hoth, and Woolley), or the use of mitomycin C in squamous cell carcinoma of the cervix (Baker and Miyamoto), or on the clinical pharmacology of mitomycin C (Reich) will be of interest to clinicians. Moreover, several chapters are directed to recently acquired information on unusual toxicities, and these are of interest and importance to clinicians.

Chapter 1

MITOMYCIN C: AN OVERVIEW[1]

Stanley T. Crooke

I. INTRODUCTION

Mitomycin C is a highly toxic antitumor antibiotic that has demonstrated activity against a variety of human malignancies. Although mitomycin C has been studied clinically for more than 20 years, only in the recent past has information been generated that allows enhanced clinical utility. As a result, interest in mitomycin C has increased, and thus the papers presented in this symposium are particularly timely. The purpose of this paper is to provide a brief overview as an orientation for those that follow.

II. CHEMISTRY

Mitomycin C is isolated from *Streptomyces caespitosus* as blue violet crystals, and is closely related to mitomycin A and pofiromycin. The structures of mitomycin B and porfiromycin are shown in Fig. 1 (Wakaki *et al.*, 1958; Webb *et al.*, 1962). It has a molecular weight of 334, and is soluble in water and organic solvents.

[1] These studies were supported in part by Grant No. CA-10893-10, and Contract No. N01-CM-77147 awarded by the National Cancer Institute.

1

Mitomycin C is an alkylating agent, and has three potentially active groups: a quinone, a urethane, and an aziridine ring (Phillips *et al.,* 1960; Schwartz *et al.,* 1963). For antitumor activity the carbamate must be reduced and the methoxy group lost (Iyer and Szybalski, 1963; Iyer and Syzbalski, 1964). When activated it is a bifunctional or trifunctional alkylating agent.

Numerous analogs of mitomycin C have been prepared, and in subsequent papers several newer analogs will be discussed. From these studies a number of generalizations have been derived:

1. The aziridine ring is not essential for antibacterial activity, but is for antineoplastic activity.
2. Low quinone reduction potential enhances activity.
3. Increasing water solubility and decreasing lipophilic properties result in enhanced antitumor activity.
4. Decreased binding to proteins results in increased activity.
5. Substitutions on positions X, Y, or Z have significant effects on activity (Fig. 1).

III. MECHANISM OF ACTION

Mitomycin C and analogs are potent alkylating agents when activated. Recent studies have shown that mitomycin B and mitomycin C induce interstrand and intrastrand cross-links in a variety of types of DNA, and this is dependent on the base composition of the DNA (Iyer and Szybalski, 1963; Lown and Weir, 1978). In addition it has been shown to degrade DNA (Lown and Weir, 1978) and inhibit DNA synthesis (Schwartz *et al.,* 1963). It is most effective during the late G_1 and S phases of the cell cycle.

IV. PHARMACOLOGY

Although mitomycin C is absorbed after oral administration, the absorption is too variable to allow effective oral administration (Crooke *et al.,* 1976). It has also

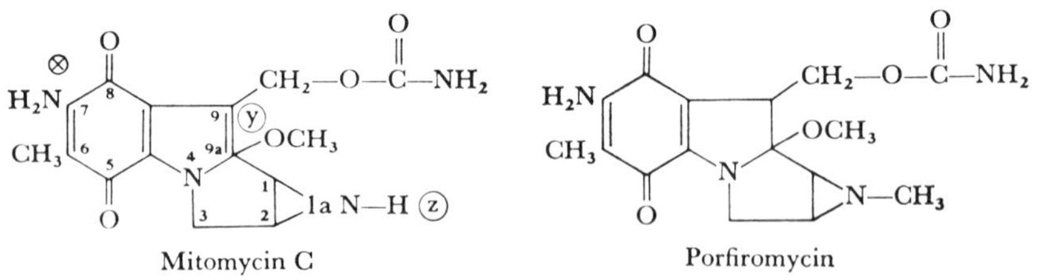

Fig. 1.   Structures of mitomycin and porfiromycin (Crooke and Bradner, 1976).

been reported to be absorbed after intrapleural and intraperitoneal administration (Fujita, 1971), but it is not absorbed after intravesical administration (Crooke *et al.*, 1978).

Surprisingly little information on the metabolism and excretion of mitomycin in humans has been published. It has been reported to be cleared rapidly from blood and to demonstrate nonlinear pharmacokinetics (Fujita, 1971). Only approximately 6% of a 20 mg intravenous dose was recovered in the urine, but little information is available concerning metabolism in humans (Fujita, 1971).

V. DOSAGE SCHEDULES

Although studies in animals demonstrated that intermittent schedules were superior, initial clinical trials employed daily dose schedules in which often mitomycin C was administered until the first evidence of myelosuppression (Crooke and Bradner, 1976). More recently, however, intermittent schedules have resulted in more manageable and predictable hematopoietic toxicities with no reduction in clinical activity (Baker *et al.*, 1976; Crooke and Bradner, 1976).

VI. CLINICAL ACTIVITIES

As a single agent mitomycin C has been shown to be active against adenocarcinomas of various sites, squamous cell carcinomas of various sites, including the cervix, and ovarian carcinomas (Crooke and Bradner, 1976). Responses induced by mitomycin C employed as a single agent have been of uniformly short duration (Crooke and Bradner, 1976).

A variety of interesting combinations have evolved during the past few years. Among the more interesting combinations are the MA (mitomycin C, adriamycin), FAM (5-fluorouracil, adriamycin, mitomycin C), and MOB (mitomycin C, oncovin, and bleomycin) regimens which have induced remissions in a variety of adenocarcinomas and in disseminated squamous cell carcinoma of the cervix.

Intravesically administered mitomycin C has also recently been reported to be highly effective against superficial transitional cell carcinomas of the bladder (Mishina *et al.*, 1975; Crooke *et al.*, 1978). Complete response rates in a phase I-II evaluation appeared to be dose responsive, and doses of 25 mg weekly for 8 weeks resulted in a complete remission rate of approximately 60% with no absorption, no systematic toxicities, and no significant local toxicities.

VII. CLINICAL TOXICITIES

The principal dose-limiting toxicity of mitomycin C is delayed cumulative myelosuppression. The nadirs of leukopenia and thrombocytopenia are typically reached more than 28 days after a single dose (Crooke and Bradner, 1976). The toxicity is so cumulative that in many regimens an automatic dose reduction is employed after two full doses. A number of compounds such as adenine and pyridoxine have been reported to rescue patients from mitomycin-C-induced myelosuppression, but the evidence is unconvincing (Fujimoto, 1966).

Alopecia, rashes, and gastrointestinal toxicities including nausea, vomiting, and diarrhea are other side effects. Extravasation at the site of injection can produce significant cellulitis. Although mitomycin C has been reported to be nephrotoxic, no careful study to determine the actual incidence has been reported. In addition, mitomycin C has been reported to induce pulmonary fibrosis, but again the incidence and severity of this toxicity. Papers in this volume will address the significance of these toxicities.

ACKNOWLEDGMENTS

I would like to thank Steven D. Reich, M.D., M. Dianne DeFuria, and Manuel L. Gutierrez, M.D. for critical review of the manuscript, and Ms. Julie Durantini for excellent typographical assistance.

REFERENCES

Baker, L. H., Izbicki, R. M., and Vaitkevicius, V. K. (1976). *Med. and Ped. Oncol. 21*, 207-213.
Crooke, S. T., and Bradner, W. T. (1976). *Cancer Treat. Rev. 31*, 121-139.
Crooke, S. T., Henderson, M., Samson, M., and Baker, L. H. (1976). *Cancer Treat. Rep. 60*, 1633-1636.
Crooke, S. T., Johnson, D. E., and Bracken, R. B. (1978). *Proc. Am. Soc. Clin. Oncol. 14*, 321.
Fujimoto, S. (1966). *Cancer Chemother. Rep. 50*, 313-318.
Fujita, H. (1971). *Jap. J. Clin. Oncol. 12*, 151-162.
Iyer, V. N., and Szybalski, W. (1963). *Proc. Nat. Acad. Sci. 50*, 355-362.
Iyer, V. N., and Szybalski, W. (1964). *Science 145*, 55-58.
Lown, S. W., and Weir, G. (1978). *Can. J. Biochem. 56*, 296-304.
Mishina, T., Oda, K., Murata, S., Ooe, H., Mori, Y., and Takahashi, T. (1975). *J. Urol. 114*, 217-279.
Phillips, F. S., Schwartz, H. S., and Sternberg, S. S. (1960). *Cancer Res. 20*, 1354-1361.
Samson, M. K., Comis, R. L., Baker, L. H., Ginsberg, S., and Crooke, S. T. (1978). *Cancer Treat. Rep. 62*, 163-165.
Schwartz, H. S., Sternberg, S. S., and Phillips, F. S. (1963). *Cancer Res. 23*, 1125-1136.
Wakaki, S., Marumo, H., Tamioka, K., Shimizu, G., Kato, E., Kamada, H., Kudo, S., and Fujimoto, Y. (1958). *Antibiot. and Chemother. 8*, 228-240.
Webb, J. S., Cosulich, D. B., Mowat, J. H., Patoic, J. B., Broschard, W., Myer, W. F., Williams, R. P., Well, C. F., Fulmer, T., Pidaks, C., and Lancaster, J. E. (1962). *J. Am. Chem. Soc. 84*, 3185.

Chapter 2

THE MOLECULAR MECHANISM OF ANTITUMOR
ACTION OF THE MITOMYCINS[1]

J. William Lown

I. INTRODUCTION

Antitumor agents currently in clinical use fall into four classes: (*a*) alkylating agents, (*b*) antibiotics, (*c*) antimetabolites, and (*d*) a miscellaneous group containing, for example, *cis*-platinum compounds (Montgomery *et al.,* 1970). There is intense interest currently in antitumor antibiotics, many of which show promising clinical properties (Montgomery *et al.,* 1970). Since bacterial infections are a major cause of mortality of cancer patients (Klatersky *et al.,* 1972) and since most chemotherapeutic agents are immunosuppressive, part of the interest in antitumor antibiotics is the expectation that they may provide a twofold action in the patient.

The University of Alberta group has been actively engaged in studying the molecular mechanism of action of a range of naturally occurring antitumor antibiotics and structurally related synthetic compounds including those listed in Fig. 1 (Lown, 1977). These inhibit nucleic acid functions in the cell by a variety of mechanisms. Despite their widely different structures and properties, recent studies, including our own (Lown, 1977), have shown some common features in their chemical modification of nucleic acid cell target sites.

[1] This research was supported by grants from the National Cancer Institute, DHEW, no. 1 R01 CA21488-01; Grant A-2305 from the National Research Council of Canada, and a grant from the National Cancer Institute of Canada.

AMINOQUINONES   ANTHRACYCLINES

MITOMYCIN C   DAUNORUBICIN
MITOMYCIN B   ADRIAMYCIN
STREPTONIGRIN   (CARMINIC ACID)
AZIRIDINOQUINONES

PEPTIDES   NITROSOUREAS

BLEOMYCIN   STREPTOZOTOCIN
NEOCARZINOSTATIN   CHLOROZOTOCIN
CARZINOPHYLLIN

Fig. 1.   Antitumor antibiotics that inhibit nucleic acid functions.

II. THE MOLECULAR MECHANISM OF ACTION OF THE MITOMYCINS

A. Properties of the Mitomycins and Activation

The mitomycin antibiotics were first isolated from *Streptomyces caespitosus* by Hata in Japan (Hata *et al.,* 1956). Mitomycin C, the most thoroughly studied example of this group, contains three recognized carcinostatic groups: aziridine, carbamate, and quinone. It is effective against a range of neoplasms including chorioepithelioma, reticulum cell sarcoma, and seminoma (Szybalski and Iyer, 1967) (see Fig. 2). Mitomycin C and porfiromycin are thus used clinically for the treatment of carcinomas of the breast, lung, colon, and stomach.

Early studies on the mechanism of action by Szybalski and Iyer (1967) established that DNA is the principal cell target site. Enzymatic reductive activation produces the hydroquinone shown which readily loses methanol to give the aziridinomitosene or "activated form" of the antibiotic. Iyer and Szybalski (1963) envisaged three possible reactive sites (indicated by arrows on Fig. 3) and considered that the antibiotic functioned by forming interstrand linkages in DNA as shown (Kirsch, 1967). It occurred to us that a more detailed biochemical study of the course of these reactions with DNA would be useful.

1. Metabolite of Streptomyces Caespitosus

2. Broad Spectrum Antitumor Activity. Especially Effective Against Chronic Myelogenous Leukemia, Epithelial Tumors, Chorioepithelioma, Reticulum Cell Sarcoma and Seminoma

3. Active Against Certain Viruses

4. Toxic, Tolerated Dose ca 40 mg per Course of Treatment

5. Requires NADPH Mediated Reductive Activation

6. Antitumor Action Exerted by Inhibition of DNA Synthesis:—
    a) Covalent Cross-Linking of Replicating DNA
    b) Degradation of DNA

Fig. 2.   Characteristics of mitomycin C.

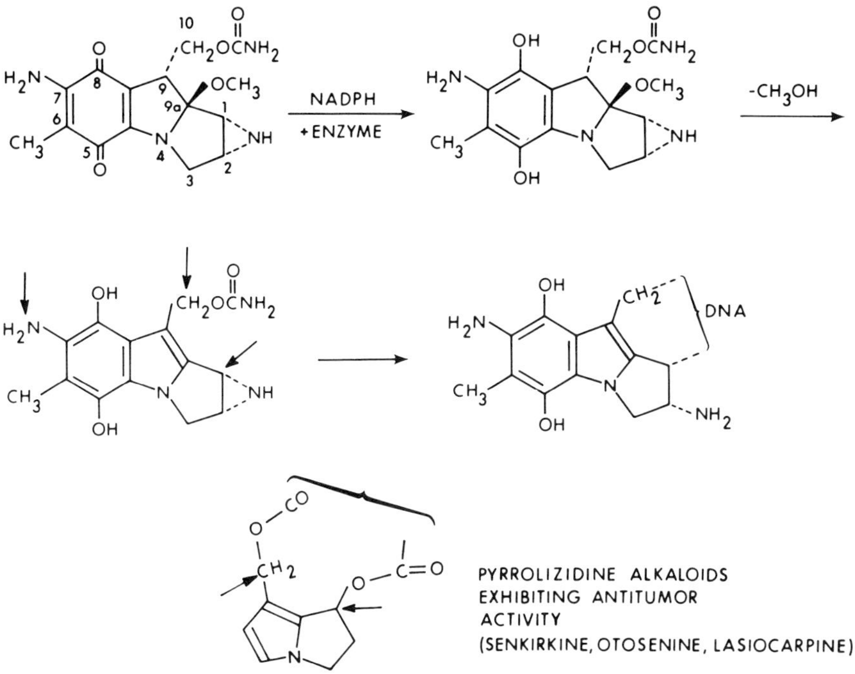

Fig. 3. A mechanism for the activation of mitomycin C with nucleic acids.

In addition other aspects of the mechanism, such as the degradation of DNA by the mitomycins, required investigation (Reich *et al.*, 1960; Wakaki, 1961). Figure 3 also shows the analogy with the pyrrolizidine antitumor alkaloids which also act by alkylating nucleic acids (Culvenor *et al.*, 1969).

B. DNA Cross-Linking and Alkylation

A reexamination of the mechanism of interstrand cross-linking was undertaken. The conventional method of establishing interstrand cross-links in DNA is by hyperchromicity (Hamaguchi and Geiduschek, 1961) or by sedimentation studies (Iyer and Szybalsky, 1963). We have developed an alternative procedure based on the fluorescence properties of the dye ethidium (see Fig. 4) (Lown *et al.*, 1976). This planar molecule is used to stain DNA on gels and binds by intercalation into duplex DNA. When it does so it suffers an enhancement of fluorescence since the quenching of fluorescence that occurs in polar water is removed as it enters the hydrophobic region of the duplex (Morgan and Paetkau, 1972). In the control experiment heat denaturation separates the strands, and provided one uses high pH to prevent formation of regions of self-complementarity, the fluorescence will fall to zero (Morgan and Paetkau, 1972). If, however, one introduces a cross-link by the action of an antibiotic such as mitomycin C or carzinophillin, this serves as a nucleation site for

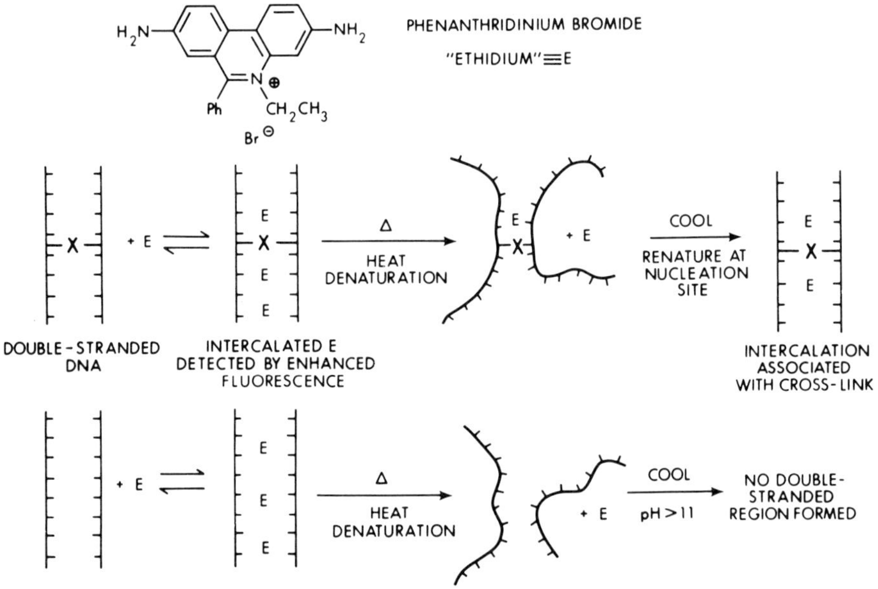

Fig. 4. Ethidium fluorescence assay for determining DNA interstrand cross-linking.

subsequent renaturation after a heating and cooling cycle (Lown *et al.,* 1976). In addition one may readily quantify interstrand cross-linking. Using this method one can detect interstrand cross-linking of DNA by mitomycin C reduced with, for example, sodium borohydride. In addition by using DNAs of different base composition, one can establish that the extent of cross-linking increases with the (G + C) content (Fig. 5) (Lown *et al.,* 1976) suggesting, as was found by Szybalski and Iyer (1967), that there is a preferential reaction of the aziridinomitosene with guanosine groups. We will return to this point later.

It was deemed necessary to have independent confirmation that the fluorescence measurements are recording the extent of cross-linking. This can be done using an S_1-endonuclease (see Fig. 6) which specifically degrades single-stranded DNA but has minimal effect on double-stranded DNA (Lown *et al.,* 1976).

In the control experiment heat-denatured DNA (*Escherichia coli* DNA has a suitable C_0t value) is readily degraded by the enzyme to mononucleotides, and therefore all potential intercalation sites for the ethidium are destroyed. When a cross-link is introduced by activated mitomycin C, again this acts as a nucleation site and promotes rapid renaturation. The resultant duplex DNA is resistant to action by the S_1-endonuclease.

Figure 7 compares the two methods of estimating DNA interstrand cross-linking for three separate runs using mitomycin C (Lown *et al.,* 1976). The agreement is quite good except in run 3 where extended exposure of the duplex DNA to the endonuclease results in more degradation, presumably because of the natural "breathing" of the DNA which momentarily exposes single-stranded regions.

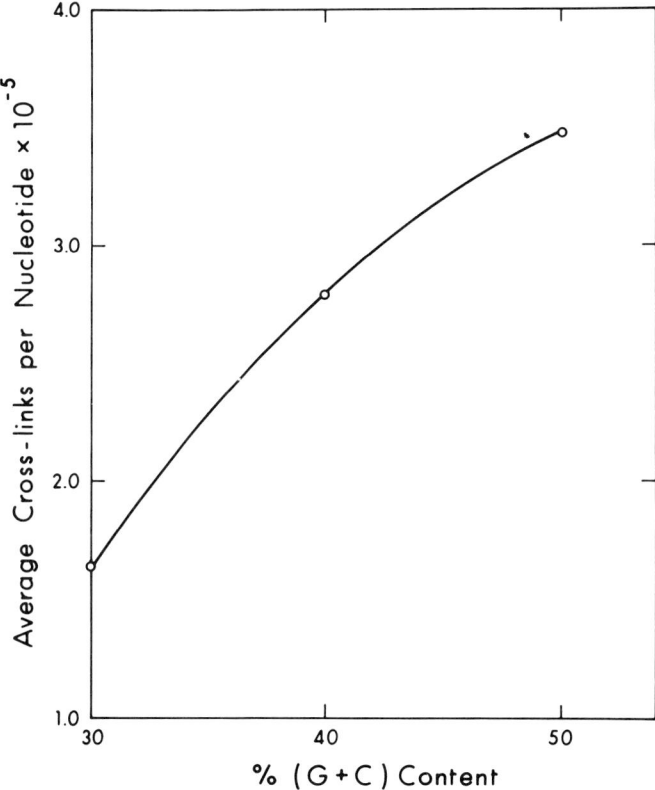

Fig. 5. (G + C) dependence of the efficiency of cross-linking of DNA by mitomycin.

Using the ethidium assay we could also show that mitomycin C will cross-link DNA at somewhat lower pHs but without reductive activation (Fig. 8) (Lown *et al.,* 1976). We will refer to this again later since this may be significant biochemically because tumor tissue is characterized by a somewhat lower pH than normal tissue (Conners *et al.,* 1970). One can refine the assay to obtain information about the position on the base attacked by mitomycin C (Hsiung *et al.,* 1976). Dimethyl sulfate is known to alkylate the N-7 position of guanine (Lawley, 1966) producing a quaternary salt. The latter is sensitive to base and is converted to the zwitterion, then the imidazolium ring is opened and the net effect is to remove the positive charge (Hsiung *et al.,* 1976). Since ethidium itself is positively charged, this process removes the electrostatic repulsion and allows more ethidium to flood back in. The result is a time-dependent increase in the fluorescence readings (Fig. 9). The rate at which this process occurs exactly parallels the rate of the chemical reaction measured independently (Hsiung *et al.,* 1976). In contrast mitomycin C, which certainly alkylates guanosine in DNA, shows no such time dependence. One may conclude that alkylation on guanine takes place at a position other than N-7, probably the 0-6 position. This result agrees with the recent results of Tomasz,

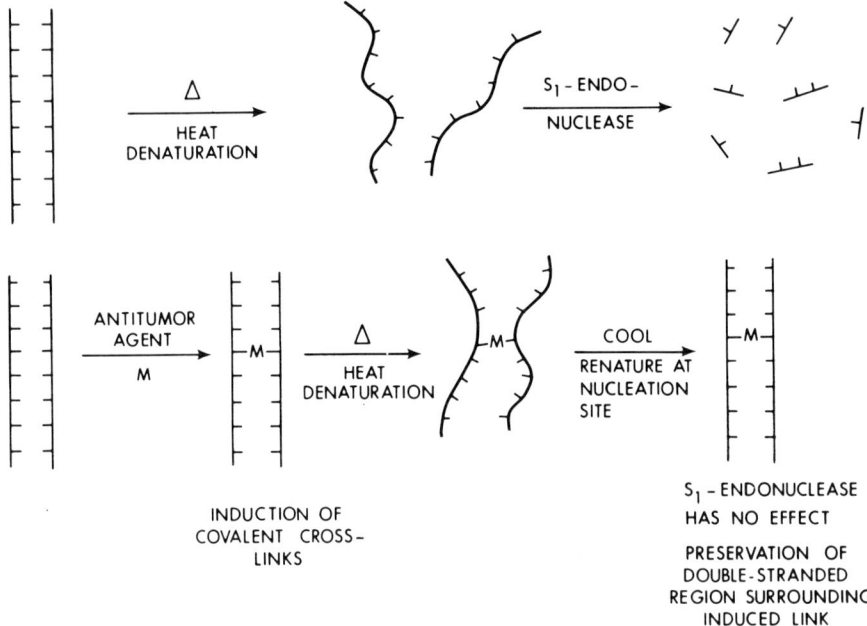

Fig. 6. Confirmation of induction of interstrand cross-linking of λ-DNA by antitumor agents using S_1-endonuclease.

Assay	% Cross-Linked		
Run No.	1	2	3
Ethidium fluorescence – Before dialysis	34	48	61
After dialysis	39	51	60
S_1 Endonuclease – After dialysis	32	51	44

*Runs 1, 2 and 3 contained 0.06, 0.15 and 0.2 mM mitomycin respectively with a constant molar ratio of 96:1 of sodium borohydride to mitomycin.

Fig. 7. Comparison of the cross-linking of *E. coli* DNA assayed by ethidium fluorescence and by S_1-endonuclease sensitivity. Runs 1, 2, and 3 contained 0.06, 0.15 and 0.2 mM mitomycin C respectively with a constant molar ratio of 96:1 of sodium borohydride to antibiotic.

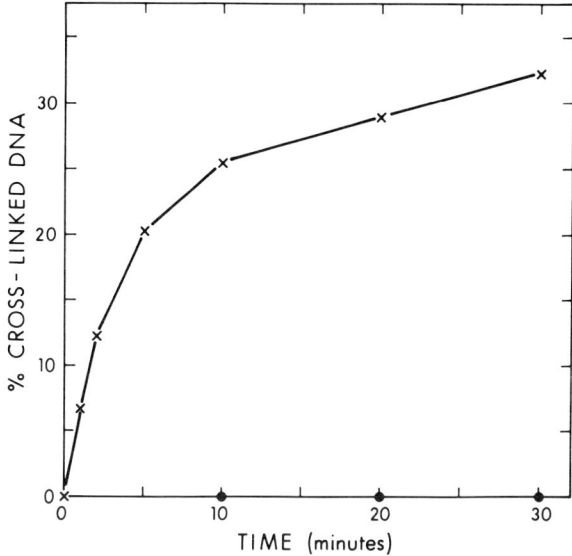

Fig. 8. Cross-linking of DNA by mitomycin C without reductive activation.

who, by using a tritium exchange out procedure, concluded that mitomycin C does not alkylate at N-7 of guanine (Tomasz *et al.*, 1974).

When mitomycin C is attached covalently to DNA it impedes the intercalation of ethidium sterically, and this is revealed by a suppression of the fluorescence which is proportional to the amount bound (Lown *et al.*, 1976). The extent of alkylation thus measured increases markedly as the pH decreases in accord with an initial protonation of the aziridine (Fig. 10). The lower pH of tumor tissue compared with normal tissue referred to earlier (Connors *et al.*, 1970) may again result in preferential reaction here. A similar pH dependence on the rate and extent of DNA interstrand cross-linking is also observed (Lown *et al.*, 1976) (Fig. 11). This suggested to us that the cross-linking proceeds in a stepwise fashion that we could confirm as follows (Fig. 12). Mitomycin C is covalently attached to DNA by a pulsed low pH treatment that produces about 50% cross-linking. The unreacted antibiotic was removed by dialysis which did not affect the extent of cross-linking. The purified antibiotic-DNA complex was then subjected to reduction by $NaBH_4$. An immediate increase in the number of interstrand cross-links was observed confirming the stepwise nature of the cross-linking (Lown *et al.*, 1976). This mitomycin C-DNA complex is of interest itself since it has been found recently that complexes of anthracyclines with DNA show greater clinical effectiveness than the free antibiotic (DiMarco *et al.*, 1975).

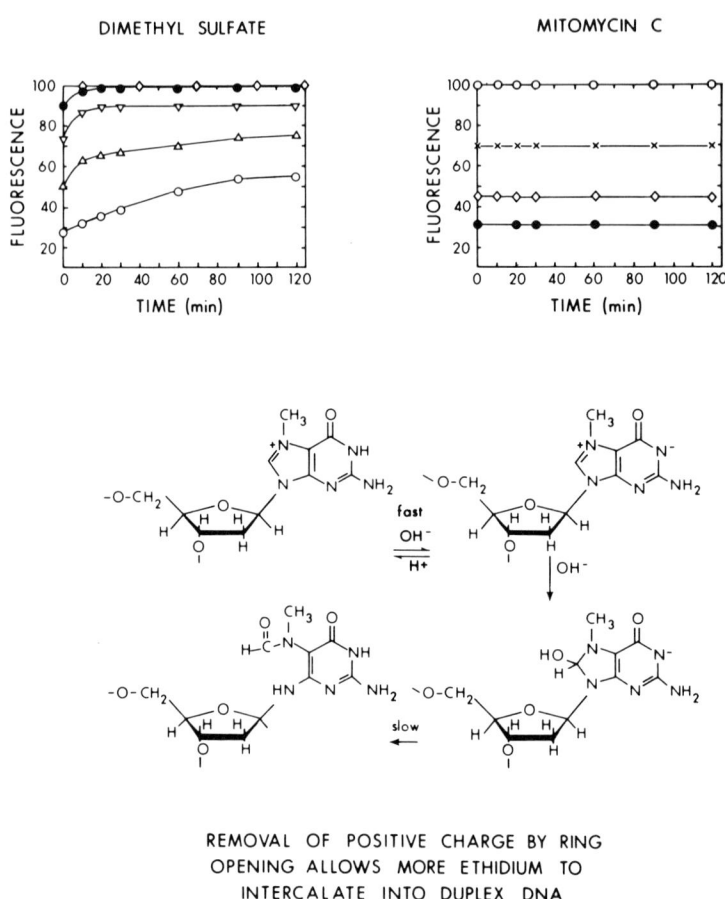

Fig. 9.   Time dependence of ethidium λ-DNA fluorescence at pH 11.8 after alkylation.

C.   Kinetic Assessment of Positional Activity in Mitomycin C

The results indicate that activated mitomycin C may be regarded as a bifunctional alkylator giving rise (Fig. 13) to two resonance-stabilized cationic centers that can react with biological nucleophiles (Lown and Weir, 1978b). The reactive portion of the antibiotic is a substituted indole. In order to establish the relative reactivities of the two C-1 and C-10 positions in the indole moiety as well as the relative ease of displacement of the two leaving groups we prepared the model indoles shown in Fig. 13. Comparison of the rates of displacement in the first two compounds shows that the carbamate is displaced more readily than the quaternary ammonium group by a factor of ≈10 (Lown and Weir, 1978b). When the same leaving group is used in the two different positions it is clear that the 3-position of the indole is more reactive by a factor of about 10. Thus the natural antibiotic places the more reactive

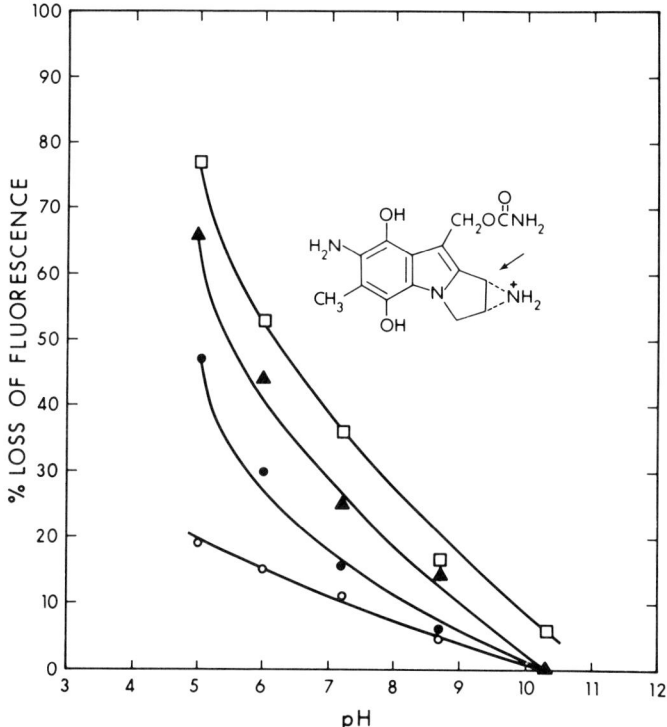

Fig. 10. Acid catalysis of alkylation of DNA by mitomycin C.

group, the carbamate, in the more reactive C-10 position. The fact that we observe that the aziridine group reacts first with DNA (Lown *et al.*, 1976) indicates that these tendencies are overcome by the release of ring strain in the aziridine. The last model compound is of interest in that it is very reactive and alkylates DNA readily at physiological pH (Lown and Weir, 1978b). This analysis suggests it might be possible to design simpler analogs of mitomycin C that may exhibit antitumor properties.

D. Correlation of DNA Cross-linking with Antileukemic Activity

Since DNA interstrand cross-linking is a lethal event to the cell compared with alkylation, which is more easily repaired, we attempted to establish a correlation between antileukemic activity of mitomycin C and some aziridinoquinones and their efficiency of DNA cross-linking (Fig. 14) (Akhtar *et al.*, 1975). The correlation is fair and suggests this assay may be useful in the prescreening of antitumor agents.

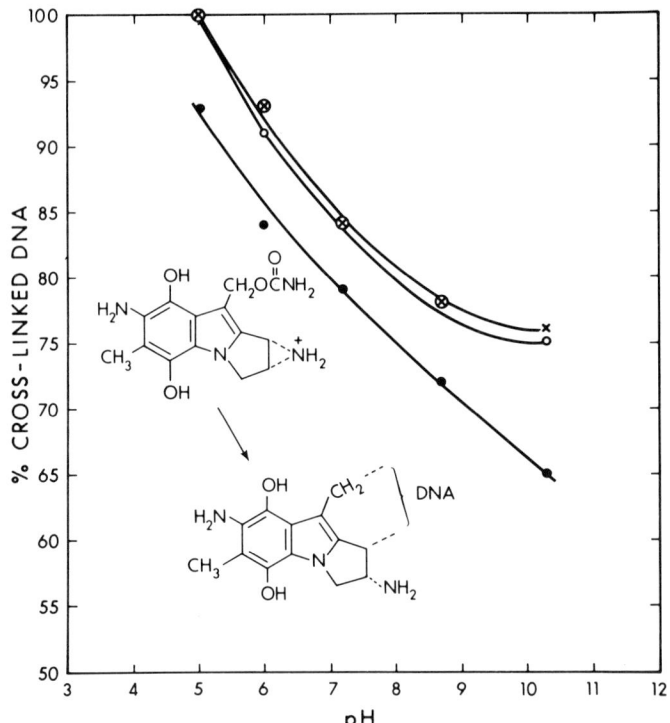

Fig. 11.   Acid catalysis of cross-linking of DNA by mitomycin C.

STEP–WISE CROSS–LINKING OF λ–DNA BY MITOMYCIN C

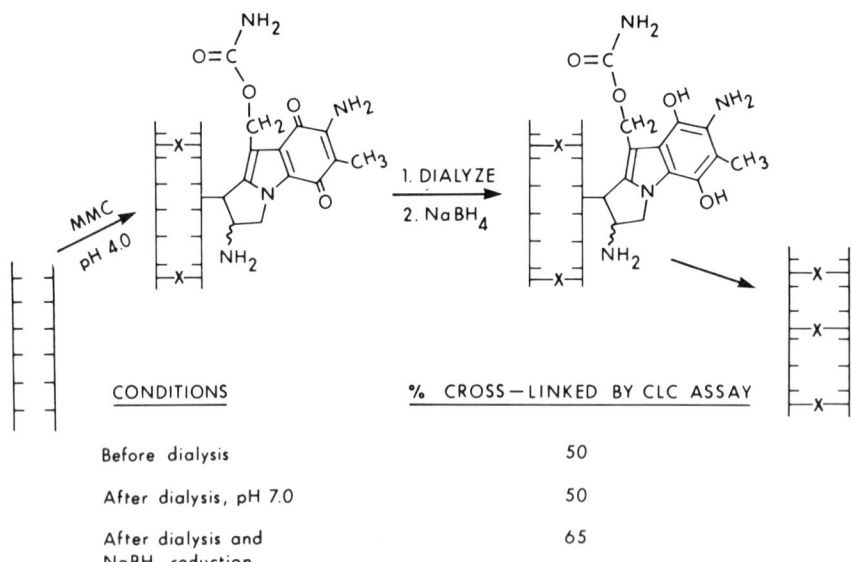

CONDITIONS	% CROSS–LINKED BY CLC ASSAY
Before dialysis	50
After dialysis, pH 7.0	50
After dialysis and NaBH$_4$ reduction	65

Fig. 12.   Step-wise cross-linking of λ-DNA by mitomycin C.

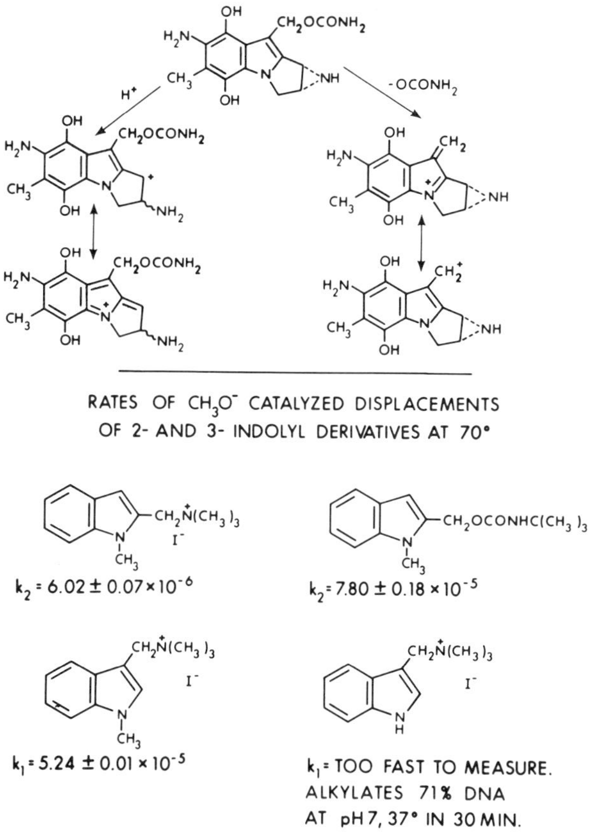

RATES OF CH_3O^- CATALYZED DISPLACEMENTS
OF 2- AND 3- INDOLYL DERIVATIVES AT 70°

$k_2 = 6.02 \pm 0.07 \times 10^{-6}$

$k_2 = 7.80 \pm 0.18 \times 10^{-5}$

$k_1 = 5.24 \pm 0.01 \times 10^{-5}$

$k_1 = $ TOO FAST TO MEASURE.
ALKYLATES 71% DNA
AT pH 7, 37° IN 30 MIN.

Fig. 13. Activated mitomycin C as a bifunctional alkylation.

E.   Degradation of DNA by Mitomycin

We remarked earlier that mitomycin C, in addition to alkylating and producing cross-links in DNA, is also observed to degrade DNA *in vivo* like the anthracycline antibiotics (Reich *et al.*, 1960; Wakaki, 1961). Hitherto this had been attributed to the stimulation of exonucleases in the repair cycle (Kersten, 1962; Nakata *et al.*, 1961). Recently, however, Bachur has demonstrated that these antibiotics actually inhibited nuclease action (Goodman *et al.*, 1974) so that we sought an alternative explanation. Our experience of the mechanism of action of the structurally related antibiotic streptonigrin (Cone *et al.*, 1976) led us to explore a free radical mechanism.

1.   PM2 Assay for DNA Degradation

In order to detect the degradation of DNA we developed a fluorescence assay that employs negatively supercoiled PM2 phage covalently closed circular (CCC)

	L 1210		λ – DNA CROSS–LINKING	
	OD	ILS	* %	TIME (min)
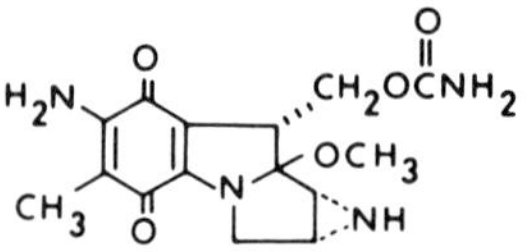 H_2N, CH_2OCNH_2, OCH_3, CH_3 (mitomycin C structure)	1.5	60	100	4
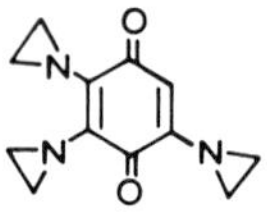 (aziridinyl benzoquinone structure)	0.1	47	100	10
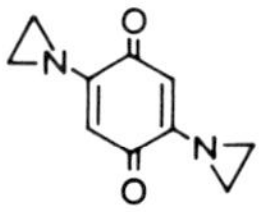 (aziridinyl benzoquinone structure)	0.5	26	92	10
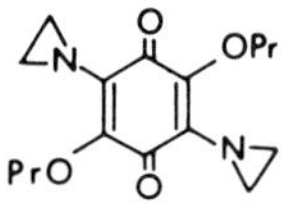 (OPr, PrO aziridinyl benzoquinone structure)	4.0	50	80	60
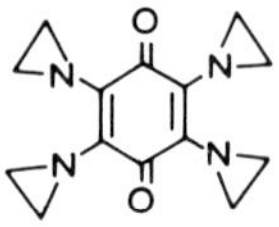 (tetra-aziridinyl benzoquinone structure)	0.01	39	82	100
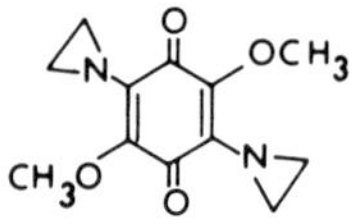 (OCH_3, CH_3O aziridinyl benzoquinone structure)	2.0	36	82	120
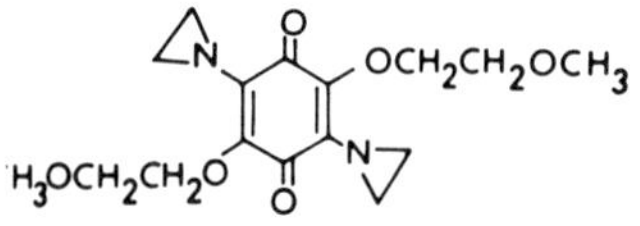 ($OCH_2CH_2OCH_3$, $H_3OCH_2CH_2O$ structure)	2.0	7.0	55	255
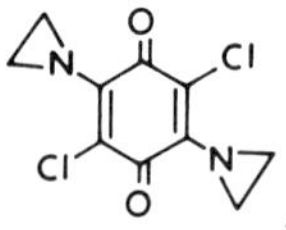 (Cl, Cl aziridinyl benzoquinone structure)	11.0	0	18	120

* CONCENTRATION OF AGENTS 0.04 g/litre
ILS INCREASED LIFE SPAN OF MICE OVER CONTROLS

Fig. 14. Correlation of λ- DNA cross-linking by mitomycin C and other bifunctional agents with anticancer activity.

DNA (Cone *et al.*, 1976) (Fig. 15). If such a DNA is nicked it produces the open circular form. Since the latter is subject to fewer topological constraints than the supercoiled form, it accepts more ethidium, and so one sees a characteristic 30% rise in fluorescence before heat denaturation. After heating, the strands separate and

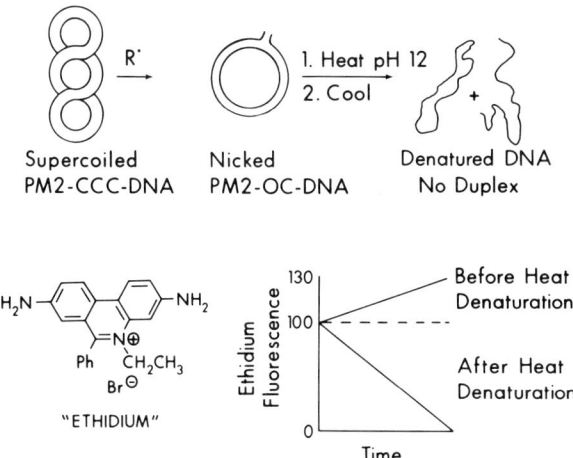

Fig. 15. Fluorescence assay for detecting single-strand cleavage of covalently closed circular DNA. The release of topological constraints upon nicking the DNA allows more dye to intercalate and gives a 30% increase in fluorescence intensity. Denaturation at pH 12 prevents duplex formation and the fluorescence falls to zero.

the fluorescence falls to zero. A particular advantage of this assay is that by adding selective inhibitors one may examine the chemical mechanism of the scission process. Row (a) in Fig. 16 represents the basic scission assay just described. This is complicated, however, in the case of mitomycin C because of the concomitant cross-linking—row (b). This holds the strands together and ensures renaturation so that the fluorescence is maintained at a high value. By adding selective enzymatic and chemical inhibitors (row c), one can prevent scission and thereby establish the chemical mechanism of cleavage.

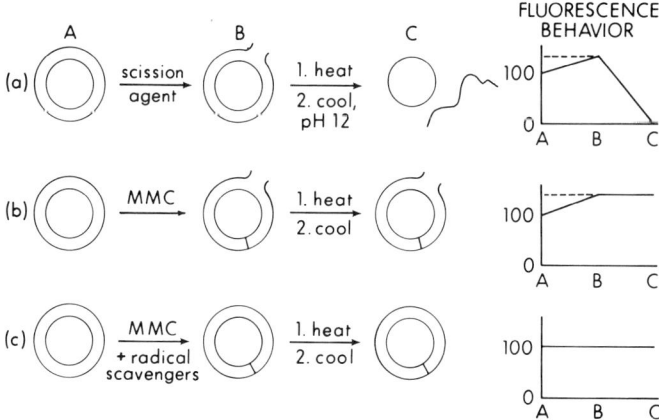

Fig. 16. Modification of fluorescence assay for determining DNA scission by concomitant cross-linking.

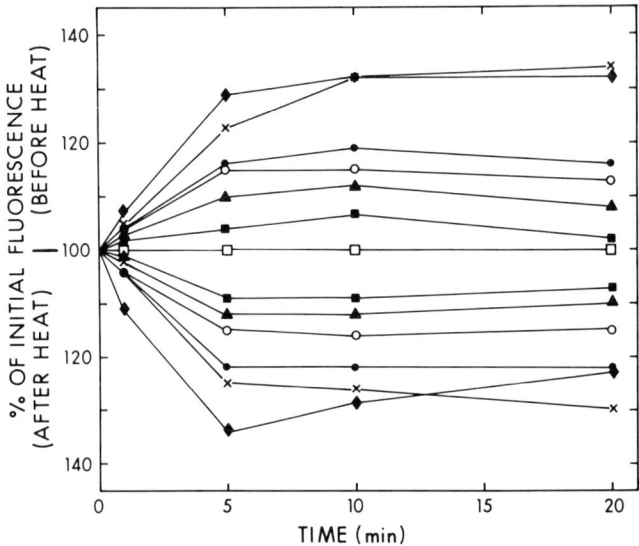

Fig. 17.   Nicking of PM2-CCC-DNA by reduced mitomycin and its inhibition.

Figure 17 shows the action on PM2-CCC-DNA of 10 μM mitomycin C reduced with NaBH$_4$. The (♦) symbols indicate rapid scission. Upon adding superoxide dismutase (●) one obtains suppression of the scission implicating the superoxide anion as an intermediate. Similarly, addition of catalase (○) also suppresses the DNA cleavage proving the intermediacy of H$_2$O$_2$. More efficient suppression is obtained by general free radical scavengers like mannitol (■) or sodium benzoate (□) which suggests the intermediacy of hydroxyl radicals.

2.   Proposed Mechanism of DNA Cleavage

On the basis of these results we can formulate a mechanism for the cleavage of DNA by activated mitomycin C (Fig. 18) (Lown *et al.*, 1976). The antibiotic is first reduced to the hydroquinone form MH$_2$.The latter is oxidized to produce the semiquinone and hydroperoxy radical. The latter species is in equilibrium with the superoxide anion. The cell is normally protected from the latter by the action of the enzyme superoxide dismutase (Fridovich, 1972). Similarly, the cell protective enzyme catalase removes H$_2$O$_2$ in step 5. The action of free radical scavengers implicates the hydroxyl radical as an intermediate. The Haber-Weiss reaction 6 was until recently regarded as the primary source of OH˙ radicals *in vivo*, but is now generally regarded as being too slow to compete with reactions 4 and 5 (van Hemmen, 1977; McClune and Fee, 1976; Halliwell, 1976). The consensus is that OH˙ radicals are generated by reaction of H$_2$O$_2$ with traces of Fe complexed either with protein or with ATP in a Fenton reaction (Czapski and Ilan, 1977) (steps 7 and 8). The

$$M + NADPH \xrightarrow{H^+} MH_2 + NADP^+ \qquad 1$$

$$MH_2 + O_2 \longrightarrow MH^. + HO_2^. \qquad 2$$

$$HO_2^. \rightleftharpoons H^+ + O_2^{.} \qquad 3$$

$$2O_2^{.} + 2H^+ \xrightarrow{SOD} H_2O_2 + O_2 \qquad 4$$

$$2H_2O_2 \xrightarrow{Catalase} 2H_2O + O_2 \qquad 5$$

$$H_2O_2 + O_2^{.} \longrightarrow OH^. + OH^- + O_2(^1\Delta g + ^3\Sigma g) \qquad 6$$

$$ATP.Fe^{3+} + O_2^{.} \longrightarrow ATP.Fe^{2+} + O_2 \qquad 7$$

$$ATP.Fe^{2+} + H_2O_2 \longrightarrow ATP.Fe^{3+} + OH^. + OH^- \qquad 8$$

$$OH^. + DNA \longrightarrow Strand\ Breakage \qquad 9$$

M = Mitomycin C
SOD = Superoxide Dismutase

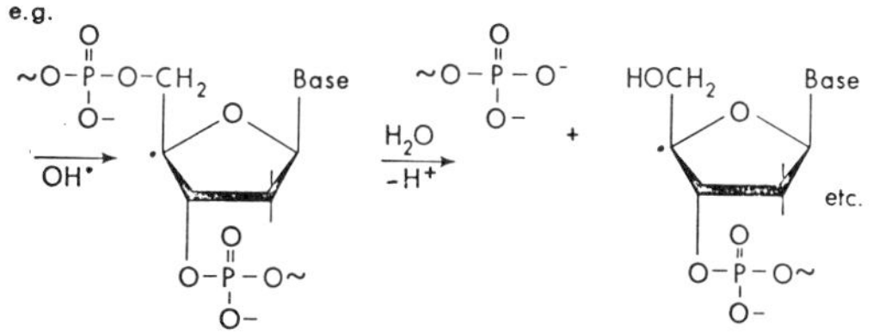

Fig. 18. Proposed chemical mechanism of DNA degradation by reduced mitomycin C.

$OH^.$ radical is known to degrade DNA in a series of reactions involving initial hydrogen abstraction from position 4 of the ribose (Dizdaroglu *et al.*, 1975).

3. Electrochemical Studies of Intermediates

Fast responding electrochemical techniques applied to the mitomycins allowed the measurement of redox potentials of the various participating species (Rao *et al.*, 1977). Examination of authentic samples of the compounds in Fig. 19 confirmed their intermediacy in the decomposition of activated mitomycin C. The results per-

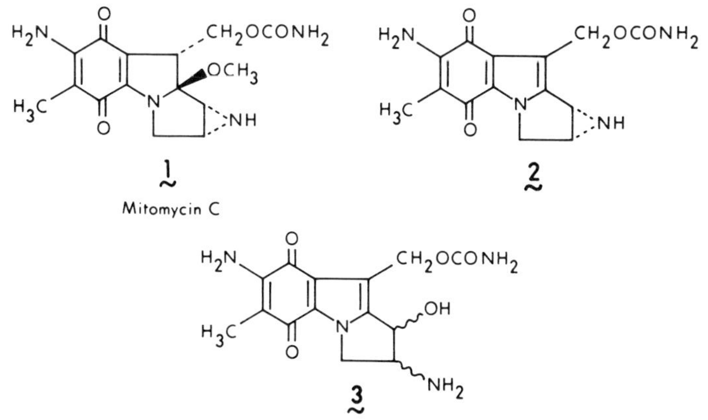

Fig. 19. Structures of mitomycin C derivatives studied electrochemically.

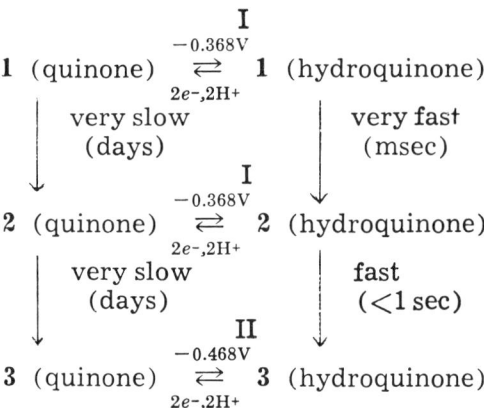

$$
\begin{array}{ccc}
 & \text{I} & \\
 & -0.368\text{V} & \\
\mathbf{1}\ (\text{quinone}) & \rightleftarrows & \mathbf{1}\ (\text{hydroquinone})\\
 & 2e\text{-},2\text{H}+ &
\end{array}
$$

Fig. 20. Redox behavior of mitomycin C derivatives determined electrochemically.

mit the establishment of redox potentials for the intermediate species and an estimate of their lifetimes (Rao *et al.*, 1977b)(Fig. 20). These results are significant in the light of the recent proposal by Moore (1977) for the mechanism of action of mitomycin C. This mechanism differs from the earlier one of Iyer and Szybalski (1963) in the postulated oxidation level of the activated mitomycin species. The idea that after initial 2-electron reduction, the mitomycin C hydroquinone is converted to a new quinone by elimination of aziridine and carbamate receives confirmation by our electrochemical studies (Rao *et al.*, 1977b). When the mitomycins are reduced, there takes place an initial 2-electron-2-proton reduction which corresponds in potential (−0.368 V) to a quinone-hydroquinone conversion. A second 2-electron-2-proton reduction then occurs, the potential of which corresponds to that of an indoloquinone-indolohydroquinone reduction of the elimination product 2 (Fig. 19). Additional evidence for a second reducible species other than the original quinone being the biologically active state of the mitomycins has been obtained by Tomasz by sequential reduction (Tomasz *et al.*, 1974; 1976). Similar electrochemical investigation was made of mitomycin B, (which also degrades DNA by a free radical pathway) and the corresponding aziridine ring opened species and eliminated product (Rao *et al.*, 1977a)(Fig. 21). This established (as shown in Fig. 22) the existence of an analogous second reducible species in the decomposition of activated mitomycin B.

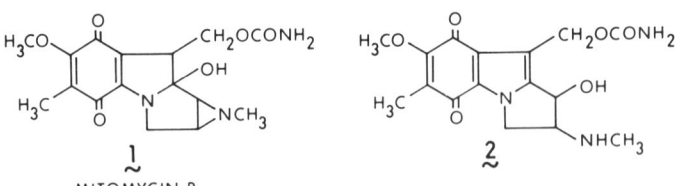

Fig. 21. Structures of mitomycin B derivatives studied electrochemically.

$$
\begin{array}{ccc}
& I & \\
& -0.200\,\text{V} & \\
\mathbf{1}\ (\text{quinone}) & \underset{2e^-,2H^+}{\overset{}{\rightleftharpoons}} & \mathbf{1}\ (\text{hydroquinone})
\end{array}
$$

| slow | | fast |
| (days) | | (sec) |

$$
\begin{array}{ccc}
& II & \\
& -0.320\,\text{V} & \\
\mathbf{2}\ (\text{quinone}) & \underset{2e^-,2H^+}{\overset{}{\rightleftharpoons}} & \mathbf{2}\ (\text{hydroquinone})
\end{array}
$$

Fig. 22. Redox behavior of mitomycin B derivatives studied electrochemically.

4. Epr Studies of Intermediates

Our proposed mechanism of degradation of DNA by the mitomycins requires the intermediacy of the semiquinone species. Epr signals have been detected *in vivo* following the administration of the antibiotic by the Lederle group and more recently by Bachur in Baltimore (Goodman *et al.*, 1974; Bachur *et al.*, 1977). These signals had been tentatively ascribed to the semiquinones, but definite assignment

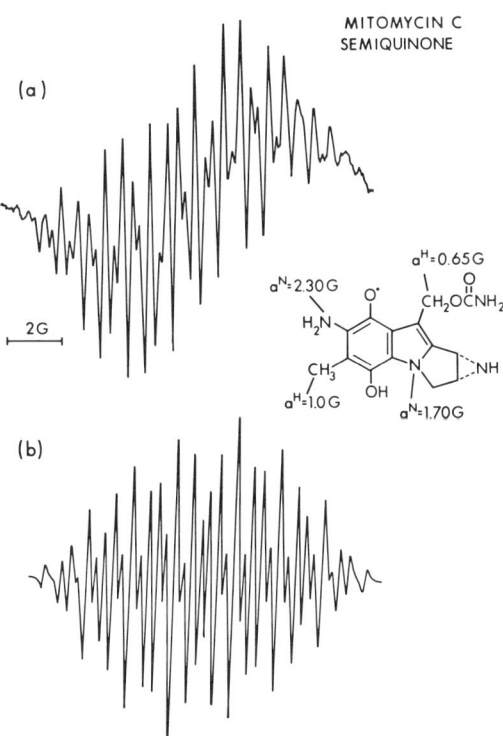

Fig. 23. Electron spin resonance spectrum of mitomycin C semiquinone: (a) observed spectrum (b) computer simulation with the hyperfine couplings indicated.

was difficult because of poor resolution. We examined the oxidized mitomycin C hydroquinone by epr. In Fig. 23, (a) is the experimentally observed spectrum and (b) a computer simulation employing the values of the hyperfine couplings shown (Lown *et al.*, 1978b). This definitely identifies the antibiotic semiquinone as a viable reaction intermediate and allowed us to estimate the lifetime. Similar examination of mitomycin B gave the experimentally observed spectrum, Fig. 24 (a), and the computer simulation, Fig. 24 (b), using the values of the hyperfine couplings shown (Lown *et al.*, 1978b) The epr spectrum of mitomycin B is simpler than that of mitomycin C since the coupling from the 7-NH$_2$ group has been removed. The latter group which we mentioned previously had been considered by Iyer and Szybalski (1963) as a possible reaction site. However, we demonstrated that the aziridine ring opened mitomycin B, which lacks a 7-NH$_2$ group, will alkylate DNA (Lown and Weir, 1978a). This definitely confirms the carbamate group as the second reactive site after the aziridine in these antibiotics. Our proposed mechanism also requires the production of hydroxyl radicals. Although it is not possible to detect this species directly because of its transient nature, we confirmed its generation using spin trapping techniques (Lown *et al.*, 1978b) (Fig. 25). The spin-trapped and relatively stable nitroxide radical has been identified as the OH˙ radical. The work of von Sonntag has demonstrated that OH˙ radicals generated by radiation

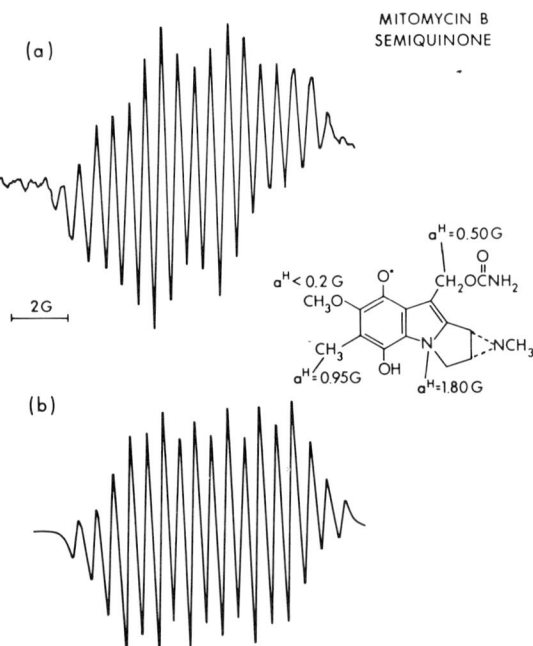

Fig. 24. Electron spin resonance spectrum of mitomycin B semiquinone: (a) observed spectrum (b) computer simulation with the hyperfine couplings indicated.

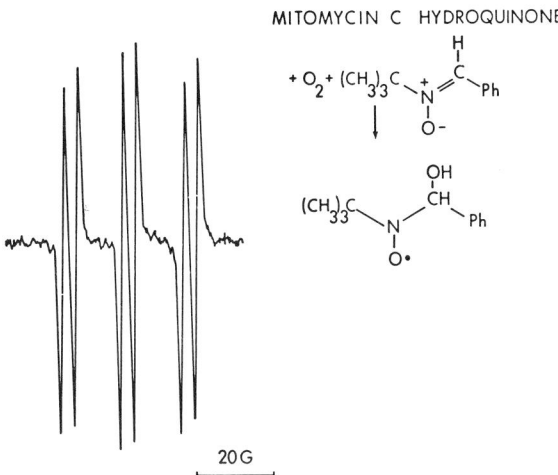

MITOMYCIN C HYDROQUINONE

Fig. 25. Electron spin resonance detection of spin-trapped hydroxyl radical from reduced mitomycin C.

degrade DNA by the mechanism shown in Fig. 26 (Dizdaroglu *et al.*, 1975). It remains to be demonstrated if treatment of DNA with reduced mitomycin C gives rise to sugar fragments of this type.

5. Comparison with other Antitumor Antibiotics

It was mentioned at the outset that many antitumor antibiotics of widely different structures nevertheless show some common aspects of their mechanism of action. In Fig. 27 are several antibiotics that we have found to degrade DNA by this superoxide anion-hydroxyl radical pathway. These include the two mitomycins C (Lown *et al.*, 1976) and B (Lown and Weir, 1978a), the clinically important anthra-

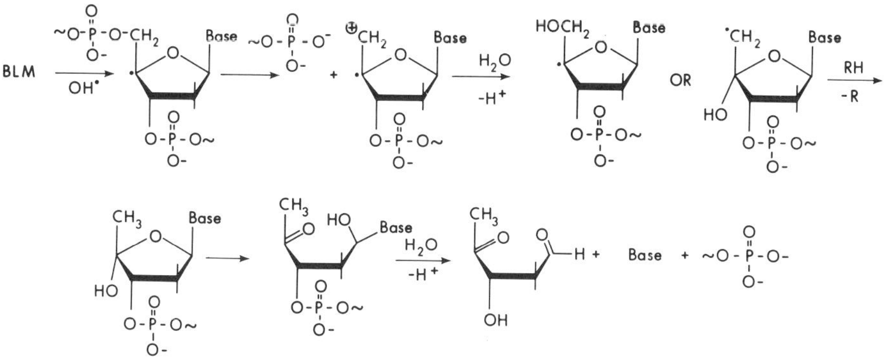

Fig. 26. DNA strand breakage by hydroxyl radical (von Sonntag *et al.*, 1975).

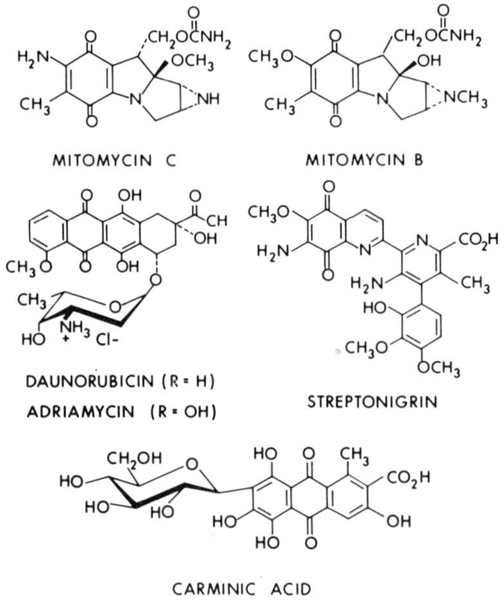

MITOMYCIN C

MITOMYCIN B

DAUNORUBICIN (R = H)
ADRIAMYCIN (R = OH)

STREPTONIGRIN

CARMINIC ACID

Fig. 27. Additional antitumer antibiotics which degrade DNA by the superoxide-hydroxyl radical pathway.

cyclines daunorubicin and adriamycin (Lown *et al.*, 1977), streptonigrin (Cone *et al.*,1976), carminic acid (Lown *et al.*, 1978a), and (not shown) the peptide antibiotic neocarzinostatin (Sim and Lown, 1978), bleomycin (Lown *et al.*, 1977), and tallysomycin. For streptonigrin, which shows the highest redox potential, the work of White, Laszlo, Hochstein, and of ourselves established that the O_2^- —OH$^{\bullet}$ degradation pathway is the principal mechanism of action (Cone *et al.*, 1976). The effects on the cell are more pronounced since streptonigrin inactivates superoxide dismutase. The cyclic generation of O_2^- *in vivo* has been observed in the case of mitomycin C and of the anthracyclines (Bachur *et al.*, 1977). In the latter case there is evidence linking O_2^- production directly to the cardiotoxicity. Regarding the latter, cardiac tissue is known to be deficient in superoxide dismutase (Hien *et al.*, 1975), and the cardiotoxicity of the anthracyclines may be suppressed by coadministration of a radical scavenger α-tocopherol (Meyers *et al.*, 1976).

III. DISCUSSION

Figure 28 attempts to summarize our findings on those chemical transformations that are significant in the antitumor action of the mitomycins. It shows how species

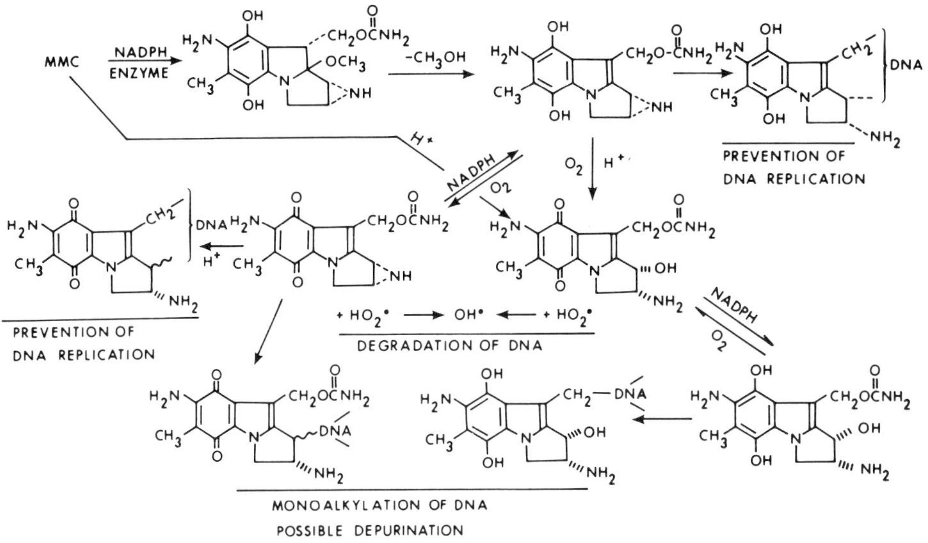

Fig. 28. Chemical transformations involved in the antitumor action of mitomycin C.

are formed which can (*a*) alkylate, (*b*) cross-link, (*c*) depurinate, and (*d*) cleave DNA in cyclic redox processes. As our understanding of the molecular transformations of sensitive cell target sites induced by the mitomycins increases, the prospects of rational synthetic design of clinically effective and less toxic analogs of these important antineoplastic agents should improve.

ACKNOWLEDGMENTS

I should like to acknowledge the outstanding research efforts of Dr. Asher Begleiter and Mr. Gordon Weir.

REFERENCES

Akhtar, M. H., Begleiter, A., Johnson, D., Lown, J. W., McLaughlin, L. W., and Sim, S. K. (1975). *Can. J. Chem. 53,* 2891-2905.
Bachur, N. R., Gordon, S. L., and Gee, M. V. (1977). *Molecular Pharmacol. 13,* 901-910.
Cone, R., Hasan, S. K., Lown, J. W., and Morgan, A. R. (1976). *Can. J. Biochem. 54,* 219-223.
Connors, T. A., Mitchley, B. C. V., Rosenoer, V. M., and Ross, W. C. J. (1970). *Biochem. Pharmacol. 13,* 395-400.
Culvenor, C. C. J., Downing, D. T., and Edgar, J. A. (1969). *Ann. N. Y. Acad. Sci. 163,* 837-847.
Czapski, G., and Ilan, Y. A. (1977). Abstract C-11, International Conference on Singlet Oxygen and Related Species in Chemistry and Biology, August 21-26, Pinawa, Manitoba.

Di Marco, A., Arcamone, F., and Zunino, F. (1975). *In* "Antibiotics III. Mechanism of Action of Antimicrobial and Antitumor Agents" (J. W. Corcoran and F. E. Hahn, eds.), pp. 101-128. Springer-Verlag, New York.

Dizdaroglu, M., von Sonntag, C., and Schulte-Frohlinde, D. (1975). *J. Am. Chem. Soc. 97,* 2277-2278.

Fridovich, I. (1972). *Acc. Chem. Res. 5,* 321-326.

Goodman, M. F., Bessman, M. J., and Bachur, N. R. (1974). *Proc. Nat. Acad. Sci. 71,* 1193-1196.

Halliwell, B. (1976). *F. E. B. S. Let. 72,* 8-10.

Hamaguchi, K., and Geiduschek, E. P. (1961). *J. Am. Chem. Soc. 84,* 1329-1338.

Hata, T., Sano, Y., Sugawara, R., Matsumae, A., Kanamori, K., Shima, T., and Hoshi, T. (1956). *J. Antibiot.* (Tokyo) Ser. A., *9,* 141-146.

Hien, P. V., Kovacs, K., and Matkovics, B. (1975). *Enzyme 19,* 1-4.

Hsiung, H., Lown, J. W., and Johnson, D. (1976). *Can. J. Biochem. 54,* 1047-1054.

Iyer, V. N., and Szybalski, W. (1963). *Proc. Nat. Acad. Sci. 50,* 355-362.

Kersten, W. (1962). *Biochem. Biophys. Acta. 55,* 558-560.

Kirsch, E. J. (1967). *In* "Antibiotics II—Biosynthesis" (D. Gottlieb and P. D. Shaw, eds.), pp. 66-76. Springer-Verlag, New York.

Klatersky, J., Daneau, D., and Verherst, S. (1972). *Europ. J. Cancer 8,* 149-154.

Lawley, P. D. (1966). *In* "Progress in Nucleic Acid Research and Molecular Biology" (W. E. Cohn, ed.), Vol. V, pp. 89-162. Academic Press, New York.

Lown, J. W. (1977). *In* "Bioorganic Chemistry" (E. E. van Tamelen, ed.), Vol. III, pp. 95-121. Academic Press, New York.

Lown, J. W., Begleiter, A., Johnson, D., and Morgan, A. R. (1976). *Can. J. Biochem. 54,* 110-119.

Lown, J. W., Sim, S. K., Majumdar, K. C., and Chang, R. Y. (1977). *Biochem. Biophys. Res. Commun. 76,* 705-710.

Lown, J. W., Chen, H. H., Sim, S. K., and Plambeck, J. A. (1978a). *Bioorganic Chem.,* in press.

Lown, J. W., Sim, S. K., and Chen, H. H. (1978). *Can. J. Biochem., 56,* 1042-1047.

Lown, J. W., and Sim, S. K. (1977). *Biochem. Biophys. Res. Commun. 77,* 1150-1157.

Lown, J. W., and Weir, G. L. (1978a). *Can. J. Biochem. 56,* 296-304.

Lown, J. W., and Weir, G. L. (1978b). *Can. J. Chem. 56,* 249-257.

McClune, G. J., and Fee, J. A. (1976). *F. E. B. S. Lett. 67,* 294-298.

Meyers, C. E., McGuire, W., and Young, R. (1976). *Cancer Treat. Rep. 60,* 961-692.

Moore, H. W. (1977). *Science 197,* 527-532.

Montgomery, J. A., Johnson, T. P., and Shealy, Y. F. (1970). *In* "Drugs for Neoplastic Diseases," Medicinal Chemistry Part I (A. Burger, ed.), pp. 680-783. Wiley, New York.

Morgan, A. R., and Paetkau, V. (1972). *Can. J. Biochem. 50,* 210-216.

Nakata, Y., Nakata, K., and Sakamoto, Y. (1961). *Biochem. Biophys. Res. Commun. 6,* 339-343.

Rao, G. M., Begleiter, A., Lown, J. W., and Plambeck, J. A. (1977a). *J. Electrochem. Soc. 124,* 199-202.

Rao, G. M., Lown, J. W., and Plambeck, J. A. (1977b). *J. Electrochem. Soc. 124,* 195-198.

Reich, E., Shatkin, A. J., and Tatum, E. L. (1960). *Biochem. Biophys. Acta. 45,* 608-610.

Sim, S. K., and Lown, J. W. (1978). *Biochem. Biophys. Res. Commun., 81,* 99-105.

Szybalski, W., and Iyer, V. N. (1967). *In* "Antibiotics Mechanism of Action" (D. Gottlieb and P. D. Shaw, eds.), pp. 211-245. Springer-Verlag, New York.

Tomasz, M., Mercado, C. M., Olson, J., and Chatterjee, N. (1974). *Biochem. 13,* 4878-4887.

van Hemmen, J. J., and Meuling, W. J. S. (1977). *Arch. Biochem. Biophys. 182,* 743-748.

Wakaki, S. (1961). *Cancer Chemother. Rep. 13,* 79-86.

Chapter 3

MITOMYCIN C AND ANALOG DEVELOPMENT

William A. Remers

I. INTRODUCTION

Mitomycins were discovered first in Japan. In 1956 T. Hata and collaborators at the Kitasato Institute isolated two compounds, which they called mitomycins A and B, from the culture fluid of *Streptomyces caespitosis* (Hata, 1956). These compounds were highly potent antibacterial and antitumor agents, but they were very toxic in mice. Working with the same organism, S. Wakaki and co-workers at the Kyowa Fermentation Industry isolated mitomycin C, which proved to be superior in antitumor activity to the other mitomycins (Wakaki *et al.,* 1958). Mitomycin C was rapidly developed and established by clinical trials in Japan, where it became widely prescribed during the 1960s (Frank and Osterberg, 1960). In contrast the initial trials on mitomycin C in the United States were disappointing (Jones, 1959), and it was not approved for standard clinical practice until 1974 when Bristol Laboratories introduced it as Mutamycin.®

Meanwhile, mitomycin isolation shifted to the United States. Porfiromycin, the N-methyl homolog of mitomycin C, was discovered in 1960 by a group at the Upjohn Company (De Boer *et al.,* 1961). Porfiromycin became a U. S. adopted name, and the compound was developed for phase I clinical trials (Izbicki *et al.,* 1972), but it proved to be less effective than mitomycin C and it has not been marketed. A group led by N. Bohonus at Lederle Laboratories isolated mitomycins A, B, and C, porfiromycin, and a poorly active compound named mityromycin from *Streptomyces verticillatus* (Lefemine *et al.,* 1962). Lederle made a massive investment in the structure elucidation of the mitomycins. By 1962 their team, directed by J. S. Webb (Webb *et al.,* 1962), was able to publish the complete structures of all the mitomycins (Fig. 1). These structures were confirmed by A. Tulinsky's xray crystallographic analysis (Tulinsky, 1962) and by Stevens' independent elucidation (Stevens *et al.,* 1964).

Because the mitomycins are highly potent against tumors, but also highly toxic, medicinal chemists realized the importance of preparing analogs and derivatives that might have improved therapeutic ratios. With an established large-scale commercial process for mitomycin C, Kyowa was in a position to utilize this compound and other mitomycins for the convenient preparation of numerous semisynthetic analogs (Kinoshita *et al.,* 1970; Matsui *et al.,* 1968; Kinoshita *et al.,* 1971; Kojima *et al.,* 1972). Lederle scientists chose to develop totally synthetic analogs directed toward new antibacterial agents. The antitumor activity was secondary to this goal, although a number of the compounds were screened against the 72j mammary adenocarcinoma in mice. Since it was known that aziridinomitosenes, prepared by catalytic reduction and reoxidation of mitomycins (Scheme 1), had nearly the same antibacterial and antitumor activities as the mitomycins themselves (Patrick, 1964), aziridinomitosenes became target compounds for the total synthesis. The possibility that deletion of the aziridine ring from the mitomycin structure would reduce the cytotoxicity led to the selection of simple mitosenes as target compounds. Mitosenes with opened aziridine rings (Scheme 2) had been prepared by treatment of mitomycins with acid (Webb *et al.,* 1962; Stevens *et al.,* 1964), and they showed antibacterial activity and weak antitumor activity (Oboshi *et al.,* 1967).

A group led by M. J. Weiss first synthesized the mitosene-with no substituents in ring C (Fig. 2) (Allen *et al.,* 1964). It had activity against Gram (+) bacteria in culture and in mice, but no antitumor activity. They next prepared the indoloquinone analog in which ring C had been cleaved (Fig. 2) (Allen and Weiss, 1967). This type of analog was equal in activity to the one with an intact ring C and it was much easier to synthesize. Thus, the Lederle group was able to prepare a series of indoloquinones in which substituents around the indole nucleus were varied systematically (Weiss *et al.,* 1968). The best compounds to emerge from these studies were one in which the carbamate nitrogen was substituted with an hydroxyethyl group (Allen *et al.,* 1968) and one in which this feature was combined with an ethylenimino substit-

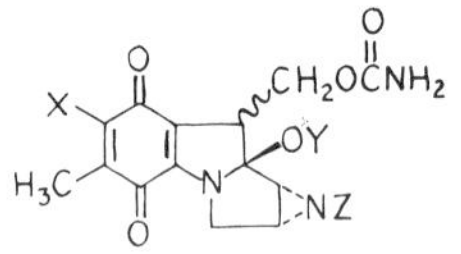

		X	Y	Z
MITOMYCIN	A	CH_3O	CH_3	H
	B	CH_3O	H	CH_3
	C	H_2N	CH_3	H
PORFIROMYCIN		H_2N	CH_3	CH_3

Fig. 1. Structures of the natural mitomycins.

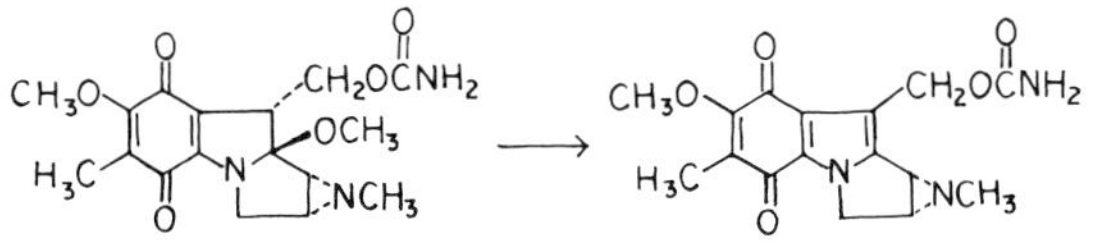

Scheme 1.   Aziridinomitosene formation.

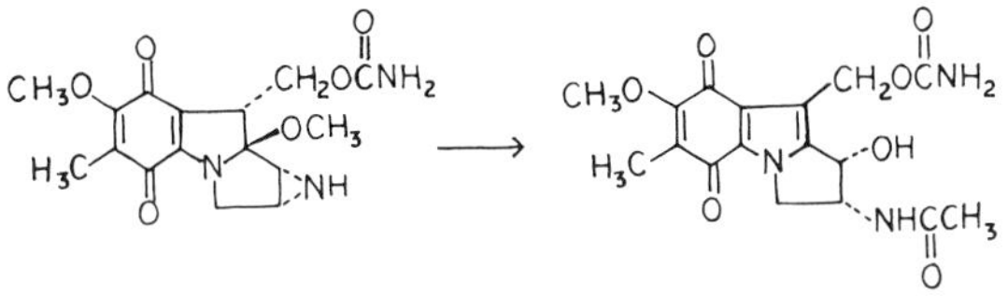

Scheme 2.   Formation of a 1, 2-disubstituted mitosene.

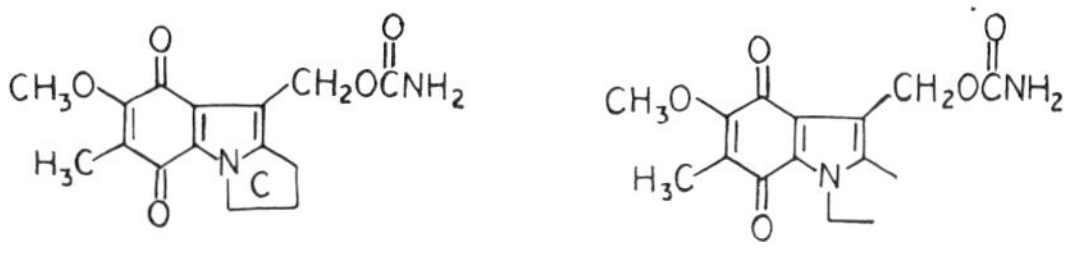

Fig. 2.   Synthetic mitosene and its indoloquinone analog.

uent in the quinone ring (Fig. 3) (Remers and Weiss, 1968). The latter compound had good activity against a variety of Gram (+) bacteria in mice, but it was not active against tumors and it was highly toxic (Weiss *et al.,* 1968). It should be noted, however, that these substituents gave good antitumor activity when applied to the mitomycins (Kojima *et al.,* 1972).

During the course of this research and afterward, mitomycin mode of action studies were conducted (Iyer and Szybalski, 1964; Tomasz *et al.,* 1974; Lown, 1976). They led to a fascinating, but incompletely established, picture of the biochemical transformations and covalent bonding steps involved in the mitomycin-DNA interaction. According to this picture (Scheme 3) mitomycins are first reduced with the aid of NADPH to the semiquinone radical. This species binds noncovalently to DNA. Further reduction converts it into the hydroquinone, which readily loses methanol (water in the case of mitomycin B) to give the aziridinomitosene hydroquinone. Because the alkylating functional groups are now in conjugation with the indole nitrogen, they have become highly activated and are able to covalently bind the DNA. Carbon 1 appears to bind first as the aziridine ring opens, followed by carbon 10, which loses the carbamoyloxy substituent (Lown *et al.,* 1976). Sartorelli has derived the name "bioreductive alkylation" for an overall process of this type (Lin *et al.,* 1974). The two alkylating centers of mitomycins enable them to cross-link DNA, and this effect is thought to be the lethal one to cancer cells (Iyer and Szybalski, 1964). An additional lethal effect

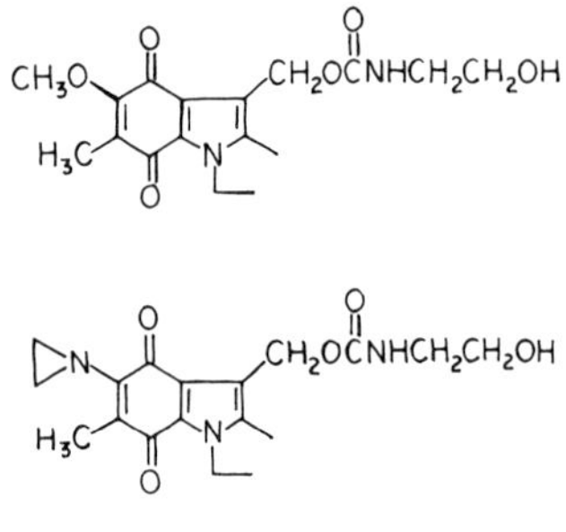

Fig. 3.   Synthetic indoloquinones.

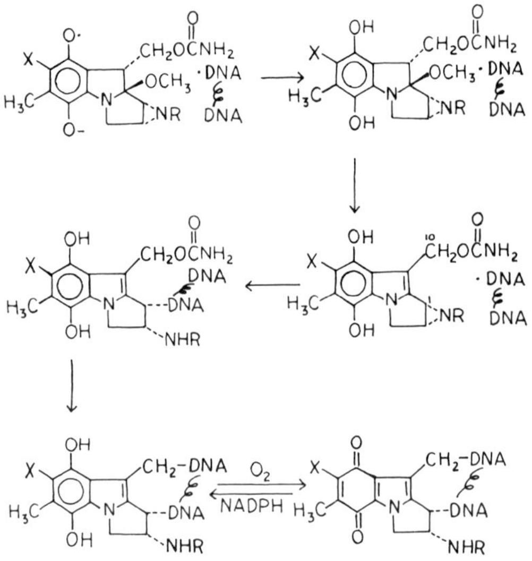

Scheme 3.   Mitomycin activation and binding with DNA.

might be the liberation of hydrogen peroxide that occurs when mitomycins, especially when bound to DNA, go through successive redox cycles (Tomasz, 1976).

II. RESULTS AND DISCUSSION

With this view of the mode of action, and of mitomycin structure-activity relationships derived mainly by the Japanese group (Kinoshita *et al.*, 1971; Matsui *et al.*, 1968; Kojima *et al.*, 1972), investigators are now in a position to consider a more rational design of mitomycin analogs. The following factors appear to be most significant in designing an analog with good antitumor activity: (*a*) Analogs must have two functional groups capable of alkylation. Ideally these groups are

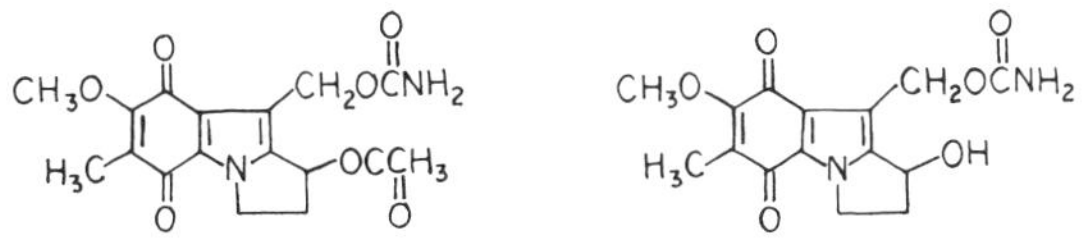

Fig. 4. 1-substituted mitosenes.

inactive when the molecule is in the quinone form, but activated when it is reduced to the hydroquinone. (*b*) The quinone reduction potential should be optimum in order to take advantage of any difference that might exist between the reducing capability of normal and cancer cells. (*c*) Analogs should be relatively hydrophilic, at least for antileukemia activity (Remers and Schepman, 1974).

Based on these factors, Remers and co-workers have designed and synthesized 1-acetoxy-7-methoxy mitosene (Fig. 4), a compound in which the second alkylation site is afforded by elimination of the acetoxy group (Leadbetter *et al.*, 1974). It is active against P388 murine leukemia, although less so than the natural mitomycins. However, this compound is inactivated by serum esterases, and it is possible that less-readily hydrolyzed esters will show better activity. With the interest and support of Bristol Laboratories and the National Cancer Institute, Remers' group is preparing a large number of semisynthetic mitomycins based on mitomycin C. Although the results of this study are too preliminary to report at this time, the basis for their design can be described. As shown in Fig. 5, the key points of variation on the mitomycin or aziridinomitosene molecules are the quinone ring substituent (X), the aziridine-ring substituent (Y), and the carbamate substituent (R). The X substituent is very important since it influences both the quinone reduction potential and the lipophilicity of the analog. Y substituents influence the reactivity of the aziridine ring and they also affect the lipophilicity. The R group is presumably lost during the course of alkylation, but it can influence lipophilicity and perhaps initial binding to DNA.

A number of outstanding organic chemists have recently been engaged in the total synthesis of mitomycins. The objective of their work is to develop methodology for the preparation of complex mitomycin analogs that can not be made semisynthetically. This approach has been highlighted by Kishi's syntheses of mitomycins A and C and porfiromycin (Nakatsubo *et al.,* 1977; Fukuyama *et al.,* 1977).

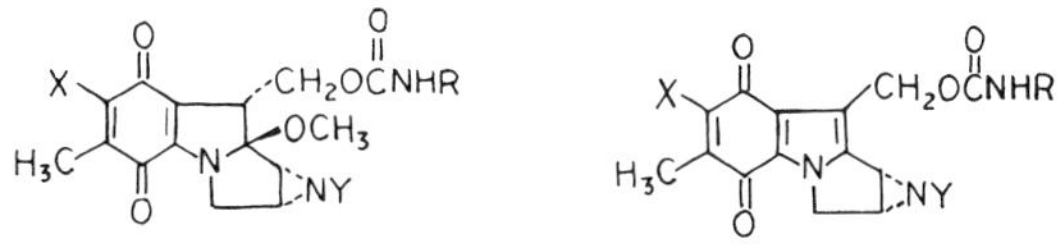

Fig. 5.   New mitomycin derivatives.

REFERENCES

Allen, G. R., Jr., Poletto, J. R., and Weiss, M. J. (1964). *J. Am. Chem. Soc. 86,* 3877.

Allen, G. R., Jr., and Weiss, M. J. (1967). *J. Med. Chem. 10,* 1.

Allen, G. R., Jr., Poletto, J. F., and Weiss, M. J. (1968). *J. Med. Chem. 11,* 822.

DeBoer, C., Dietz, A., Lummus, N. E., and Savage, G. M. (1961). "Antimicrobial Agents: Annual 1960," pp. 17-22. Plenum Press, New York.

Frank, W., and Osterberg, A. E. (1960). *Cancer Chemother. Rep. 9,* 114.

Fukuyama, T., Nakatsubo, F., Cocuzza, A. J., and Kishi, Y. (1977). *Tetrahedron Lett.* 4295.

Hata, R., Sano, Y., Sugawara, R., Matsume, A., Kanamori, K., Shima, T., and Hoshi, T. (1956). *J. Antibiot.* (Tokyo) Ser. A. *9,* 141.

Iyer, V. N., and Szybalski, W. (1964). *Science 145,* 55.

Izbicki, R., Al-Sarraf, M., Reed, M. L., Vaughn, C. B., and Vaitkevicius, V. K. (1972). *Cancer Chemother. Rep. 56,* 615.

Jones, R. Jr. (1959). *Cancer Chemother. Rep. 2,* 3.

Kinoshita, S., Uzu, K., Nakano, K., Shimizu, M., Takahasi, T., Wakaki, S., and Matsui, M. (1970). *Progr. Antimicrobial Anticancer Chemother. 2,* 1058.

Kinoshita, S., Uzu, K., Nakano, K., Shimizu, M., and Takahasi, T. (1971). *J. Med. Chem. 14,* 103, 109.

Kojima, R., Driscoll, J., Mantel, N., and Goldin, A. (1972). *Cancer Chemother. Rep., Part 2 3,* 121.

Leadbetter, F., Fost, D. L., Ekwuribe, N. N., and Remers, W. A. (1974). *J. Org. Chem. 39,* 3508.

Lefemine, D. V., Dann, M., Barbatschi, F., Hausmann, W. K., Zbinovsky, V., Monnikendam, P., Adam, J., and Bohonus, N. (1962). *J. Am. Chem. Soc. 84,* 3184.

Lin, A. J., Cosby, L. A., and Sartorelli, A. C. (1974). *Cancer Chemother. Rep. 4,* 23.

Lown, J. W., Begleiter, A., Johnson, D., and Morgan, A. R. (1976). *Can. J. Biochem. 54,* 110.

Matsui, M., Yamada, Y., Uzu, K., and Hirata, T. (1968). *J. Antibiot.* (Tokyo) *21,* 189.

Nakatsubo, F., Fukuyama, T., Cocuzza, A. J., and Kishi, Y. (1977). *J. Am. Chem. Soc. 99,* 8115.

Oboshi, S., Matsui, M., Masago, N., Wakaki, S., and Uzu, K. (1967). *GANN 58,* 315.

Patrick, J. B., Williams, R. P., Meyer, W. E., Fulmor, W., Cosulich, D. B., Broschard, R. W., and Webb, J. S. (1964). *J. Am. Chem. Soc. 86,* 1889.

Remers, W. A., and Schepman, C. S. (1974). *J. Med. Chem. 17,* 729.

Remers, W. A., and Weiss, M. J. (1968). *J. Med. Chem. 11,* 737.

Stevens, C. L., Taylor, K. G., Munk, M. E., Marshall, W. S., Noll, K., Shah, G. D., Shah, L. G., and Uzu, K. (1964). *J. Med. Chem. 8,* 1.

Tomasz, M. (1976). *Chem.-Biol. Interact. 13,* 89.

Tomasz, M., Mercado, C. M., Olson, J., and Chatterjie, N. (1974). *Biochem. 13,* 4878.

Tulinsky, A. (1962). *J. Am. Chem. Soc. 84,* 3188.

Wakaki, S., Marumo, H., Tomioka, K., Shimizu, G., Kato, E., Kamada, H., Kudo, S., and Fujimoto, Y. (1958). *Antibiot. and Chemother. 8,* 228.

Webb, J. S., Cosulich, D. B., Mowat, J. H., Patrick, J. B., Broschard, R. W., Meyer, W. E., Williams, R. P., Wolf, C. F., Fulmor, W., Pidacks, C., and Lancaster, J. E. (1962). *J. Am. Chem. Soc. 84,* 3185, 3186.

Weiss, M. J., Redin, G. S., Allen, G. R., Jr., Dornbush, A. C., Lindsay, H. L., Poletto, J. F., Remers, W. A., Roth, R. H., and Sloboda, A. E. (1968). *J. Med. Chem. 11,* 742.

Chapter 4

IN VIVO EVALUATION OF ANALOGS

William T. Bradner

I. INTRODUCTION

Mitomycin C (MMC) is a very active antitumor agent in animal tumor systems and in man (Crooke and Bradner, 1976). It is also severely myelosuppressive, a toxicity that has limited its clinical utility. Thus, in the search for new analogs with improved therapeutic properties, we have developed our evaluation capability at Bristol Laboratories along lines that would permit us to screen for toxic side effects at a very early stage of compound development. The central features of our current methodology are the use of P-388 leukemia as a primary antitumor screen and a test for leukopenia in the BDF_1 mouse as a critical toxicity screen before further work is done.

II. PROCEDURES

Table I shows an outline of the sequence of procedures for screening a new mitomycin analog.

TABLE I.   Screening of New Mitomycins

A.	*In vitro* tests (antimicrobial and ILB).
B.	P-388 leukemia, single dose.
C.	Compound purity check.
D.	LD_{50}—heavy BDF_1 males, ip.
E.	Leukopenia.
F.	Nephrotoxicity, BUN.
G.	Dose schedules, L-1210 leukemia.
H.	B16 melanoma, Lewis lung carcinoma, other tumors.
I.	Other blood chemistry tests—SGPT, CPK-MB.

A. In Vitro Tests

Two tests that can be performed with microgram quantities are antimicrobial, using *Bacillus subtilis* and induction of lysogenic bacteria (Price *et al.*, 1964). *In vitro* tests are very useful in establishing starting dose levels since they correlate rather well with toxicity (Bradner, 1958). Such testing is not essential when the chemical formula of a new material is very close to an analog previously studied. In such cases a reasonable prediction can be made of *in vivo* potency.

B. In Vivo P-388 Leukemia

Although mitomycin C is effective against a broad spectrum of experimental tumors many of which have been used for analog screening, we have chosen P-388 leukemia because it is highly sensitive, quite uniform in reproducibility of results, and reasonably fast growing. P-388 and other tumors are described in the test protocol publication of the National Cancer Institute (Geran *et al.*, 1972). We have now standardized on a single dose, day 1 treatment since mitomycins generally are highly active on the regimen of widely spaced dosing (Hata *et al.*, 1961; Kojima *et al.*, 1972a), and much higher doses can be given when the compound is in short supply.

C. Check for Compound Purity

Although most samples are reasonably pure from the chemical standpoint (95 to 98%), this is sometimes insufficient for unambiguous biological results, especially with synthetic routes involving mitomycin A (MMA). Because of the high potency of MMA even trace amounts could influence the experimental results with compounds that are much less potent. TLC bioautographs and liquid chromatography can quantitate MMA presence. These analyses, of course, are only performed on active compounds.

D. LD_{50} in Mice

Those compounds having acceptable antitumor characteristics and available in sufficient quantity and purity are tested to establish single dose intraperitoneal LD_{50} in heavy BDF_1 male mice.

E. Leukopenia

In order to screen for myelosuppressive effects, we inject groups of BDF_1 mice with an LD_{50} dose of the candidate drug and incremental lower doses. Using the ocular bleeding technic, serial samples of blood are taken from individual animals and total white blood cell count (WBC) determined in a Coulter Model S automated counter. The data are entered into a computer which determines significant changes in WBC from a pretreatment control measurement for each animal. By using the LD_{50} as a starting point and titrating down, it is possible to compare analogs that vary widely in potency.

F. Nephrotoxicity, BUN

There have been scattered reports that mitomycin C is nephrotoxic in some clinical circumstances, although there is little evidence for this in animals. In the original New Drug Application to the Food and Drug Administration, 23 of 1281 patients had significant BUN rises from pretreatment measurements during MMC therapy. This is an incidence of 1.8%. However, the condition, when observed, appeared to be delayed in onset and associated with high total doses. Assessment of renal toxicity by automated BUN measurement is easy to perform with mice and considered important in the evaluation of new mitomycin analogs since we do not wish to enhance kidney damage while gaining other therapeutic attributes.

G. Dose Schedules, L-1210 Leukemia

Once we have found a new analog that has favorable characteristics in comparison with MMC, we proceed to route and regimen studies with L-1210 leukemia in ascitic form. This tumor is more resistant to MMC and faster growing than P-388 and is well suited for such studies. We are particularly interested in determining schedule dependence in preparation for tumor spectrum or panel studies. Occasional compounds that are somewhat weaker on the P-388 test and are available in quantity are passed by the toxicity testing directly to L-1210 and possibly other tumors. This is done to establish some efficacy advantage before studying side effects.

H. Tumor Spectrum

We have available B16 melanoma and Lewis lung carcinoma, both of which respond to MMC. These and additional tumors used by extramural investigators are available for further study of analogs to determine any possible advantages.

III. CHEMICAL EXAMPLES

The three compounds selected as examples to demonstrate our screening procedures are: MMC, the clinical compound; MMA, the most potent known mitomycin;

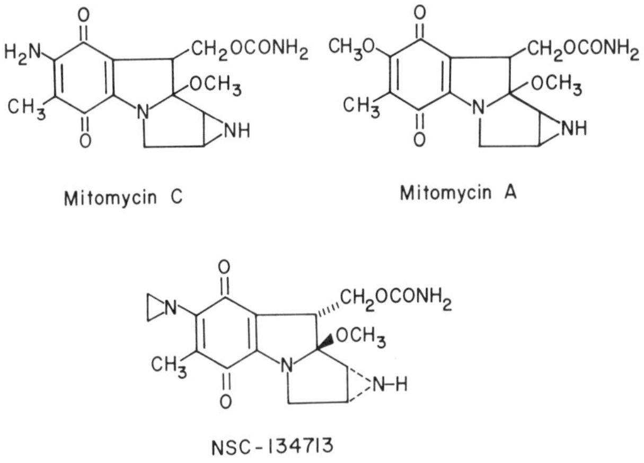

Fig. 1.   Chemical structures of mitomycin C, mitomycin A, and NSC-134713.

and NSC-134713, a highly potent 7-aziridinomitosane prepared by Matusi *et al.*
(1968) and found to be active on L-1210 leukemia (Kojima *et al.*, 1972b). The
structures are shown in Fig. 1.

IV. ANTITUMOR TESTING

The results of antitumor tests of the three demonstration compounds are summarized in Table II. It is clear that MMA and NSC-13413 are 2 to 4 times more
toxic than MMC. Based on the minimum effective dose, that is, the lowest dose
tested producing greater than T/C 125%, both MMA and NSC-134713 are 16 times
more potent than MMC.

TABLE II.   Effect of Mitomycin Analogs
on P-388 Leukemia

Dose[a]	Effect, MST % T/C[b]		
mg/kg	MMC	MMA	NSC-134713
6.4	206	–	Tox
3.2	300	–	78
1.6	161	233	266
0.8	156	228	222
0.4	133	183	189
0.2	117	156	178
0.1	111	156	150
0.05	111	144	144
0.025	–	133	139
0.0125	–	–	117

[a]Single dose, ip., day 1.
[b]T/C 125 considered significant tumor inhibition.

TABLE III.   Single Dose LD_{50}

Compound	Dose mg/kg
Mitomycin C	7.5
Mitomycin A	1.7
NSC-134713	3.0

Mice: heavy BDF_1 males.
Route: ip.
Evaluation time: day 14.
Calculation: Weil (1952).

V.   ACUTE TOXICITY AND LEUKOPENIA

A.   Acute Toxicity

Results of the LD_{50} determination are shown in Table III. MMA and NSC-134713 are clearly more toxic than MMC as initially revealed in the antitumor test.

B. Leukopenia

Fig. 2 shows in graphic form the percentage change in total WBC following an LD_{50} dose of 7.5 mg/kg and .75 increments of the LD_{50}. All MMC doses were significantly leukopenic through day 5 with some evidence of recovery on day 7. In tests performed in a similar manner with MMA (Fig. 3) and NSC-134713 (Fig. 4), significant leukopenia was not observed.

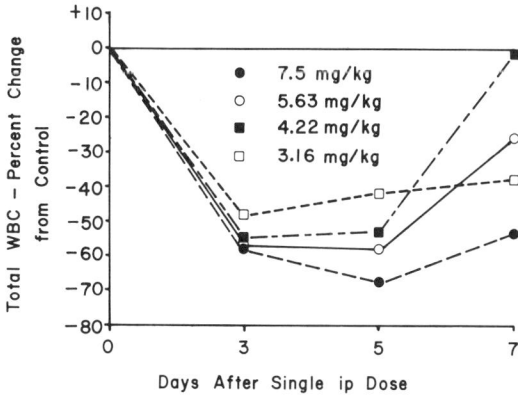

Fig. 2.   Effect of mitomycin C on total white blood cell count in male BDF_1 mice.

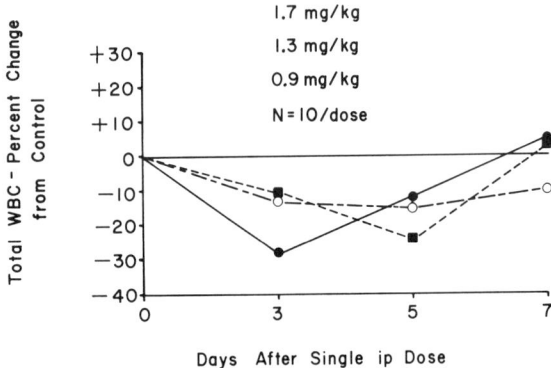

Fig. 3. Effect of mitomycin A on total white blood cell count in male BDF₁ mice.

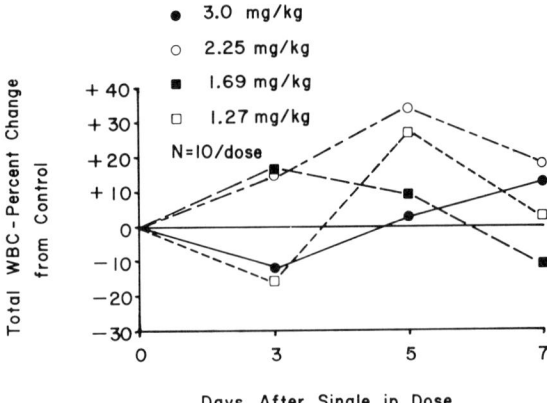

Fig. 4. Effect of NSC-134713 on total white blood cell count in male BDF₁ mice.

VI. RENAL, HEPATIC, AND OTHER TOXICITIES

A. Renal Toxicity

Fig. 5 shows in bar-graph form the effects of an LD_{50} dose of MMC, MMA, and NSC-134713 on BUN. For comparison, a nephrotoxic compound cis-platinum (cis-DDP) is shown as a positive control. MMC and MMA did not affect BUN in any animal, whereas cis-DDP was severely nephrotoxic. NSC-134713 caused no change at the lower doses, but 2/9 animals surviving the LD_{50} dose had significant BUN elevation.

B. Hepatic Toxicity

Fig. 6 shows data on SGPT. In this case, the mycotoxin sterigmatocystin was used a positive control. Though some increase was observed with the mitomycins, it cannot be considered clinically meaningful.

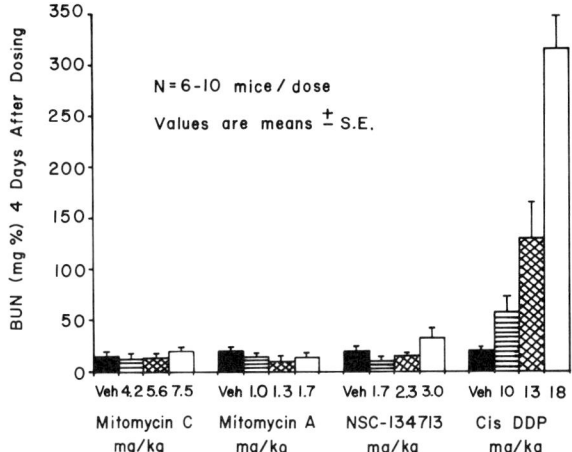

Fig. 5. Effect of mitomycin analogs and *cis*-DDP (single dose IP) on BUN in male BDF₁ mice.

C. Other Tests

We have under development tests in mice for both cardiac and pulmonary toxicity. Although these organ sites have not been a problem with MMC used as a single agent, such toxicities might be revealed in combination therapy regimens, and scattered clinical reports have suggested this possibility. Thus, the availability of simple tests for these side effects would permit us to screen new analogs in combination with putatively cardiotoxic and pulmonary toxic drugs and to determine whether or not the side effect is enhanced.

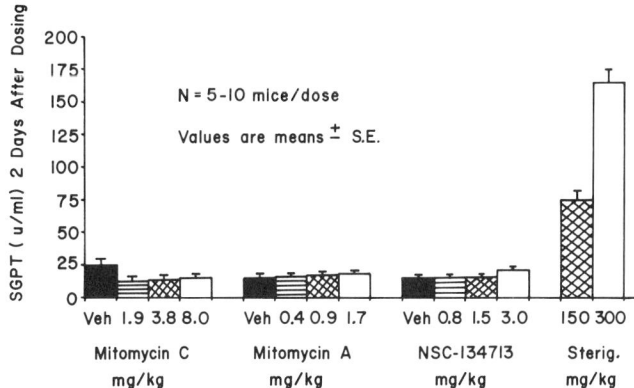

Fig. 6. Effect of mitomycin analogs and sterigmatocystin (single dose IP) on SGPT in male BDF₁ mice.

VII. DISCUSSION

All the tests performed so far with the more potent mitomycins could be run with less than 100 mg of compound. Resynthesis of a promising compound is usually required at this point so that treatment schedule studies, tests against other tumors, and further side effects evaluation can be carried out. Now that we have these simple and rapid test tools for screening of new mitomycin candidates, we believe greater progress can be made in identifying a second generation of mitomycins with improved therapeutic potential.

REFERENCES

Bradner, W. T. (1958). *Ann. N. Y. Acad. Sci. 76*, 469-474.
Crooke, S. T., and Bradner, W. T. (1976). *Cancer Treat. Rev. 3*, 121-139.
Geran, R. I., Greenberg, N. N., MacDonald, M. M., Schumacher, A. M., and Abbott, B. J. (1972). *Cancer Chemother. Rep. 3*, 1-103.
Hata, T., Hossenlopp, C., and Takita, H. (1961). *Cancer Chemother. Rep. 13*, 67-77.
Kojima, R., Goldin, A., and Mantel, N. (1972a). *Cancer Chemother. Rep. 3*, (Part 2), 111-119.
Kojima, R., Driscoll, J., Mantel, N., and Goldin, A. (1972b). *Cancer Chemother. Rep. 3*, (Part 2), 121-135.
Matsui, M., Yamada, Y., Uzu, K., and Hirata, T. (1968). *J. Antibiot. 22*, 189-198.
Price, K. E., Buck, R. E., and Lein, J. (1964). *Appl. Microbial. 12*, 428-435.
Weil, C. S. (1952). *Biometrics 8*, 249-263.

Chapter 5

MORPHOLOGICAL EFFECTS OF MITOMYCIN C ON CELLULAR FINE STRUCTURE[1]

Yerach Daskal
Stanley T. Crooke

I. INTRODUCTION

There are not many data available on the precise ultrastructural lesions induced by mitomycin C (MC). Of the few available morphological studies, Lapis and Bernhard (1965) and Simard and Bernhard (1966) have described the nucleolar lesion induced by the drug. Most of the other studies have been carried out at the light microscopic level only.

The morphological data in the present study were obtained from several model systems, namely, Novikoff hepatoma ascites cells grown *in vitro* cell cultures, the normal rat liver, and the normal and tumorous mouse bladders. The drug treatments were all of short duration, essentially in an attempt to mimic an "acute" effect in the above systems. In addition, some studies were carried out in the scanning electron microscopic modality in order to determine whether any topological manifestations of MC action were present.

[1] These studies were supported by the Cancer Center Grant CA-10893, P. 5, awarded by the National Cancer Institute, DHEW, and by the Bristol Fund.

41

II. THE EFFECTS OF MC ON NOVIKOFF HEPATOMA
ASCITES CELLS *IN VITRO*

A. Scanning Electron Microscopy (SEM)

Novikoff hepatoma ascites cells grown *in vitro* were treated with 10 μg/ml MC for 2 hr. As shown in Fig. 1, the surface morphology of these treated cells does not differ significantly from untreated (control) cells shown in Fig. 2. The reduction in the distribution as well as the sizes of surface filopodial extensions in the treated cells may represent a general cellular response to a large variety of cytotoxic agents rather than a specific alteration induced by mitomycin C. Moreoover, the distribution pattern of some structural markers such as surface blebs, ruffles, and microvilli may be frequently related to cell cycle morphological variations rather than drug-induced effects.

B. Transmission Electron Microscopy (TEM)

In contrast to SEM, TEM has revealed that within 1-2 hr after drug treatment (3-10 μg/ml), the nucleolus of the cell is a prime site for a defined subcellular lesion. Under these conditions (10 μg/ml for 1 hr), nucleoli assume a compact configuration and are clearly segregated (Fig. 3) into granular (G) and fibrillar (F) components. At higher magnifications (Fig. 4a, inset), it can be seen that in addition to the segregation of the nucleolar components, electron-dense microspherules (Unuma and Busch, 1967; Goldblatt and Sullivan, 1970) are present in various stages of extrusion. The formation of micropherules, concomitant with nucleolar segregation, has been observed also after actinomycin D treatments (Simard and Bernhard, 1966; Unuma and Busch, 1967) and after class II anthracyclines (Daskal *et al.,* 1978), and acridine orange dyes (Recher *et al.,* 1973). Neither the composition, origin, nor function of the microspherules is known at present. It may be speculated, however, that these represent specific chromatin segments sequested from the nucleolar DNA.

Within 2 hr after 10 μg/ml MC, nucleoli reach their most compact configuration (Fig. 4) and, in addition to the extrusion of nucleolar microspherules, components of the nucleolar organizer elements (NOR) are segregated from the nucleolar bodies. To date, no clear relationship has been established between the nucleolar organizer regions, seen as patches of low electron density, and the rest of the nucleolar components (Goesens *et al.,* 1974). Furthermore, the precise mechanism by which MC may induce the segregation of the NOR components is not clear.

Finally, the segregation of the nucleolar components proceeded to the point

---

Figs. 1, 2. Scanning electron micrographs of Novikoff hepatoma cells grown *in vitro* after treatment with 10 μg/ml mitomycin C for 2 hr (1) and control untreated cells (2). The only putative changes as a result of the drug treatments may be manifested in the form of reduced elaborations of the cellular surface in the treated cells.

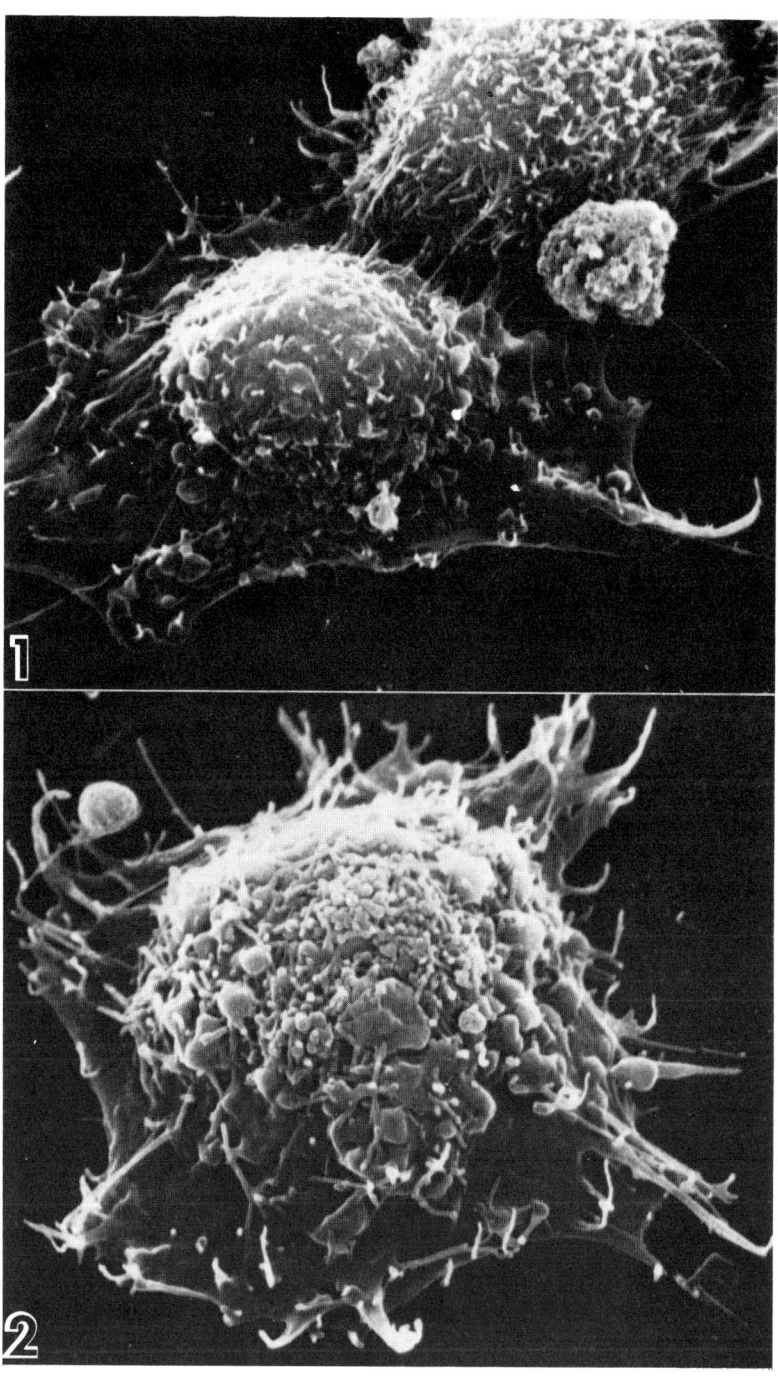

where ring-shaped nucleoli were formed (Fig. 5) after more than 2 hr of MC (10 μg/ml) treatment. Since the presence of segregated nucleoli is the ultrastructural manifestation of the complete inhibition of ribosomal RNA synthesis in the nucleolus, it may be concluded that mitomycin C, either directly or indirectly, will ultimately inhibit nucleolar DNA transcription (Crooke and Bradner, 1976). Since nucleolar DNA is enriched with GC sequences, it is most interesting that mitomycin C apparently has a "homing" capability toward such sequences, as is detailed by Lown (this volume).

Although similar results have been reported by Lapis and Bernhard (1965) in another cell line, when KB cells were treated with MC for up to 72 hr nucleolar microspherules were not induced. Whether these morphological differences observed in the two cell lines represent variations in the effects of MC *in vitro* and *in vivo* will be discussed below.

III. EFFECTS OF MITOMYCIN C ON THE MORPHOLOGY OF THE NORMAL LIVER OF THE RAT

Within 2 hr after the IP injections of 2.5 mg/kg of MC, the onset of what appears to be a transient but characteristic drug-induced hepatitis is evident (Fig. 6a). The patchy cytoplasm of the hepatic parenchyma cells is depleted of glycogen and mitochrondrial condensation is evident. In addition, a general reduction in the distribution of rough ER is clearly seen. Only restricted regions of the cytoplasm still contain patches of mature, well-developed rough ER (Fig. 6a) mainly around the cell nucleus. Increased vesiculation of the cytoplasm was present (Fig. 6b). Increasing the concentration of MC to 5 mg/kg resulted in further cytoplasmic injury (Fig. 7) with further reduction in the presence of rough ER even around the nuclear peripheries. Furthermore, instead of the numerous cytoplasmic vesicles previously ob-

---

Fig. 3. Transmission electron micrograph of hepatoma cell *in vitro* after treatment with 10 μg/ml mitomycin C for 1 hr. All nucleoli in these cells are totally segregated into the fibrillar (F) and granular (G) components.

Fig. 4. Nucleolus of hepatoma cell 2 hr after treatment with mitomycin C (10 μg/ml). The dense bodies with the segregated nucleolus (4a-M) are microspherules. These may be observed to be extruded from the nucleolar body. NOR—nucleolar organized components also segregate from the main nucleolar body into distinct patches of low electron density.

Fig. 5. Final stages in the inactivation of the nucleolus after mitomycin C treatment, resulting in a ring-shaped nucleolus, totally inactive in rRNA synthesis.

Fig. 6. Rat hepatocyte after 2.5 mg/kg mitomycin C (2 hr). Vesiculation of the cytoplasm is evident. In addition to glycogen depletion (pointers), the rough ER is restricted to some focal regions in the cytoplasm (Fig. 6a and b). Cytoplasmic vesiculation is most evident in Fig. 6b (arrows). Even at this low magnification, nuclear changes are distinct in the form of an increase in the number of perichromatin granules (PCG) within the chromatin clusters. (Fig. 6b pointers).

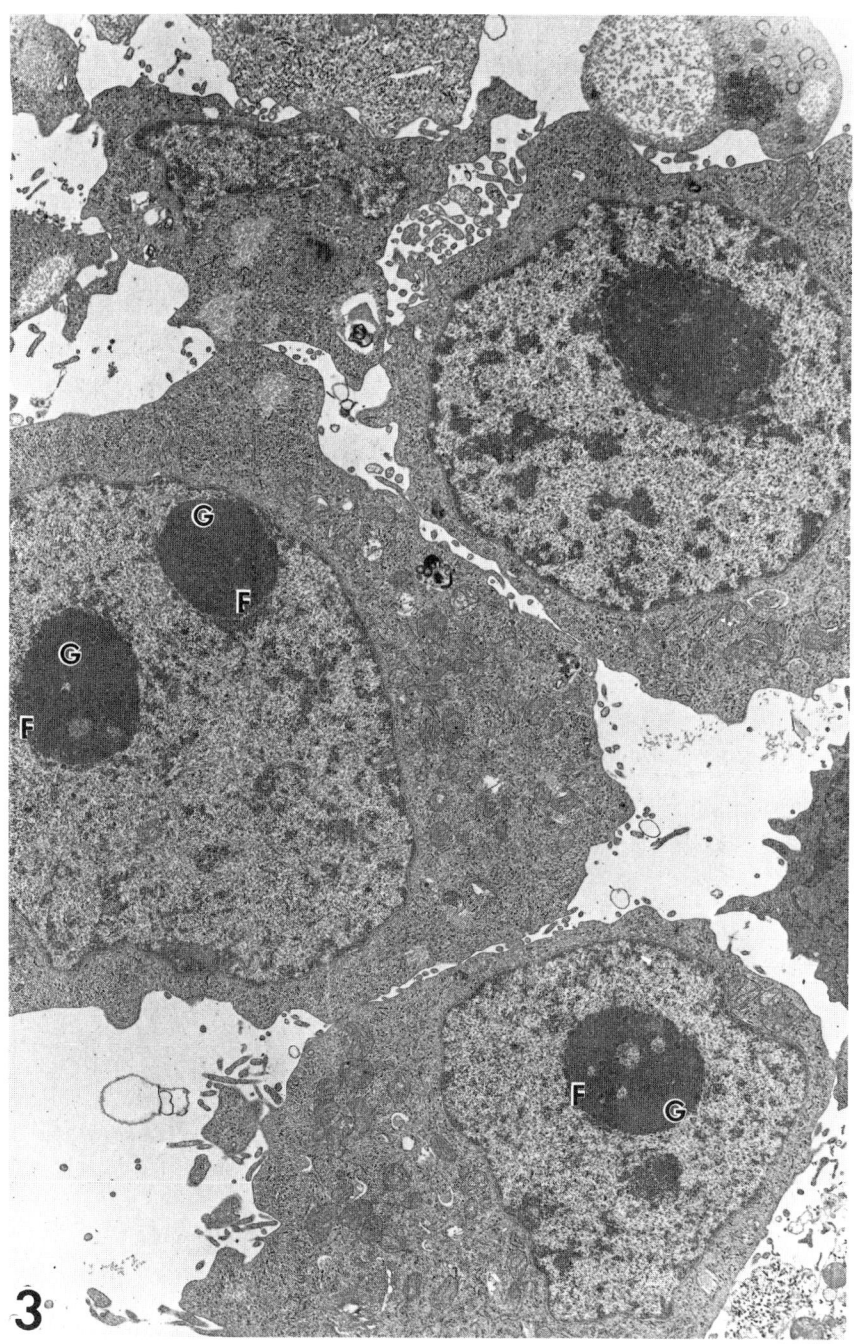

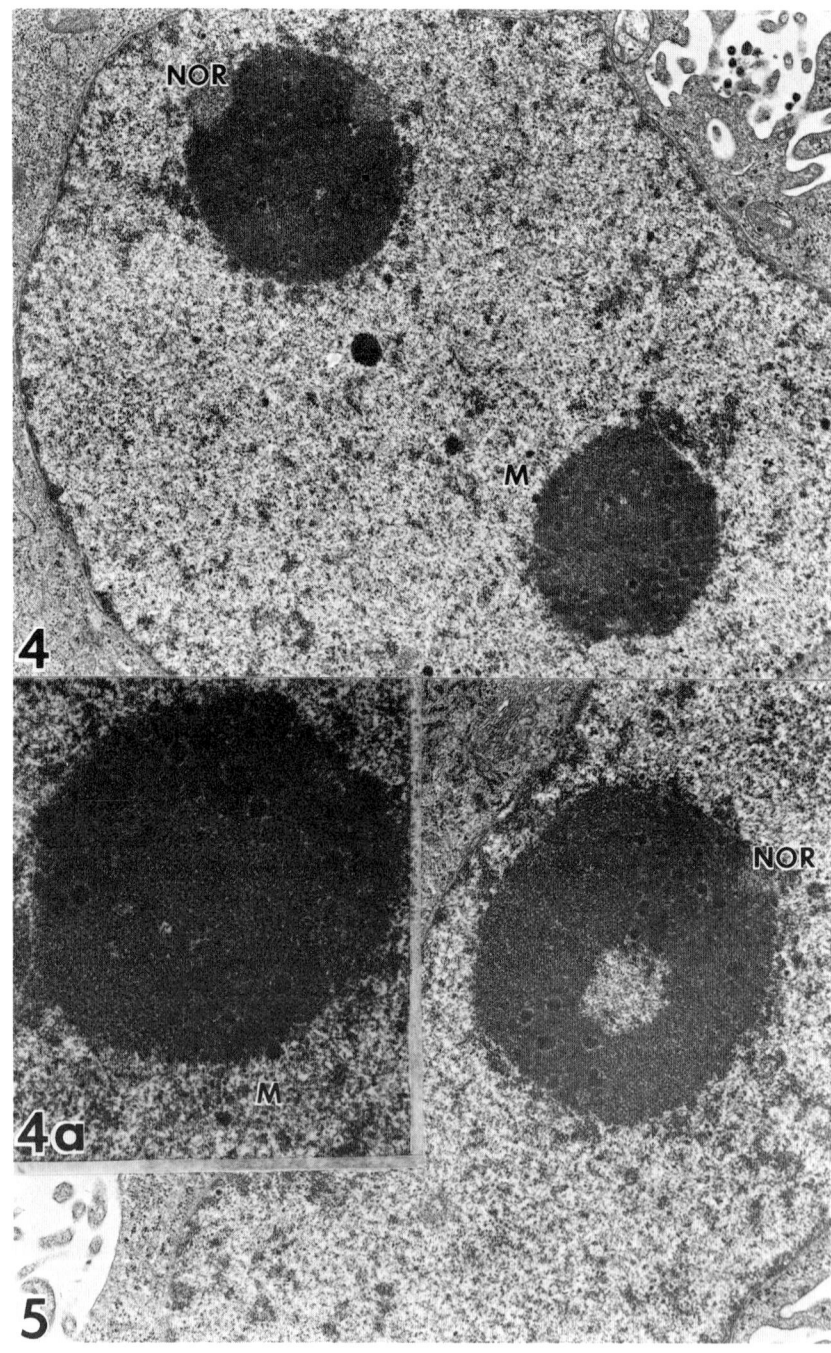

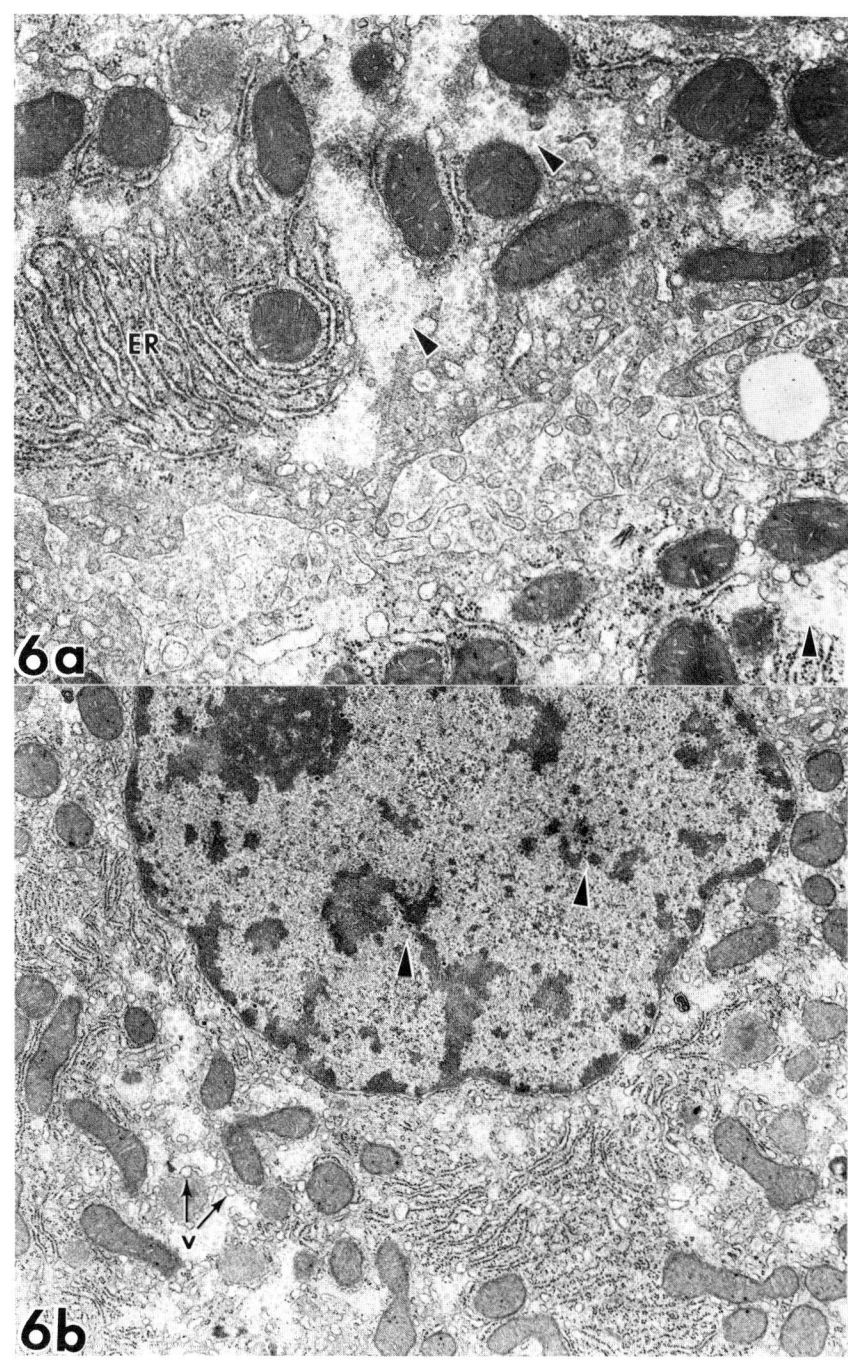

served, myelin figures (pointers, Fig. 7) seemed to accumulate. Distinct islands of electron-dense matrix (ground substance) in the hepatocytes around mitochondria are distributed within the liver in a focal fashion.

With respect to the effects of MC on the rat liver nucleus, specific lesions were observed 1 hr after a dose of 5 mg/kg IP. Rather than affecting the nucleolus as was shown in Novikoff hepatoma ascites cells *in vitro* (Figs. 3-5), MC seemed to affect the number of perichromatin granules (PCG) with the nucleus (arrows, Fig. 7) and around the nucleolus as well as to increase chromatin hypercondensation (inactivated chromatin clumps). Dramatic increases in PCG numbers were observed 3 hr after the injection of 5 mg/kg MC (Fig. 8a). The distribution pattern of the PCG within the nucleus is similar to that observed after cycloheximide (Daskal *et al.*, 1975; Moyne *et al.*, 1977), that is, frequently associated with a clump of heterochromatin (pointers and Fig. 8a inset).

Within the cytoplasm, 3 hr after treatment with 5 mg/kg of mitomycin C (Fig. 8b), the accumulation of myelin figures (membrane whorls) continued. Again, neither the function, origin, nor composition of the PCG is precisely known. Some data are available (Watson, 1962; Vasquez-Nin and Bernhard 1971), and they indicate that PCGs are excised chromatin-containing structures (Daskal *et al.*, 1978). If this is the case, then a possible analogy may exist between the sequestering of nucleolar microspherules by MC in Novikoff cells *in vitro* and the increase of PCGs in the rat liver nuclei.

Furthermore, the difference in the subcellular lesion induced by MC *in vivo* and *in vitro* may possibly reflect variations in the activation of the three alkylation sites in the MC molecule, in the rat liver *in vitro* and Novikoff ascites cells.

IV. EFFECTS OF MC ON THE MOUSE BLADDER EPITHELIUM

The intravesicular administration of MC was shown to yield undetectable serum concentrations and induce significant response rates in lower-grade tumors (Crooke and Bradner, 1976). To further evaluate whether some localized cytotoxic effects occur after the intravesicular administration of MC, both light microscopic and analyses of treated mouse bladders were undertaken.

In this study, MC was instilled in varying concentrations via a catheter to fasted mice. The catheter was clamped, and the MC solution allowed to remain in the bladder for 2 hr. Immediately after the instillation, the bladder was drained, the animals sacrificed, and the bladders excised. The bladders were washed thoroughly with normal saline, cut into hemispheres, and fixed for microscopy. The concentrations and instillation times were chosen to be comparable to those employed in current clinical trials studying intravesically administered MC (see Bracken and

---

Fig. 7. Rat hepatocyte after 5 mg/kg mitomycin C. Cytoplasmic lesions increase in severity concomitant to the appearance of myelin figures (pointers). Nucleolar condensation occurs and there is increase in perichromatin granules (arrows) within the condensed chromocenters.

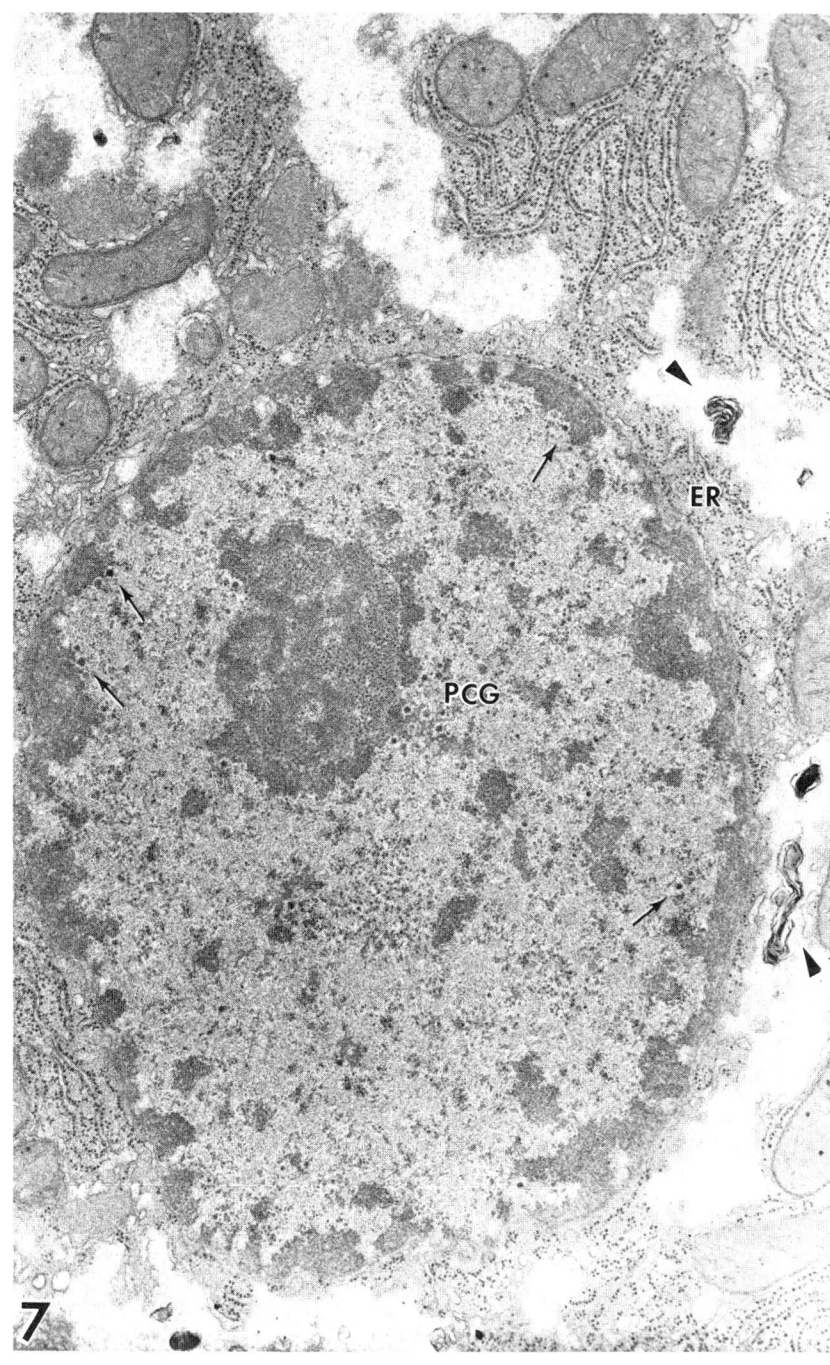

Johnson, this volume).

Examination by light microscopy of either the normal (Fig. 9a) or the tumor-bearing mouse bladder (Fig. 9b) after intravesicular administration of 5 mg/ml of MC shows that focal changes in the transitional epithelium are present. In the normal bladder (Fig. 9a), heteropyknotic nuclei can be clearly seen. In addition to the presence of these "washed out" nuclei, the cytoplasm of these cells appears hypervacuolated. These changes are consistent with the possible onset of cell necrosis. In the FANFT-induced, tumor-bearing bladders (Fig. 9b), a similar focal distribution of what appears to represent drug-induced cell necrosis may be observed as well. Transmission electron microscopy of similar specimens confirmed the data obtained from light microscopy. Examination of tumor-bearing MC-treated bladders (Fig. 10) as well as untreated ones (Fig. 11a) clearly showed the loss in nuclear matrix density as well as a general loss in cytoplasmic architecture and organization, formation of large vacuoles, and an increase in the intercellular spaces. These features were not present in the untreated samples (Fig. 11b).

The nuclei of the treated tumor cells did not show the normal chromatin distribution. Nucleoli were compact with a possible indication for the onset of segregation (Fig. 10). Cytoplasmic lipid inclusion vacuolation, vesiculation, and increases in the intercellular spaces were also observed (compare Fig. 9, 10, 11). Examination of the surfaces of either the normal or tumorous bladder before and after mitomycin C treatments yielded additional information on the topological effects of mitomycin C on the transitional epithelium of the bladder. The surface of the normal bladder consists of well-defined hexagonal sections delimited by ridges (Fig. 12a). The transitional epithelium may possess very short microvilli (Fig. 12a) or, depending on the state of contraction, elongated small ridges (Fig. 13a).

After the intravesicular administration of 5 mg/ml of mitomycin C. the general appearance of the surface of the transitional epithelium differed from that of the normal untreated one (Fig. 12a). Although the dividing ridges were still present, no other topological substructural detail was observed. The differences of the fine surface structure of the untreated (Fig. 13a, normal control) and the treated (Fig. 13b, normal) are more evident at higher magnifications. In addition to the disappearance of the short microvilli (observed also in transmission electron microscopy [Fig. 11]) in the treated (Fig. 13b), the formation of indentations or clefts along

---

Fig. 8. Rat liver nucleus, 3 hr after mitomycin C treatments. The dramatic increase of perichromatin granules is clearly demonstrated (pointers) in discrete clusters (inset 8a). Within the cytoplasm (8b) at this time point (3 hr) only restricted regions contain rough ER and the concentration of myelin figures seems to increase.

Fig. 9. Light micrographs of normal (9a) and tumor-bearing (9b) mouse bladders' transitional epithelium regions after the intravesicular administration of 5 mg/ml mitomycin C. The affected cells can be seen by their lucid nuclei both in the normal and FANFT-induced tumor-bearing bladders. In addition, the differential pyknosis of the cells and the increased vacuolation of the cytoplasm of the transitional epithelial cells represent focal areas of mitomycin C cytotoxicity (Lu-Luminal space).

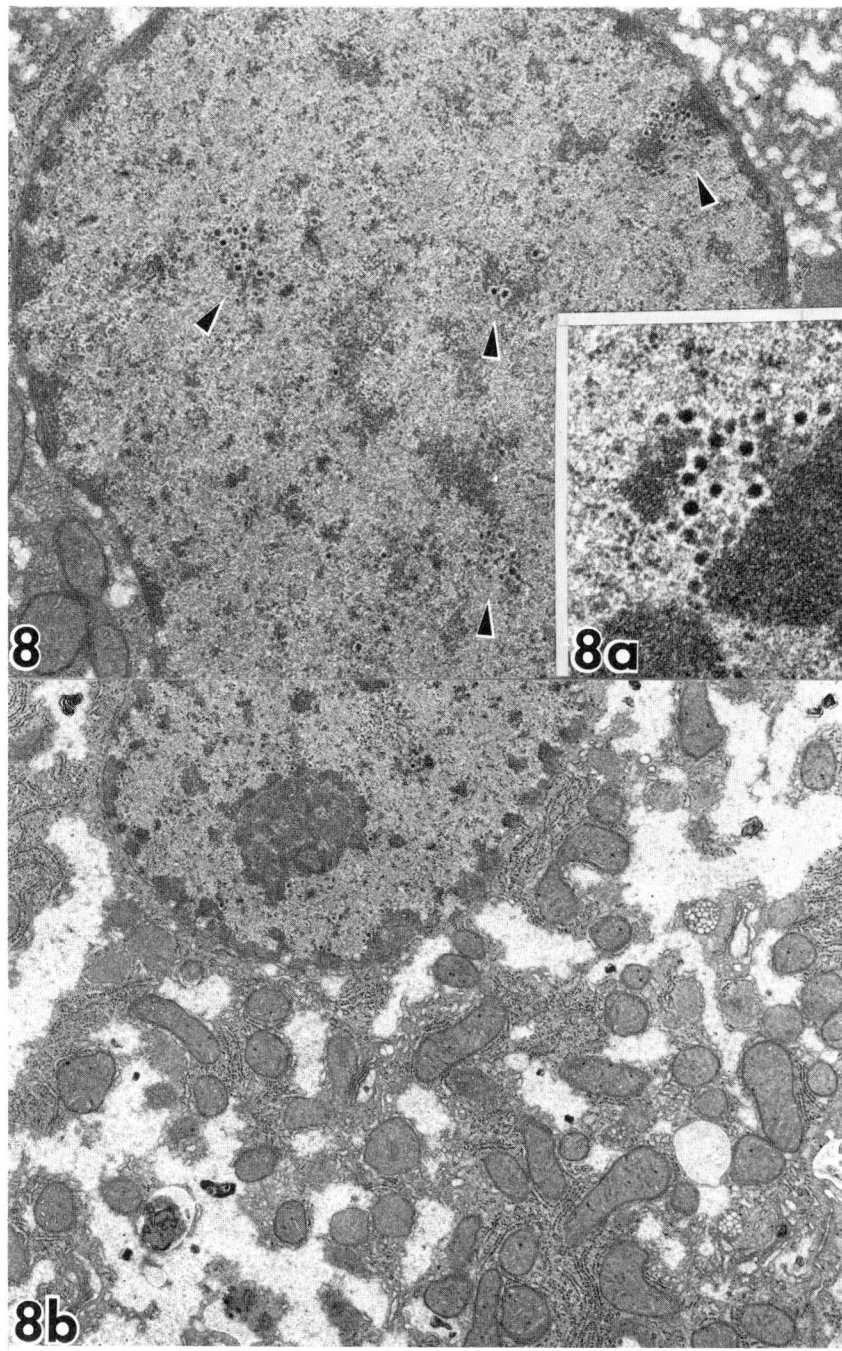

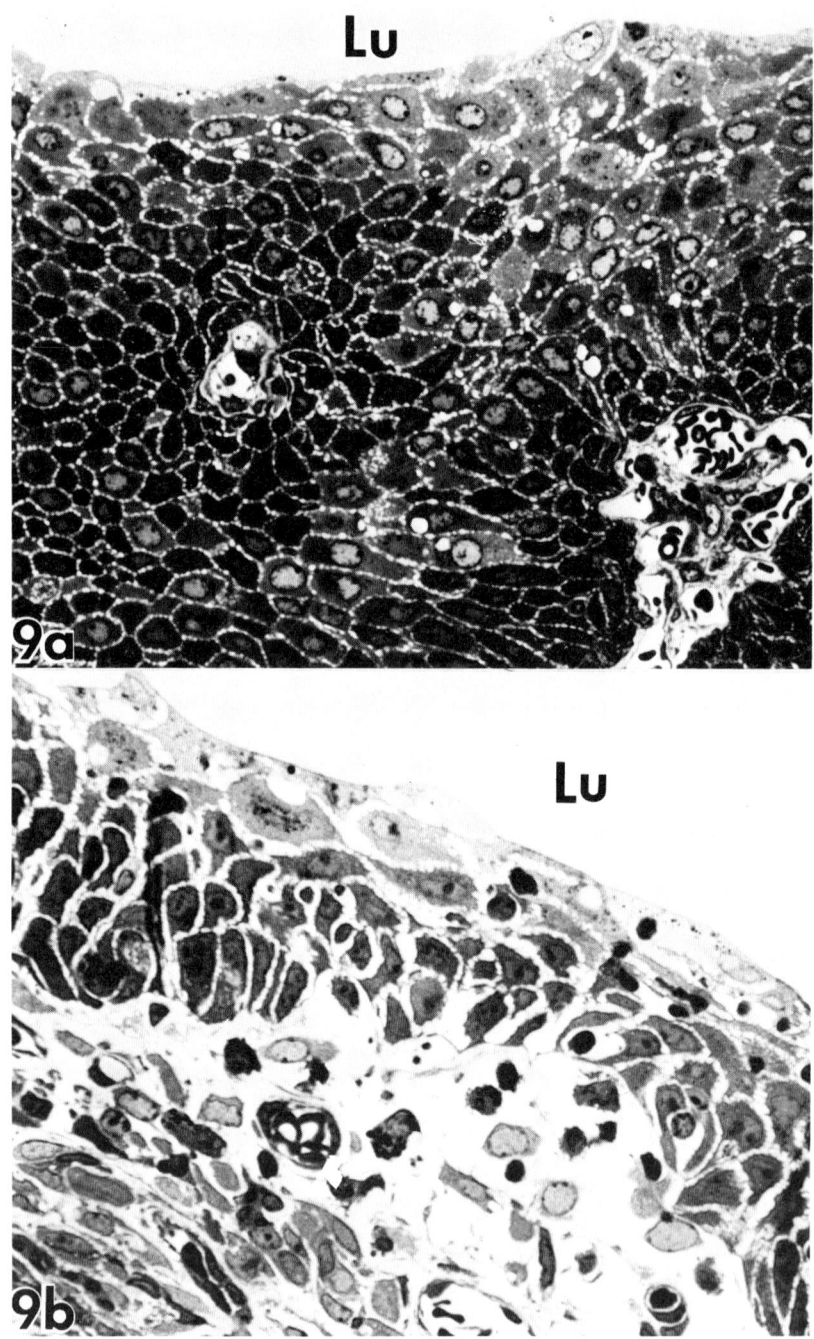

the dividing ridges can be observed. Similar data were obtained also when bladders containing FANFT-induced tumors were examined before and after mitomycin C treatments (Fig. 14 and 15). The fine structural features of the untreated tumor cells, that is the elaborated microvillar complexes and the cell-to-cell interactions (Fig. 14) were lost after mitomycin C treatments. Instead, the tumor cells appeared collapsed (Fig. 15), evidenced little if any surface substructures (Fig. 15a and b), and intercellular spaces appeared to be increased. These features are consistent with the onset of cell death probably mediated by the exposure of the tumor cells to mitomycin C. It should be noted that some of these effects were of a focal distribution probably due to either lack of complete contact with mitomycin or a non-homogeneous distribution of the drug.

Future studies using similar multimodal morphological evaluation of drug treatments should be able to assist, clarify, and determine optimal routes, schedules, and doses for drug administration.

Fig. 10. Survey electron micrograph of the transitional epithelial region of tumor-being mouse bladder after intravesicular administration of 5 mg/ml mitomycin C. General cell necrosis is evident, manifested in the form of excess cytoplasmic vacuolation (V), increased intercellular spaces, nuclei of low electron density, contracted chromatin, and hypercondensed nucleoli (Lu-Luminal space).

Fig. 11. Electron (11a) and light micrographs (11b) of tumor-bearing but untreated mouse bladders, for comparative purposes with Figs. 9 and 10. Note electron density of the tumor nuclei (Figure 11a), the intercellular interactions and (11b) the configuration of the chromatin and nucleoli within the untreated cells. Both micrographs are on the immediate proximity of the luminal region.

Fig. 12. Scanning electron micrograph of the normal bladder surface before (12a) and after (12b) mitomycin C intravesicular administration (5 mg/ml). The fine surface detail such as complex ridge morphology, topical short villi, and microridges were not apparent after drug treatments.

Fig. 13. A higher magnification of areas similar to those shown in Fig. 12. Surface elaboration present prior to drug exposure (13a) is lost after treatment (13b). Note the discrete changes in the morphology and intercellular contacts in the ridge regions, and distinct loss of topical villi.

Fig. 14. Scanning electron micrograph at low (14a) and higher magnifications (14b) before drug treatments. Note elaborate cellular surfaces. In the distant background the "normal" bladder surface may be observed consisting of distinct ridges with the characteristic short patchy microvillar-bearing transitional epithelial cells.

Fig. 15. Similar tumor to that seen in Fig. 14 but after treatment with mitomycin C (intravesicular administration of 5 mg/ml). Note the altered cellular surface, denudation of surfaces both of the tumor cells and the bladder surfaces (15a). At higher magnifications the reduced elaborations, the mottled appearance of the cellular surfaces, and increases in intercellular spaces are evident. These changes are consistent with the onset of drug-induced cellular necrosis.

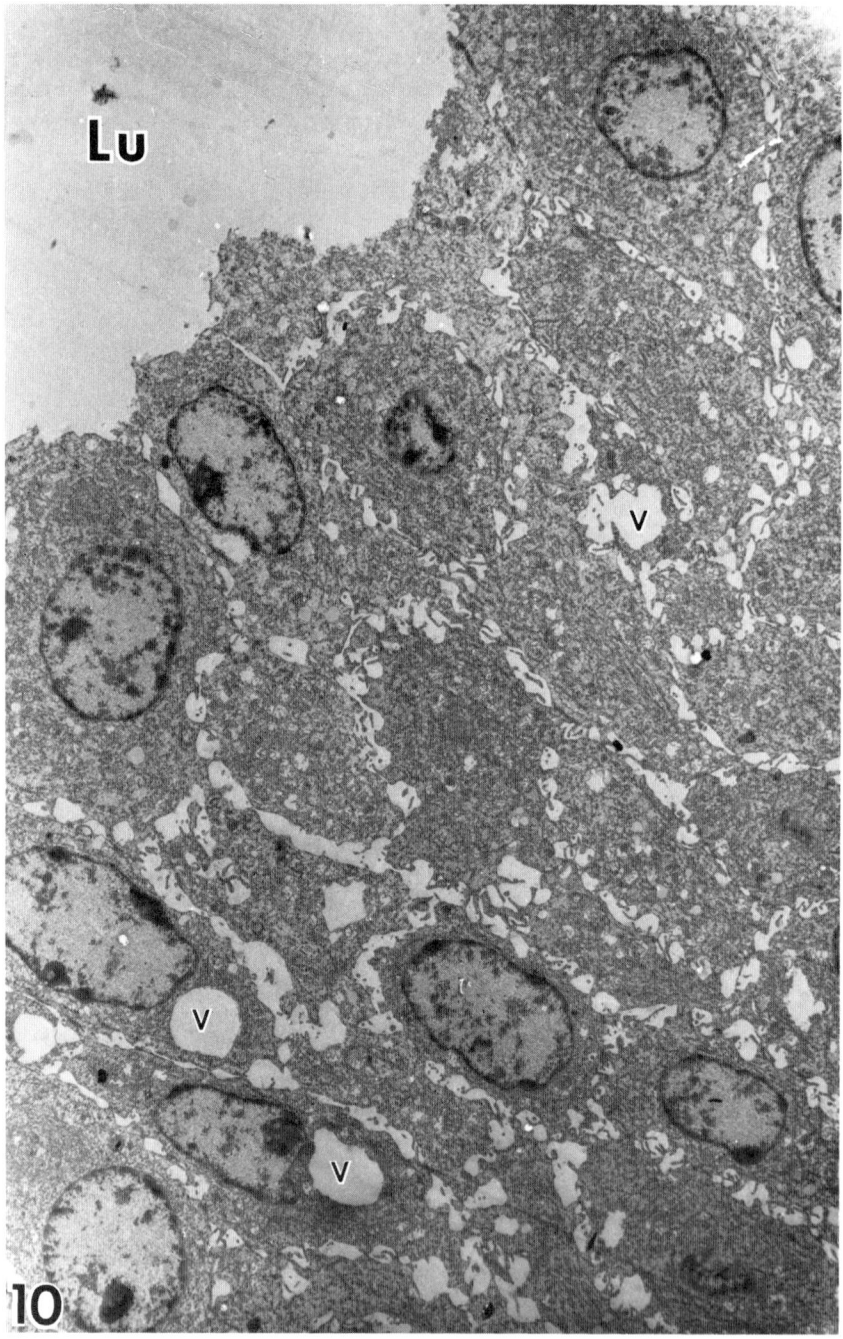

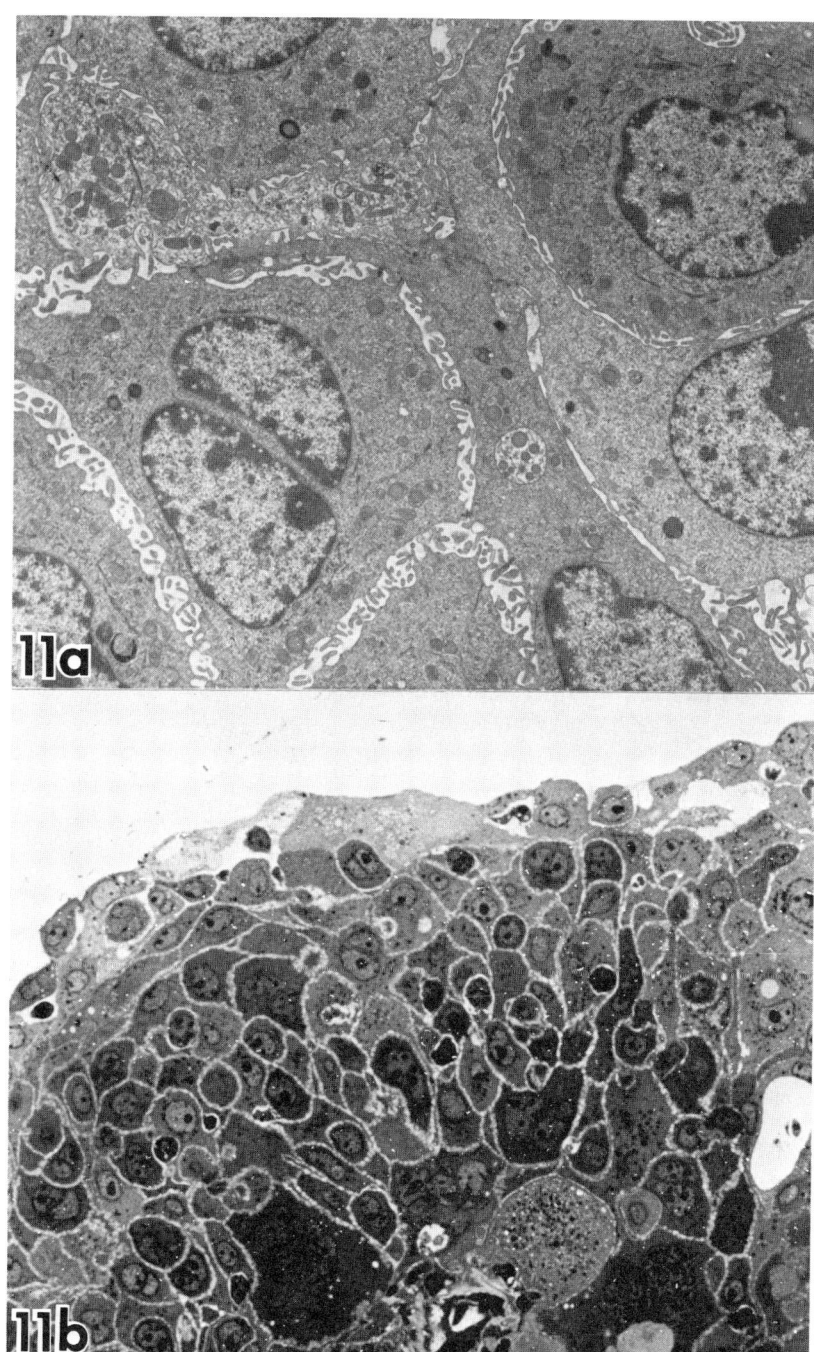

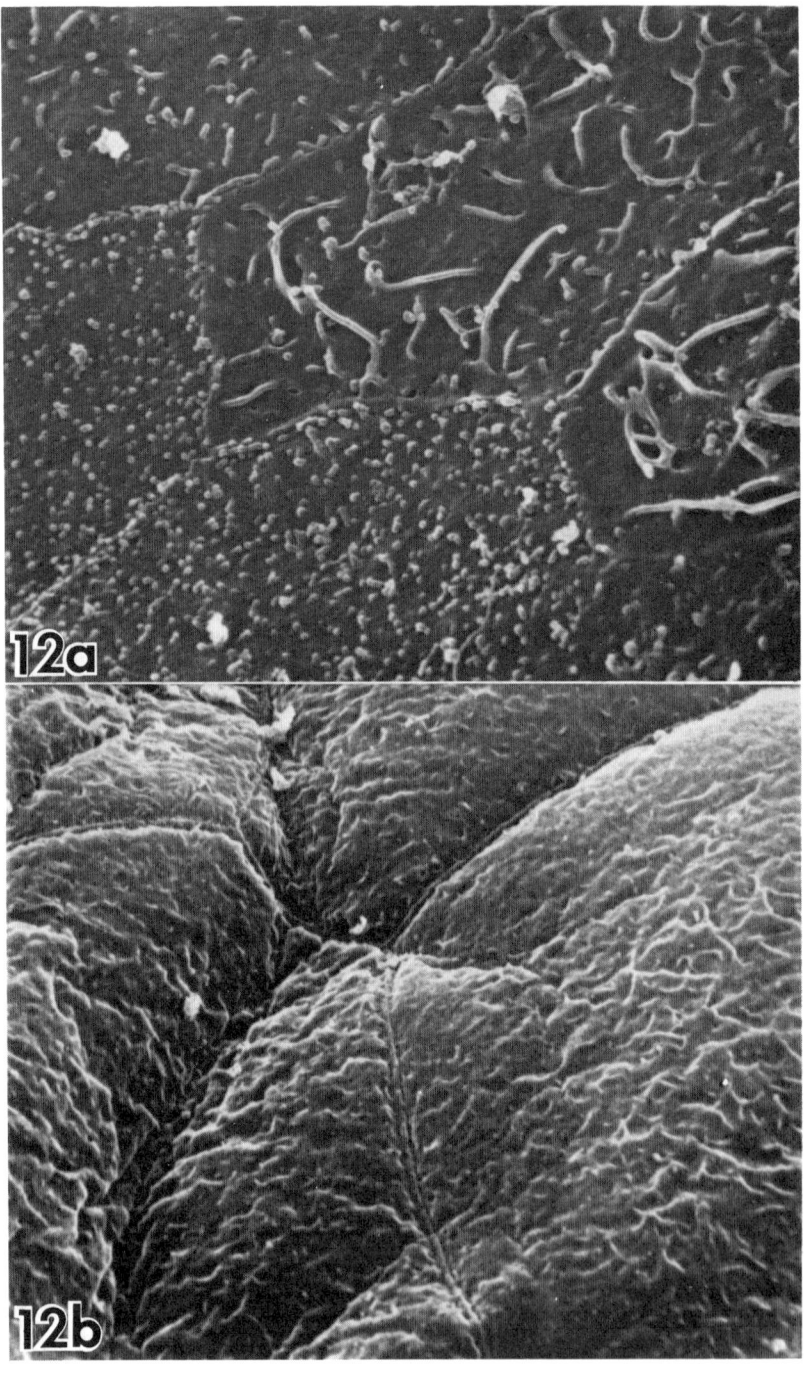

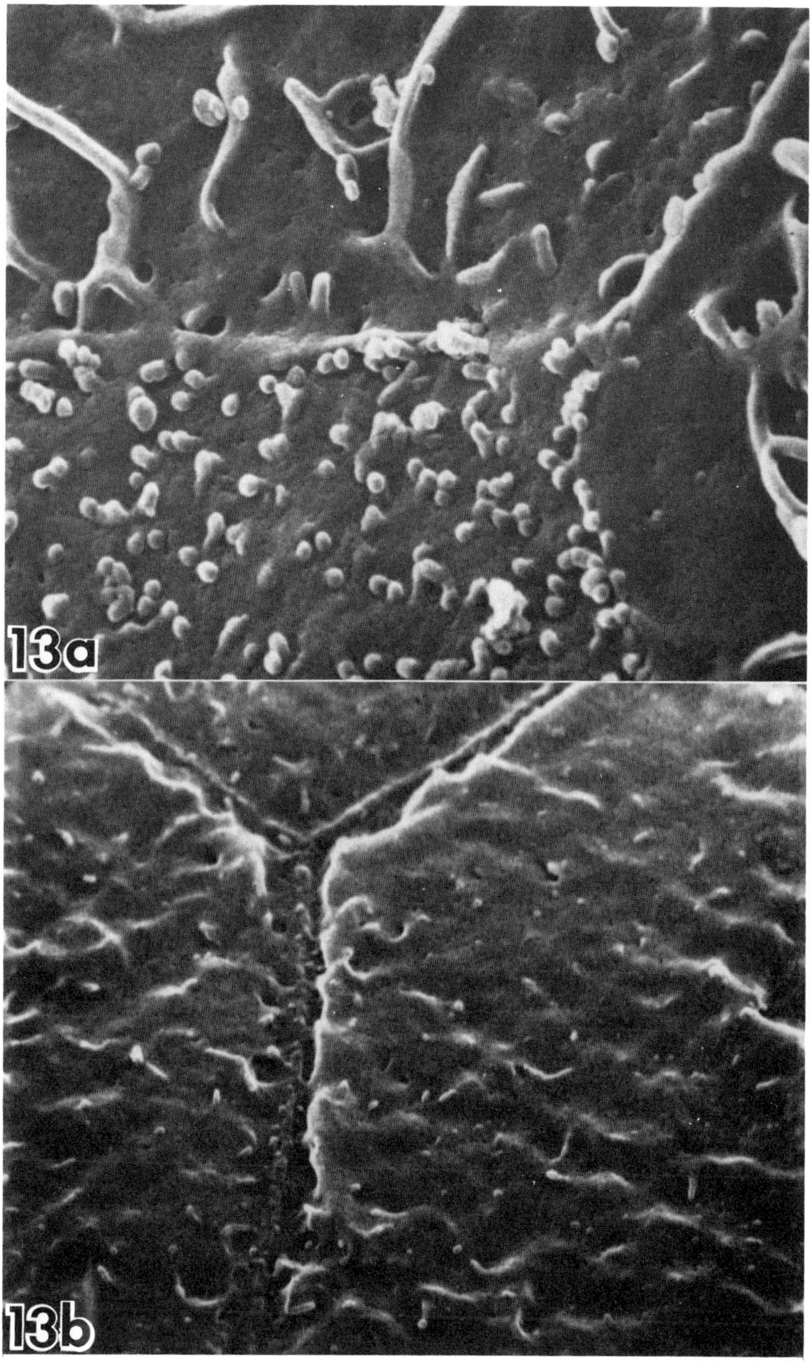

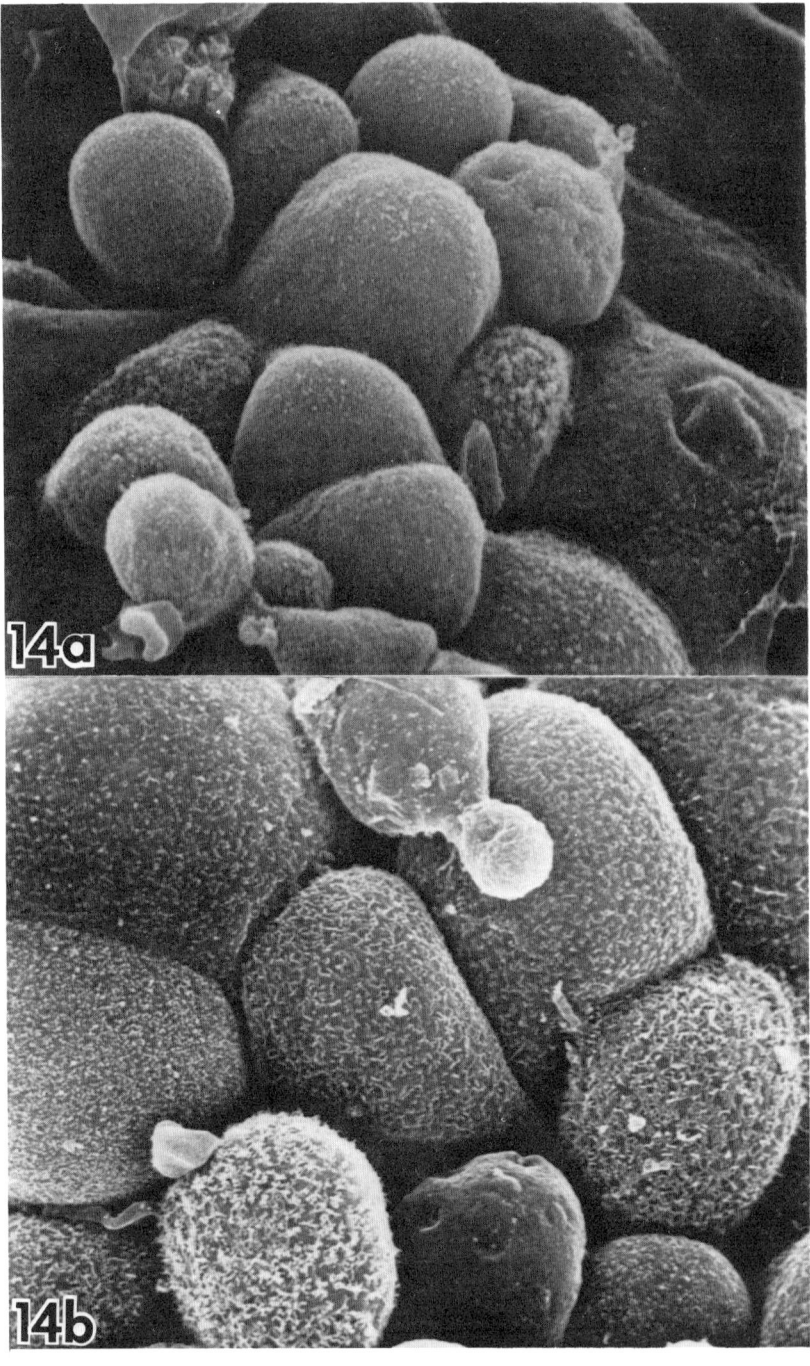

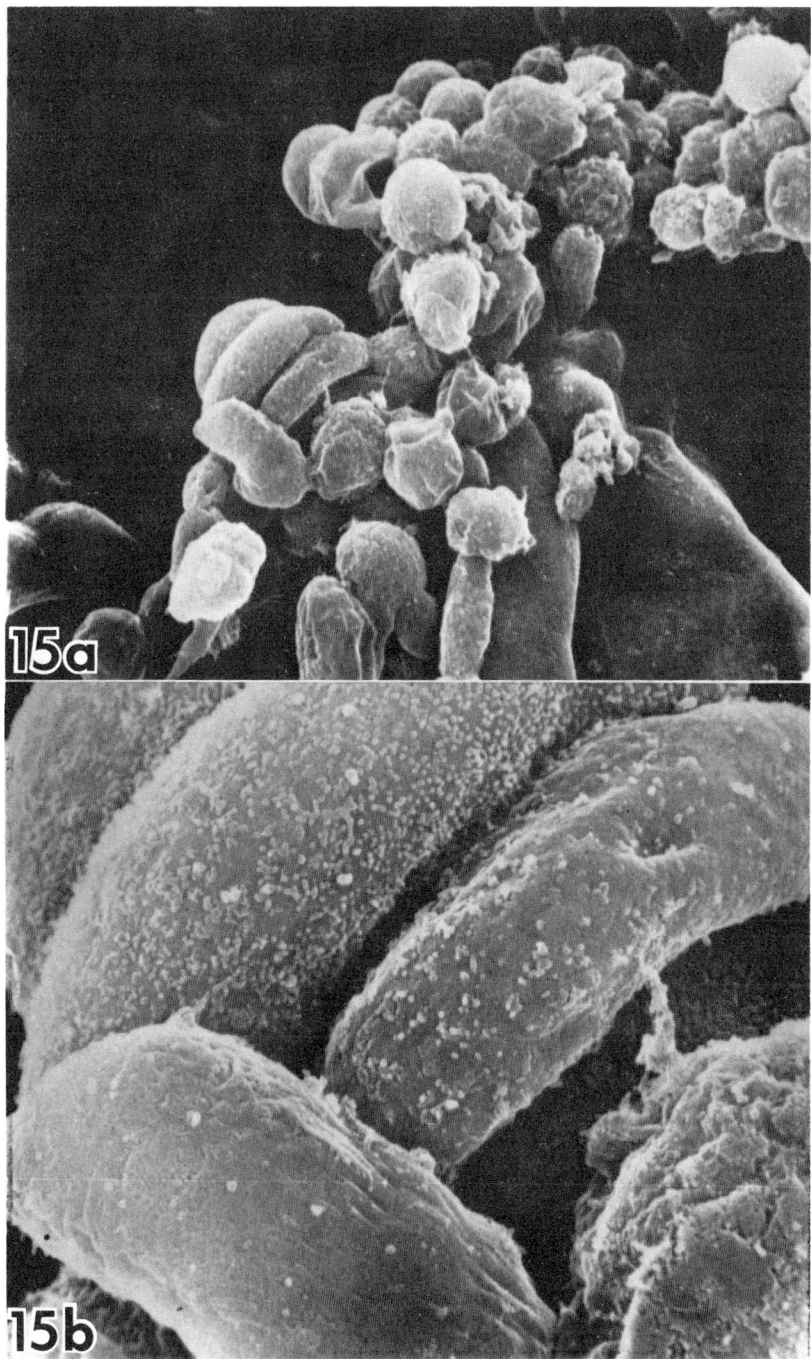

ACKNOWLEDGMENTS

The authors are grateful for the collaboration of Dr. M. Soloway, Memphis Medical Center, for the FANFT-induced bladder tumors and the excellent technical assistance of Mr. C. Woodard.

REFERENCES

Crooke, S. T., and Bradner, W. T. (1976). *Cancer Treat. Rep. 3,* 121-139.

Daskal, Y., Merski, J. A., Hughes, J. B., and Busch, H. (1975). *Expt. Cell Res. 93,* 395-401.

Daskal, Y., Komaromy, L., and Busch, H. (1978). *J. Cell Biol. 79,* (part 2), 122.

Goessens, G., and Lepoint, A. (1974). *Exptl. Cell Res. 87,* 63-72.

Goldblatt, P. J., and Sullivan, R. J. (1970). *Cancer Res. 30,* 1349-1356.

Lapis, K., and Bernhard, W. (1965). *Cancer Res. 25,* 628-643.

Moyne, G., Nash, R. E., and Puvion, E. (1977). *J. Biol. Cellul. 30,* 5-16.

Recher, L., Chan, H., and Sykes, J. A. (1973). *J. Ultrast. Res. 44,* 347-354.

Simard, R., and Bernhard, W. (1966). *Int. J. Cancer 1,* 463-479.

Unuma, T., and Busch, H. (1967). *Cancer Res. 27,* 1232-1242.

Vasquez-Nin, G., and Bernhard, W. (1971). *J. Ultrast. Res. 36,* 842-860.

Watson, M. L. (1962). *J. Cell. Biol. 13,* 162-167.

Chapter 6

SUPPRESSOR ACTIVITY IN THE SPLEEN OF TUMOR-BEARING MICE[1]

Bertie F. Argyris

I. INTRODUCTION

It is well known that many tumors carry tumor-specific transplantation antigens (Klein, 1968) that can activate an immune response in the tumor-bearing host. This immune response can take place via cytotoxic T cells (Cerottini and Brunner, 1974), armed macrophages (Lohmann-Matthes, 1976), antibody-producing B cells (Berger and Amos, 1977), or F c-receptor-positive null cells (Perlmann, 1976; Haller et al., 1977).

The presence of cytotoxic cells in a tumor-bearing host raises the question of why tumors are not rejected by these hosts. The growth of tumors, in spite of an immune response, could be due to the fact that (a) tumors can proliferate faster than they are destroyed by the cytotoxic cells; (b) tumor-specific antigens can activate B cells to produce blocking antibodies (Hellstrom and Hellstrom, 1974)—these blocking antibodies combine with the tumor antigen, and the resulting blocking factor can enhance tumor growth (Hellstrom and Hellstrom, 1976); (c) tumor cells can activate suppressor cells, which can inhibit the immune response and encourage tumor growth.

A number of reports have appeared recently in the literature which indicate that tumors can activate suppressor cells (Nordlund and Gershon, 1975; Manor et al.,

[1] Supported by P. H. S. Research Grant CA15462 from the National Cancer Institute and by a University Award from the Research Foundation of SUNY.

1976; Takei *et al.,* 1976; Fujimoto *et al.,* 1976a; Fujimoto *et al.,* 1976b). In the experiments we discuss here we will show that P-815 mastocytoma, transplanted subcutaneously into syngeneic DBA/2 mice, can activate splenic suppressor cells. These suppressor cells are capable of inhibiting the proliferation of normal spleen cells responding in mixed lymphocyte culture (MLC) to alloantigens. MLC is an *in vitro* assay for cell-mediated immunity (Bach *et al.,* 1969), and the results therefore suggest that tumors activate suppressor cells that inhibit the cell-mediated immune response.

II. MATERIALS AND METHODS

The P-815 mastocytoma is an ascites tumor, syngeneic for DBA/2 mice, and carried in these mice by weekly serial intraperitoneal (IP) passage of 4×10^6 cells. Solid subcutaneous (SC) tumor transplants are produced by SC injection of 10×10^6 P-815 cells into DBA/2 mice. Fifteen or 20 days later the spleen of the tumor-bearing animal is removed and tested for hyporesponsiveness (Argyris and DeLustro, 1977) and suppressor activity (Argyris, 1977) in MLC. Details of these techniques are described in previous publications (Argyris, 1977; Argyris, 1978).

Removal of glass-adherent cells from tumor-sensitized spleen is carried out by three 1-hour cycles of adsorption on a glass surface as described previously (Argyris, 1977). Theta-positive cells are removed by treatment with antitheta serum and complement. This procedure and the preparation of antitheta serum is described in one of our previous publications (Argyris, 1977).

Cell-impermeable diffusion chambers are constructed from 4 mm-thick slices of plastic tubing (8 mm diam.), sealed on each side with a Millipore GS filter (pore size, 0.22 μm). The sterile chambers are filled with 10×10^6 tumor cells/0.1 ml via a small hole on the side of the chamber, which is sealed with a hot needle before the chambers are implanted in the peritoneal cavity through a midventral incision. Control mice carry empty chambers (Argyris, 1978).

III. RESULTS

The experiment presented in Table I tests the MLC reactivity of spleen cells from DBA/2 mice implanted for 20 days with a SC transplant of P-815 tumor cells. The incorporation of ^{3}H-thymidine (^{3}H-TdR) in nonsensitized (NS) spleen cells in MLC is used as positive control and set as 100% response. The data indicate that spleen cells from tumor-bearing mice (SS) are hyporesponsive in MLC when incubated with both BALB/C or C57BL/6 stimulating cells.

Hyporesponsiveness in MLC can be the result of a decrease in reactive cells or the presence of suppressor cells. To distinguish between these two alternatives, the experiments presented in Table II have been carried out. In these experiments, 5×10^5 spleen cells from tumor-bearing mice have been added to normal MLC or

TABLE I. MLC Reactivity of Spleen Cells from DBA/2 Mice Carrying a 20-Day Old SC Transplant of Syngeneic P-815 Mastocytoma[a]

Responding spleen (3×10^5)	Stimulating spleen (3×10^5)	^{3}H-TdR INCORPORATION (CPM $\pm$ SE)			
		AA_m	AB_m	SI	% Response
DBA/2 NS	BALB/C	$29,397 \pm 2177$	$107,910 \pm 8476$	3.7	100
SS		$15,781 \pm 806$	$37,034 \pm 2732$	2.3	27
DBA/2 NS	C57BL/6	$18,495 \pm 942$	$43,112 \pm 2630$	2.3	100
SS		$13,115 \pm 1800$	$20,185 \pm 1806$	1.5	29

[a]NS = nonsensitized spleen cells; SS = sensitized spleen cells; AA_m represents background proliferation of responding cells incubated with syngeneic mitomycin-treated cells; AB_m represents thymidine (^{3}H-TdR) incorporation in responding cells incubated with allogeneic mitomycin-treated stimulating cells; SI = stimulation index obtained by dividing the AB_m counts by the AA_m counts; % response is calculated according to the formula

$$\frac{AB_m - AA_m \text{ (experimental)}}{AB_m - AA_m \text{ (control)}} \times 100$$

where control cultures are those in which NS are used as responding cells. All cultures are done in triplicate. For further details, see Argyris (1977 and 1978).

DBA/2 nonsensitized spleen (NS) responding to allogeneic mitomycin-treated BALB/C stimulating spleen cells. Control cultures receive an equivalent number of added nonsensitized spleen cells. To prevent the added cells from participating in the proliferative process of MLC, they are pretreated with mitomycin.

The data in the top half of Table II establish again that spleen cells from tumor-bearing mice (SS) are hyporesponsive in MLC. In the bottom half of Table II, one can see that this hyporesponsiveness is due to suppressor activity. The addition of mitomycin-treated spleen cells from tumor-bearing mice (SS_m) greatly suppresses the proliferation of normal DBA/2 spleen cells (NS) responding in MLC to allogeneic BALB/C stimulating spleen cells. To control for crowding of the cultures, control cultures receive an equivalent number of mitomycin-treated nonsensitized spleen cells (NS_m) and the ^{3}H-TdR incorporation in these cultures is set as 100% response.

The above results suggest that the spleen of tumor-bearing mice contains suppressor cell activity. In addition, the data show that mitomycin treatment does not prevent suppressor activity. This indicates that DNA synthesis is not required for the expression of suppressor activity.

The next series of experiments was designed to test the nature of the suppressor cells. Glass-adherent cells were removed by three 1-hour periods of adsorption on glass. The data in Table III indicate that glass-adsorbed (NA) spleen cells from tumor-bearing mice still have suppressor activity.

In the next experiments, spleen cells from tumor-bearing mice were pretreated with antitheta serum and complement. The data in Table IV indicate that removal

TABLE II.   Suppressor Activity of Spleen Cells from DBA/2 Mice Carrying a 20-Day Old
Transplant of Syngeneic P-815 Mastocytoma[a]

Responding spleen (3×10^5)	Stimulating spleen (3×10^5)	Added (5×10^5)	^{3}H-TdR INCORPORATION (CPM ± SE)			
			AA_m	AB_m	SI	% Response
DBA/2 NS	BALB/C	—	23,234 ± 2273	83,139 ± 3725	3.6	100
SS		—	26,570 ± 1877	39,790 ± 2154	1.5	22
DBA/2 NS	BALB/C	DBA/2 NS_m	12,798 ± 1002	60,032 ± 1770	4.6	100
		DBA/2 SS_m		11,849 ± 2768	0.9	0

[a]Abbreviations: see Table I. Added cells were treated with 50 mg mitomycin (Bristol Laboratories, Syracuse, New York) by incubating 100 x 10^6 cells/2 ml for 20 min in a 37° water bath. The cells were washed 3 times before addition to the MLC.

of theta-positive cells results in a loss of suppressor activity. These data indicate that suppressor activity in spleen from tumor-bearing mice depends primarily on the activity of theta-positive T cells.

In the following experiment we tested whether the tumor is able to activate suppressor cells in the host via a soluble factor. P-815 tumor cells were implanted in cell-impermeable diffusion chambers in the peritoneal cavity of DBA/2 mice. The data in Table V indicate that P-815 tumor cells implanted in cell-impermeable diffusion chambers can cause MLC hyporesponsiveness of the host spleen cells. Empty chambers have no effect. These results suggest that a soluble product from the tumor cells can activate suppressor cell activity in the spleen of the tumor-bearing host.

IV. DISCUSSION

Previously (Argyris, 1977) we have reported that *allogeneic* P-815 tumor transplants can activate suppressor cells in the spleen of C57BL/6 mice. In the present

TABLE III.   Suppressor Activity of Spleen Cells from DBA/2 Mice with 20-Day SC
Transplants of P-815 Mastocytoma, After Removal of Glass-Adherent Cells[a]

Responding spleen (3×10^5)	Stimulating spleen (3×10^5)	Added (5×10^5)	^{3}H-TdR INCORPORATION (CPM ± SE)			
			AA_m	AB_m	SI	% Response
DBA/2 NS	BALB/C	—	23,234 ± 2273	83,139 ± 3725	3.6	100
SS		—	26,570 ± 1877	39,790 ± 2154	1.5	22
NS		NS_m	12,798 ± 1002	60,032 ± 1770	4.6	100
		SS_m		11,849 ± 2768	0.9	0
		SS_m-NA		7,292 ± 188	0.6	0

[a]Abbreviations: see Table I. One part of added cells was adsorbed for three 1-hr periods on glass to remove glass-adherent cells. All added cells were treated with mitomycin before addition to the cultures; NA = nonadherent.

TABLE IV.   Loss of Suppressor Activity after Treating Spleen Cells from P-815 Tumor-Bearing DBA/2 Mice with Antitheta Serum and Complement[a]

Responding spleen (3×10^5)	Stimulating spleen (3×10^5)	Added (5×10^5)	^{3}H-TdR INCORPORATION (CPM ± SE)			
			AA_m	AB_m	SI	% Response
DBA/2 NS	BALB/C	NS	1,662 ± 207	38,977 ± 2015	23.4	100
		SS_m-NRS		5,134 ± 1214	3.1	9
		SS_m-AΘS		31,352 ± 688	18.9	80

[a]Abbreviations: see Table I. Spleen from tumor-bearing DBA/2 mice (SS) was incubated with antitheta serum (AΘS) or normal rabbit serum (NRS) and complement (Argyris, 1977). Dead cells were removed with low ionic buffer and cotton filtration (Argyris, 1977) and cells were treated with mitomycin before addition to MLC.

studies we find that the P-815 tumor can also activate splenic suppressor cells in syngeneic DNA/2 mice.

P-815 is a long-established chemically induced laboratory tumor of mast cell origin (Dunn and Potter, 1957). Since mast cell products can inhibit the immune response (Fallah *et al.*, 1975), it is important to show that the activation of suppressor cells is not limited to the P-815 mastocytoma. In studies reported elsewhere (Argyris, 1978) we have shown that other tumors, both ascites and solid, both long-established and recently induced, can also activate suppressor cells in syngeneic mice. For these studies we used an ascites C3H-strain specific tumor, a DBA/2 solid adenocarcinoma ($CA_2 D$) and several C57BL/6 solid fibrosarcomas recently induced with methyl-cholanthrene.

Viruses have been shown to inhibit the immune response (Bonnard *et al.*, 1976). It is unlikely that tumor-associated viruses are responsible for the suppressor activity. For instance, we find (Argyris, 1977) that thymus cells from tumor-bearing mice fail to express suppressor activity. The P-815 mastocytoma we carry in our laboratory is also shown to be free of mycoplasm contamination (DeLustro and Argyris, 1976b).

TABLE V.   MLC Hyporesponsiveness of Spleen Cells from DBA/2 Mice Implanted 20 Days Previously with P-815 Tumor Cells in Cell-Impermeable Diffusion Chambers[a]

Responding spleen (3×10^5)	Stimulating spleen (3×10^5)	^{3}H-TdR INCORPORATION (CPM ± SE)			
		AA_m	AB_m	SI	% Response
DBA/2 NS	BALB/C	8,609 ± 960	76,446 ± 3464	8.9	100
NS-Empty Chamber		5,217 ± 438	67,887 ± 566	13.0	92
SS-Chamber		8,419 ± 171	11,029 ± 448	1.3	4

[a]Abbreviations: see Table I. For details of diffusion chambers see Materials and Methods or Argyris (1978).

Our data show that spleen cells from tumor-bearing mice are hyporesponsive in mixed lymphocyte culture (MLC), which is an *in vitro* assay for cell-mediated immunity (Bach *et al.*, 1969). The hyporesponsiveness is shown to be due to the presence of a suppressor cell activity because the hyporesponsiveness spleen cells can inhibit the proliferation of normal spleen cells that respond *in vitro* to alloantigens.

The suppressor cells are active after treatment with mitomycin. Since mitomycin inhibits DNA synthesis we can conclude that DNA synthesis and/or cell proliferation is not required for the expression of suppressor activity.

The suppressor cell in our studies is a theta-positive T cell. This observation agrees with the findings from a number of other laboratories (Nordlund and Gershon, 1975; Manor *et al.*, 1976; Takei *et al.*, 1976; Fujimoto *et al.*, 1976a; Treves *et al.*, 1976). This does not mean, however, that only T cells can function as suppressor cells. Indeed, a number of laboratories have reported that macrophages (Veit and Feldman, 1976; Glaser *et al.*, 1976; Kruisbeek *et al.*, 1978) or macrophages and lymphocytes (Elgert and Farrar, 1978; Pope *et al.*, 1978) can function as suppressor cells.

Tumor cells in cell-impermeable diffusion chambers can still activate splenic suppressor cells. Aside from showing that suppressor cell activation can take place via a soluble factor, these data indicate that hyporesponsiveness of suppressor cells from syngeneic tumor-bearing mice is not due to the direct presence of metastasized tumor cells in the spleen cell cultures. This is important because we have previously demonstrated that tumor cells (DeLustro, 1976) or tumor cell products (DeLustro and Argyris, 1976b) added directly to MLC can also inhibit mixed lymphocyte reactivity. The nature of this soluble factor that activates suppressor cells is not shown. It may be the same as the 50,000 molecular weight protein we obtained from P-815 tumor cell extracts which is capable of directly inhibiting lymphocyte proliferation in MLC (DeLustro and Argyris, 1976b).

Cell-mediated immunity (CMI) is largely a T-cell-mediated phenomenon (Cerottini and Brunner, 1974) but requires the cooperation of macrophages (Oppenheim and Rosenstreich, 1976; Unanue and Calderon, 1975), B cells (Berger and Amos, 1977), and possibly null cells (Bakacs *et al.*, 1977). Suppressor cells that inhibit CMI could do so by affecting any of these populations. Studies are in progress in our laboratory to determine the mechanism by which suppressor cells achieve their regulation of the immune response.

REFERENCES

Argyris, B. F. (1977). *Cancer Res. 37*, 3390-3399.
Argyris, B. F. (1978). *Cancer Res. 38*, 1269-1273.
Argyris, B. F., and DeLustro, F. (1977). *Cell. Immunol. 28*, 390-403.
Bach, F. H., Bock, H., Graupner, K., Day, E., and Klostermann, H. (1969). *Proc. Nat. Acad. Sci. 62*, 377-384.
Bakacs, T., Gergely, P., and Klein, E. (1977). *Cell. Immunol. 32*, 317-328.
Berger, A. E., and Amos, D. B. (1977). *Cell. Immunol. 33*, 277-290.
Bonnard, G. D., Manders, E. K., Campbell, D. A., Herberman, R. B., and Collins, M. J. (1976). *J. Exp. Med. 143*, 187-204.

Cerottini, J. D., and Brunner, T. K. (1974). *Adv. Immunol. 18,* 67-132.

DeLustro, F., and Argyris, B. F. (1976a). *Cell. Immunol. 21,* 177-184.

DeLustro, F., and Argyris, B. F. (1976b). *J. Immunol. 117,* 2073-2080.

Dunn, T. B., and Potter, M. (1957). *J. Nat. Cancer Inst. 18,* 587-595.

Elgert, K. D., and Farrar, W. L. (1978). *J. Immunol. 120,* 1345-1353.

Fallah, H. A., Maillard, J. L., and Voisin, G. A. (1975). *Ann. Immunol.* (Inst. Pasteur) *126C,* 669-682.

Fujimoto, S., Greene, M. I., and Sehon, A. H. (1976a). *J. Immunol. 116,* 791-799.

Fujimoto, S., Greene, M. I., and Sehon, A. H. (1976b). *J. Immunol. 116,* 800-806.

Glaser, M., Kirchner, H., Holden, H. T., and Herberman, R. B. (1976). *J. Nat. Cancer Inst. 56,* 865-867.

Haller, O., Hansson, M.. Kiessling, R., and Wigzell, H. (1977). *Nature 270,* 609-611.

Hellstrom, K. E., and Hellstrom, I. (1974). *Clin. Immunobiol. 2,* 233-264.

Hellstrom, K. E., and Hellstrom, I. (1976). *Ann. N. Y. Acad. Sci. 276,* 176-187.

Klein, G. (1968). *Cancer Res. 20,* 625-635.

Kruisbeek, A. M., Zylstra, J., and Zurcher, C. (1978). *Eur. J. Immunol. 8,* 200-206.

Lohmann-Matthes, M. L. (1976). *In* "Immunobiology of Macrophage" (D. S. Nelson, ed.), pp. 463-486. Academic Press, Inc., New York.

Manor, Y., Treves, A. J., Cohen, I. R., and Feldman, M. (1976). *Transplant. 22,* 360-366.

Nordlund, J. J., and Gershon, R. K. (1975). *J. Immunol. 114,* 1486-1490.

Oppenheim, J. J., and Rosenstreich, D. L. (1976). *Prog. Allergy 20,* 65-194.

Perlmann, P. (1976). *Clin. Immunobiol. 3,* 107-132.

Pope, B. L., Whitney, R. B., and Levy, J. G. (1978). *J. Immunol. 120,* 2033-2040.

Takei, F., Levy, J. G., and Kilburn, D. G. (1976). *J. Immunol. 116,* 288-293.

Treves, A. J., Cohen, I. R., Schechter, B., and Feldman, M. (1976). *Ann. N. Y. Acad. Sci. 276,* 165-175.

Unanue, E. R., and Calderon, J. (1975). *Fed. Proc. 34,* 1737-1742.

Veit, B. C., and Feldman, J. D. (1976). *J. Immunol. 117,* 655-660.

Chapter 7

POTENTIATION OF MITOMYCIN C BY LUCANTHONE HCl (MIRACIL D) IN TRANSPLANTED C3H MAMMARY TUMORS

Lawrence S. Koons
Darrell Q. Brown
David T. Harris
Judith S. Rubinstein

I. INTRODUCTION

A. DNA Repair

The repairability of DNA that has been alkylated by sulphur mustard has been demonstrated by Crathorn and Roberts (1966). Furthermore, it has been shown that excision repair is the first step in the cross-link repair in mitomycin-C-treated mammilian cells (Fujiwara and Tatsumi, 1975).

B. Radiation Potentiators

In vitro (Rauth, *et al.,* 1970) and *in vivo* (Gaudin and Yielding, 1969; Gaudin *et al.,* 1971; and Inaba and Sakurai, 1974) studies have demonstrated an increased cytotoxic effect of alkylated DNA when it is pretreated with DNA repair inhibitors such as caffeine and chloroquine. Bases (1970) has shown that the drug lucanthone (Miracil D) potentiates radiation damage in HELA cells. His work indicates that potentiation by lucanthone is due to inhibition of repair of radiation-induced lesions in DNA. Brown *et al.,* (1976) have demonstrated an enhancement of radiation antitumor effect using lucanthone with the C3H transplanted spontaneous mammary tumor model. There was significant potentiation effect when the drug was administered 10 hr before irradiation, but not when it was given 1 hr before treatment.

II. MATERIALS AND METHODS

A. Model

The experiments were designed using the C3H mouse mammary tumor model (Brown *et al.,* 1976) and substituting mitomycin C for radiation therapy after pretreatment with lucanthone. The original transplanted tumor was removed from the host mouse and cut into small fragments approximately 1-2 mm^3 in size. Fragments were then implanted subcutaneously into the hind leg, and the tumors were selected for treatment when the sum of their dimensions reached 15 to 20 mm. Animals were assigned randomly to the various treatment groups. The mice were ear-clipped for identification. Observations and measurements were made twice weekly. Each group of mice consisted of a minimum of 14 animals. Control animals received saline intraperitoneally and their tumors had a mean doubling time of 4.5 days ± 0.5 SEM. Measurements were made to the 1/10 mm, and the volumes were calculated from the length, width, and height. Relative volumes were calculated using the pretreatment volume as the reference tumor. Doubling times were calculated from the rate of change in tumor volume. Toxicity criteria included animal weight changes and survival.

B. Drugs

Lucanthone

Lucanthone is a heterocyclic molecule (Fig. 1) that is known to inhibit DNA and RNA synthesis and thought to interact with double-stranded DNA by intercalation (Hirschberg, 1975). It forms a solution in water and a suspension in saline. For these experiments doses of 1/2 LD$_{50}$, 1/4 LD$_{50}$, and 1/8 LD$_{50}$ were used for both the solution and the suspension preparations. The animals were treated with a single dose given IP. In one set of experiments lucanthone was given 10 hr prior to mitomycin C, and in another set it was given 1 hr prior to mitomycin C.

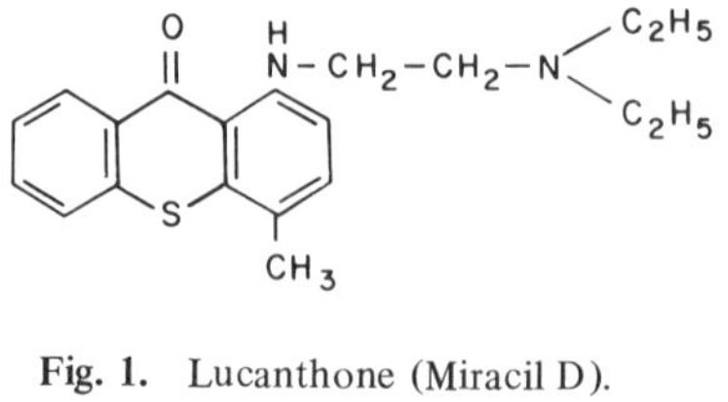

Fig. 1. Lucanthone (Miracil D).

TABLE I.   Survival of Mice Treated with Escalating Doses of Lucanthone [a]

Drug	$LD_{50\text{-}ld} \pm SE$	$LD_{50\text{-}7d} \pm SE$
IP suspension in saline	443 ± 13 mg/kg	430 ± 12 mg/kg
IP solution in H_2O	$272 \pm\ 9$ mg/kg	202 ± 12 mg/kg

[a] Survival determined after 1 day and at the end of 7 days.

Mitomycin C

Mitomycin C is a heterocyclic compound with three potentially reactive alkylating groups and is thus a polyfunctional alkylating agent when activated (Crooke and Bradner, 1976). Dose response studies were performed. In the combination treatment experiments mitomycin C was used at a dose of 4 mg/kg and was given in a single bolus intraperitoneally.

III.   RESULTS

A.   Drug Studies

Lucanthone

The results of toxicity studies for lucanthone are shown in Table I. LD_{50} studies were performed for both the solution and the suspension and the results determined after 24 hr and 7 days. The LD_{50} for lucanthone in solution is much lower than the suspension after both a 1-day and 7-day observation period.

Mitomycin C

Dose-response studies measuring tumor doubling times as a function of dose are plotted on Fig. 2. A nearly linear dose-response relationship is present.

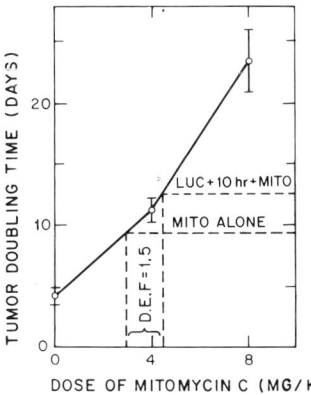

Fig. 2.   Dose-response curve for mitomycin C. Dose enhancement factor (DEF) represents ratio of intercepts on abscissa with *mito alone* as denominator (see text for explanation).

B. Tumor Measurements

Relative Tumor Volumes

In Fig. 3 is shown the plot of the relative tumor volumes versus time. Five groups of study animals are shown. There was no antitumor effect in the lucanthone-treated group. Mitomycin C at 4 mg/kg/IP caused a mild but significant antitumor effect. When the mice were pretreated with lucanthone there was significant potentiation of the mitomycin C antitumor effect. This was most pronounced during the first 2 weeks and occurred mainly during the first doubling time period. Equally good results were obtained when the animals were pretreated at 1 and 10 hr, and both the lucanthone solution and suspension produced equally effective results. Significant results were seen when the lucanthone was given at $1/2$ LD_{50} doses (100 mg/kg) but not at lower doses.

Enhancement Factor

Figure 2 is a plot of the tumor doubling time versus the dose of mitomycin C. This curve is used to interpolate a dose enhancement factor as follows: Verticals are dropped to the abscissa from the doubling time points of the groups in the current experiments; then a ratio of the two intercepts on the abscissa is calculated using the single drug value as the denominator. This ratio is called the dose enhance-

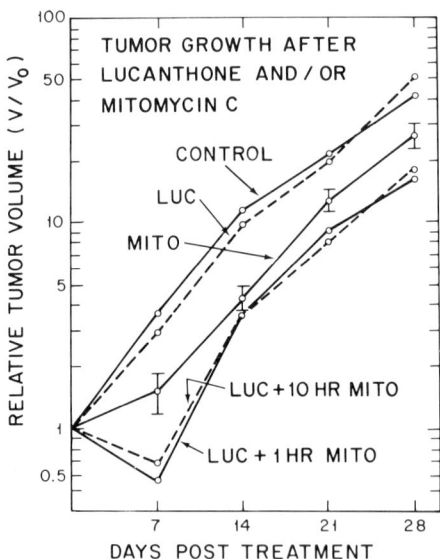

Fig. 3. Response of the mammary tumors of C3H mice after treatment. Each point represents the mean of the relative volumes of at least 12 animals. Control mice received saline IP. Mitomycin C was given at 4 mg/kg/IP, and lucanthone was administered at 100 mg/kg/IP. Only a single course of treatment was given. 1 hr mito and 10 hr mito refer to the time interval from lucanthone pretreatment to mitomycin C injection.

ment factor. When the doubling times of the lucanthone and mitomycin C groups were compared to the mitomycin C group a ratio of 1.5 was found. This means that lucanthone pretreatment resulted in an antitumor effect equivalent to that of 1.5 times the dose of mitomycin C used. In other words, giving mitomycin C at 4 mg/kg with lucanthone resulted in an antitumor effect equivalent to giving mitomycin C at 6 mg/kg as a single agent.

C. Toxicity

Mouse Weights

Treatment toxicity was evaluated by determing the relative mouse weights using the pretreatment weight as a reference (Fig. 4). The weights were adjusted for tumor size by subtracting the change in tumor weight from the start of treatment. There were no significant differences among the groups over the 28-day period.

Survival

Mean survival time for the five groups of animals in Fig. 3 is shown in Table II. There was a trend toward increased survival in the combination treatment groups but the differences were not significant.

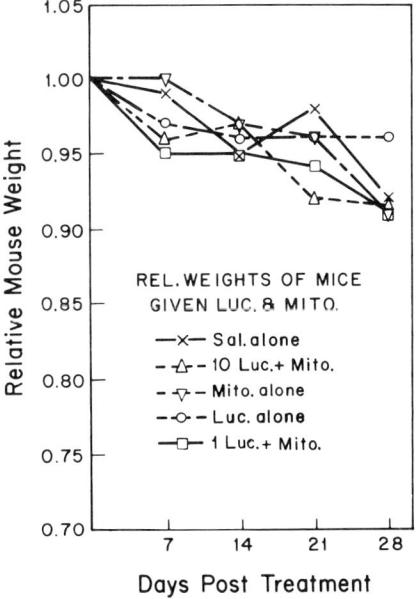

Fig. 4. Mean relative weights of the five groups of C3H mice plotted in Fig. 3. The change in tumor weight at each time point was subtracted from the total body weight before the relative weight was calculated.

TABLE II.   Mouse Survival Time Following Lucanthone
and Mitomycin C

Experimental group	Mean survival time ± SE
Saline only	33.9 ± 2.6 days
LUC* only	26.0 ± 2.9 days
MITO* only	39.0 ± 1.5 days
LUC* + 1 hr + MITO**	40.9 ± 2.5 days
LUC* + 10 hr + MITO**	45.9 ± 2.8 days

*100 mg/kg Lucanthone; ** 4 mg/kg mitomycin C.

IV. DISCUSSION

Our primary purpose was to determine whether alkylation damage can be poten-
tiated by radiation potentiators *without* an enhancement in toxicity. Using lucanthone as the potentiator and mitomycin C as the alkylator we have been able to
demonstrate this phenomenon. Our working hypothesis is that lucanthone functions
as a DNA repair inhibitor and thereby prevents the repair of mitomycin C alkylation.
Why this results in a differential antitumor effect without concomitant additive systemic toxicity is not known. Bases (unpublished observations) has studied the tissue
distribution of lucanthone in C3H HeHa mice bearing C3H-BA mammary adenocarcinomas. He was able to show enrichment of ^{3}H-lucanthone label in tumor tissue
relative to skin and muscle on the first and second day following drug injection.
Higher relative concentrations were found in liver and kidney (excretion sites), and
lung, spleen, and brain showed little difference compared to tumor tissue. Drug
levels in the bone marrow and gastrointestinal tract were not made. These are the
important sites of chemotherapy toxicity particularly with alkylating agents. It is
possible that low relative concentrations of lucanthone in these sites accounts for
the low toxicity seen. By the same token, tumor enrichment by lucanthone could
explain the enhancement effect seen when mitomycin is used as the alkylating
agent.

DNA repair processes are complicated mechanisms entailing several enzyme
systems working cooperatively (Howard-Flanders, 1973). Repair functions probably
consist of special enzymes to recognize initially specific lesions prior to more general
repair enzyme activity (Lindahl, 1976). Repair of alkylated DNA has been demonstrated (Crathorn and Roberts, 1966), but data on the specific enzymes involved are
scant. It is likely that interference in any of the numerous steps of repair synthesis
could enhance alkylation damage. Attempts at exploiting this method of combination
antitumor treatment are few (Gaudin and Yielding, 1969; Gaudin *et al.,* 1971;
Inaba and Sakurai, 1974). Although the research data show a role for lucanthone
in the interference of radiation repair (Bases, 1970), the molecular mechanisms
have not been elucidated. The current experiments suggest a similar role for lucanthone when used with mitomycin C. Further *in vitro* experiments demonstrating
DNA repair inhibition by lucanthone in the presence of alkylated DNA are necessary.

These present experiments provide a basis for further animal study and future phase I trials in human tumor situations.

REFERENCES

Bases, R. (1970). *Can. Res. 30,* 2007-2011.

Brown, D. Q., Pittock, J., Coia, L., Milligan, A., and Chalfin, L. (1976). *Rad. Res. 67,* 637.

Crathorn, A. R., and Roberts, J. J. (1966). *Nature 211,* 150-153.

Crooke, S. T., and Bradner, W. T. (1976). *Cancer Treat. Rev. 3,* 121-139.

Fujiwara, Y., and Tatsumi, M. (1975). *Biochem. Biophys. Res. Commun. 66,* 592-598.

Gaudin, D., and Yielding, K. L. (1969). *Proc. Soc. Exp. Biol. Med., 131,* 1413-1416.

Gaudin, D., Yielding, K. L., Stabler, A., and Brown, J. (1971). *Proc. Soc. Exp. Biol. Med. 133,* 202-206.

Hirschberg, E. (1975). *In* "Mechanism of Action of Antimicrobial and Anti-tumor Agents" (J. W. Corcoran and F. E. Hahn, eds.), Vol. III, pp. 274-303. Springer-Verlag, New York.

Howard-Flanders, P. (1973). *Br. Med. Bull. 29,* 226-235.

Inaba, M., and Sakurai, Y. (1974). *GANN 65,* 465-466.

Lindahl, T. (1976). *Nature 259,* 64-66.

Rauth, A. M., Berton, B., and Lee, C. P. Y. (1970). *Cancer Res. 30,* 2724-2729.

Chapter 8

THE DEVELOPMENT OF AN ACUTE INTERMITTENT SCHEDULE—MITOMYCIN C

Laurence H. Baker
Vainutis K. Vaitkevicius

I. INTRODUCTION

Mitomycin C is an anticancer agent of moderate clinical usefulness in a variety of clinical settings. However, after its initial testing in the United States following its introduction from Japan, little enthusiasm was generated for further investigations with the drug, as a result of large clinical trials conducted from 1959 to 1962 that were interpreted to show an excessive amount of toxicity. This occurred despite the apparent clinical activity of the drug in a number of far advanced cancers. These large studies utilized one of two dosage schedules: (*a*) 0.05 mg/kg daily for 6 days and then every other day until toxic signs appeared (Ansfield, 1969; Graham *et al.*, 1967; Horton *et al.*, 1968; Jones, 1959; Manheimer and Vital, 1966; Moertel *et al.*, 1968; Moore *et al.*, 1968; Reitemeier *et al.*, 1970; Watne *et al.*, 1967; Whittington and Close, 1970) or (*b*) a biweekly dose of 6-10 mg^2 (Evans, 1961; Matsunaga *et al.*, 1967). In 1968 Carter, in writing a review of mitomycin, was unable to find in the literature clinical studies using an acute intermittent dose regime.

II. MATERIALS AND METHODS

Independent of the clinical studies, several researchers were studying the drug at a more basic level. Sokoloff *et al.* (1959) described an every 3- or 4-day schedule to

TABLE I.   Influence of Dose Schedule on Treatment of
Ehrlich Ascites Tumor of Sokoloff *et al.*, 1959

Schedule	Animals dead of cancer (%)
control	100
0.04 mg/d x 7	90
0.05 mg/d x 7	60
0.04 mg/d–d1,2,5,6,9,10,13	20
0.05 mg/d–d1,2,6,8,12,13,16	all survived

be superior to a daily schedule in the Ehrlich ascites tumor system (Table I), and Hata, *et al.* (1961) reported a single treatment superior to repeated small doses, also in an Ehrlich ascites tumor system. In 1964, and again in 1969, Kenis reported that massive doses of mitomycin C appeared to be less toxic and probably more efficacious than single daily doses. The next year, Fujita, using a biological assay of E. Coli, concluded that the intermittent administration of a large dose resulted in higher total amount of mitomycin C in blood than frequent small doses Fujita (1971). Kojima *et al.* in 1972 reported some conflicting evidence suggesting that there was no real difference between an every 2-, 3-, or 4-day schedule in L1210 but that an every 8-day schedule was less effective. Additionally, they reported that their best result in L1210 occurred when a priming dose was used followed by low intermittent doses (Table II).

III. RESULTS

Whether because of these results in animal tumor models or for a variety of other reasons, at least three investigators have reported clinical development of an acute intermittent schedule with mitomycin C (Table III). In addition to some of the basic science data referred to above, it is clear that Sutow was influenced in his schedule development by work with cyclophosphamide in both the animal model (L1210) and in the clinic with children (Sutow *et al.*, 1971). He found an advantage in using an acute intermittent schedule, and thus, did develop a dose schedule

TABLE II.   Influence of Dose Schedule on
L1210 of Kojima *et al.*, 1972

Treatment schedule	Maximal ILS (%)
daily	65
every 2 days	67
every 3 days	50
every 4 days	59
every 7-8 days	34
priming dose day 1 and treatment day 8	73

TABLE III. Pediatric Phase I Study of Sutow *et al.*, 1971

Schedule	No. cancers	Leukopenia (WBC/mm^3)		Thrombocytopenia (platelets/mm^3)	
		1500-2500	<1500	50-75,000	<50,000
0.15 mg/kg x 5	12	0	5	1	6
0.4-0.6 mg/kg x 1	9	0	1	0	2

of an acute intermittent nature using 0.4 to 0.6 mg/kg, demonstrating that this was less toxic than a day x 5 schedule of equal amounts of drug. Godfrey and Wilbur (1972) later described their experiences with large, infrequent doses of mitomycin C used in adult patients. In their paper they reported that the majority of patients received 30 mg on day 1 and 20 mg 3 or 4 days later followed by additional doses of mitomycin C of 10-30 mg at 4-6 weeks. However, the total mean dose of mitomycin C was 57 mg in that series. Only 6% of their patients actually received a total dose greater than 100 mg. Godfrey concluded that his schedule did not produce a therapeutic advantage (Table IV) but was possibly less toxic and certainly more convenient.

Meanwhile, in Detroit, our interests were in the N-methyl derivative of mitomycin C, porfiromycin (Tables V and VI). In our 1967 phase I study (Loo *et al.*, 1967) and later phase II trial (Izbicki *et al.*, 1972) we reported the advantages of acute intermittent schedules of porfiromycin. Shortly thereafter, we were in the midst of developing combinations of porfiromycin using this acute intermittent schedule along with other agents when we were notified that no real advantage could be gained from the development of two very similar drugs. We therefore undertook a random prospective study of porfiromycin and mitomycin C which we initially reported in 1974 (Baker *et al.*, 1974). Our recommended dose as a result of our phase I and phase II trials with porfiromycin as a single agent was 75 mg/m^2 every 6-8 weeks. In order to do a fair comparison between mitomycin and porfiromycin we undertook a phase I study of mitomycin C trying to simulate the toxicity that we had become familiar with from porfiromycin. Patients were treated with a dose

TABLE IV. Response Rate by Tumor Type—
Study of Godfrey and Wilbur, 1972

Site	No. treated	No. responding
Stomach	9	2
Colon	29	5
Pancreas	3	1
Other GI	4	3
Breast	9	4
Sarcoma	6	1
Melanoma	15	0
Lymphoma	1	1
Others	12	2
Total	88	19 (21%)

TABLE V.   Phase I Evaluation of Porfiromycin

Schedule	No. Pts.	Hematologic toxicity		
		Mild	Moderate	Severe
30-150 ug/kg/day x 21	16	—	1	5
2 mg/kg in divided doses from 3-10 days	6	—	—	—
0.5 mg/kg weekly	10	1	1	3
0.3 mg/kg weekly	9	—	3	2
0.5 mg/kg—1st week 0.25 mg/kg weekly	11	1	2	3
0.8 mg/kg—1st week followed by 0.2 mg/kg weekly	9	—	3	1

TABLE VI.   Phase I Evaluation of Porfiromycin: Acute Intermittent Dosage

Dose mg/kg	No. Pts.	Hematologic toxicity		
		Mild	Moderate	Severe
1.0	4	—	—	—
1.2	1	—	—	—
1.5	3	—	1	1
1.8	4	—	1	2
2.0	71	20	4	6
3.0	3	—	2	—

TABLE VII.   Population Characteristics

Tumor category	No. entered	Prior therapy	Early death	Partial remission
Mitomycin-treated group				
Colorectal	12	6	1	4
Gastric	3	1	1	2
Pancreas	4	—	—	1
Gallbladder	1	—	—	—
Adrenal	1	—	—	1
Ovarian	11	8	—	3
Total	32	15	2	11
Porfiromycin-treated group				
Colorectal	12	6	1	2
Gastric	2	2	1	1
Pancreas	3	—	—	1
Gallbladder	1	—	—	—
Adrenal	1	—	—	1
Ovarian	12	7	—	5
Total	31	15	2	10

TABLE VIII.   Maximum Myelosuppression

		Leukopenia		
		$2.1\text{-}3.0 \times 10^3/mm^3$	$1.1\text{-}2.0 \times 10^3/mm^3$	$0\text{-}1.0 \times 10^3/mm^3$
Mitomycin	n = 30	7	10	2
Porfiromycin	n = 29	7	8	1
		Thrombocytopenia		
		$100\text{-}150 \times 10^3/mm^3$	$50\text{-}100 \times 10^3/mm^3$	$0\text{-}50 \times 10^3/mm^3$
Mitomycin	n = 30	4	8	8
Porfiromycin	n = 29	5	4	3

TABLE IX.   Cumulative Toxicity

		1st course		2 courses		3 or more courses	
		WBC	Platelet	WBC	Platelet	WBC	Platelet
Mitomycin	mean	3.79	192.59	3.71	126.0	2.78	59.16
	median	3.2	185.0	3.0	99.0	3.0	38.0
	range	0.3-10.0	61.0-566	1.8-6.9	25-280	0.9-3.3	15-200
		n = 30		n = 21		n = 12	
Porfiromycin	mean	4.79	204.17	3.37	118.0	1.75	44.50
	median	4.3	225.0	2.6	110.0	2.0	44
	range	0.9-9.1	70-442	2.2-5.6	31-220	0.7-2.7	10-80
		n = 29		n = 11		n = 4	

range of 10-25 mg/m² mitomycin C every 6-8 weeks.

As a result of this phase I trial we concluded that the equivalent dose of mitomycin to porfiromycin was 22.5 mg/m². Subsequently, as experience grew with mitomycin C, we recommended the reduction of the starting dose of mitomycin C to 20 mg/m² (Baker *et al.*, 1976).

Data from our initial phase II comparative trial of mitomycin C can be seen in Tables VII, VIII, and IX.

IV. DISCUSSION

As a result of our initial study with mitomycin we were able to conclude that modest clinical success was encountered against refractory and traditionally tough malignant neoplasms so as to justify further clinical trials of mitomycin C in this schedule. It appeared to us that the acute intermittent bolus schedule is a convenient one to be used in the clinic and lends itself to future combinations.

REFERENCES

Ansfield, F. J. (1969). *Cancer Chemother. Rep. 53*, 287-289.

Baker, L. H., Caoili, E. M., Izbicki, R. M., Opipari, M. I., and Vaitkevicius, V. K. (1974). *Proc. Am. Assoc. Cancer Res. 795*, (abstract), 182.

Baker, L. H., Izbicki, R. M., and Vaitkevicius, V. K. (1976). *Med. Pediatr. Oncol. 2,* 207-213.

Carter, S. K. (1968). *Cancer Chemother. Rep. 1,* (part 3), 99-114.

Evans, A. E. (1961). *Cancer Chemother Rep. 14,* 1-9.

Fujita, H. (1971). *Jap. J. Clin. Oncol. 1,* 151-162.

Godfrey, T. E., and Wilbur, D. W. (1972). *Cancer 29,* 1647-1652.

Graham, W. P., III, Ravdin, R. G., Crichlow, R. W., and Eisman, S. H. (1967). *Plast. Reconstr. Surg. 40,* 230-232.

Hata, T., Hossenlopp, R., and Takita, H. (1961). *Cancer Chemother. Rep. 13,* 67-77.

Horton, J., Olson, K. B., Cunningham, T., and Sullivan, J. (1968). *Cancer Chemother. Rep. 52,* 597-600.

Izbicki, R., Al-Sarraf, M., Reed, M. L., Vaughn, C. B., and Vaitkevicius, V. K. (1972). *Cancer Chemother. Rep. 56,* (part 1), 615-624.

Jones, R., Jr. (1959). *Cancer Chemother. Rep. 2,* 3-7.

Kenis, Y. (1969). *Recent Results Cancer Res. 21,* 54-61.

Kojima, R., Goldin, A., and Mantel, N. (1972). *Cancer Chemother. Rep. 3,* (part 2), 111-119.

Loo, R. V., Vaitkevicius, V. K., Reed, M. L., and Vaughn, C. B. (1967). *Cancer Chemother. Rep. 51,* 497-502.

Manheimer, L. H., and Vital, J. (1966). *Cancer 19,* 207-212.

Matsunaga, F., Shimoyama, T., Mikawa, K., and Ishiwata, J. (1967). *Cancer 20,* 805-808.

Moertel, C. G., Reitemeier, R. J., and Hahn, R. G. (1968). *JAMA 204,* 1045-1048.

Moore, G. E., Bross, I. D. J., Ausman, R., Nadler, S., Jones, R., Jr., Slack, N., and Rimm, A. A. (1968). *Cancer Chemother. Rep. 52,* 675-684.

Reitemeier, R. J., Moertel, C. G., and Hahn, R. G. (1970). *Cancer Res. 30,* 1425-1428.

Sokoloff, B., Nakabayashi, K., Enomoto, K., Miller, R. R., Bicknell, A., Bird, L., Trauner, W., Nisonger, J., and Renninger, G. (1959). *Growth 23,* 109-136.

Sutow, W. W., Wilbur, J. R., Vietti, T. J., Vuthibhagdee, P., Fujimoto, T., Watanabe, A. (1971). *Cancer Chemother. Rep. 55,* (part 1), 285-289.

Watne, A. L., Moore, D., and Gorgun, B. (1967). *Arch. Surg. 95,* 175-178.

Whittington, R. M., and Close, H. P. (1970). *Cancer Chemother. Rep. 54,* 195-198.

Chapter 9

THE COMBINATION OF MITOMYCIN C AND
ADRIAMYCIN (MA): TOXICITIES AND RESPONSE

Robert L. Comis
Sandra J. Ginsberg
Stanley T. Crooke

I. INTRODUCTION

Mitomycin C has exhibited antitumor activity in a variety of malignancies including adenocarcinoma of the stomach and lung (Crooke and Bradner, 1976). Initial
studies in the United States employed the drug on chronic schedules, treating
patients daily or every other day until myelotoxicity developed. Because of the
cumulative nature of mitomycin C induced myelotoxicity, profound, prohibitive
myelosuppression was dose limiting (Jones, 1959). High intermittent dose schedules
(20 mg/m^2 q 6-8 weeks) employed in recent years have yielded more manageable
myelotoxicity and mild gastrointestinal toxicity without decreased therapeutic
effects (Baker et al., 1976). Objective responses with either the chronic or high
intermittent schedule of administration have been short-lived, varying from 1 to 3
months. The cumulative nature of the myelotoxicity and short remission duration
has limited the usefulness of mitomycin C employed as a single agent.

Adriamycin is a broadly active antitumor agent with established activity in adenocarcinomas of the stomach and lung. (Blum and Carter, 1974; Moertel, 1975).
There is some evidence indicating that there may be a significant dose-response relationship for the drug (Cortes et al., 1975). Cumulative myelotoxicity is generally
not encountered employing adriamycin at a dose of 60-75 mg/m^2 every 3 weeks,

although nausea, vomiting, and stomatitis do occur.

5-fluorouracil (5-FU) is used in many combination chemotherapy programs for metastatic carcinomas. Recent evidence has indicated that intensive intravenous therapy is superior to less intensive intravenous therapy and/or oral therapy in certain tumors (Ansfield *et al.*, 1977). Low intermittent doses of 5-FU are generally employed in combination chemotherapy programs because of significant overlapping bone marrow and gastrointestinal toxicity with other drugs.

Recently MacDonald *et al.* (1976, 1977) have reported that the combination of 5-FU, adriamycin and mitomycin C (FAM) has significant antitumor activity in adenocarcinomas of the stomach and lung. In the FAM regimen, 5-FU is administered at a dose of 600 mg/m^2 on weeks 1, 2, 4, and 5 of each 8-week cycle, with adriamycin administered at a dose of 30 mg/m^2 every 4 weeks, and mitomycin C, 10 mg/m^2 every 8 weeks. Both the adriamycin dose and schedule are attenuated in this regimen because of overlapping bone marrow and gastrointestinal toxicity.

The purpose of the present investigation was to explore various doses of mitomycin C and adriamycin (MA) used in combination *without* 5-fluorouracil in an attempt to determine the maximally tolerated dose of the combination when each drug is employed on a schedule comparable to commonly used single-agent programs.

II. MATERIALS AND METHODS

Patients were eligible for the study if they had histologically documented adenocarcinoma of the stomach and lung, or other histologically documented cancer refractory to standard therapies. All patients were less than 75 years of age, and had a Karnofsky performance status of > 60%. Measurable disease was not required in the initial dose-seeking phase I study (26 patients), but was required in the 4 patients entered onto early phase II evaluation in adenocarcinomas of the stomach, breast, and lung. Pertinent patient characteristics are presented in Table I. Only 1 patient had received prior chemotherapy and 6 had received prior radiotherapy. There were 8 patients with adenocarcinoma of the stomach, 14 with adenocarci-

TABLE I.   Patient Characteristics

Entered	30
Evaluable for toxicity	27
Evaluable for response	22
Male	18
Female	12
Age	
Median 58 (range 31-71)	
Prior therapy	
Radiotherapy	6
Chemotherapy	1

TABLE II.   Planned Dose Escalations

	Mitomycin C (Every 6 weeks)	Adriamycin (Every 3 weeks)
Group I	10 mg/m^2	50 mg/m^2
Group II	12.5 mg/m^2	60 mg/m^2
Group III	15 mg/m^2	60 mg/m^2
Group IV	15 mg/m^2	75 mg/m^2

noma of the lung, and 8 with other malignancies.

Pretreatment evaluation included a complete history and physical examination, a complete blood count, platelet count, liver function tests, blood urea nitrogen, serum creatinine, electrocardiogram, chest x ray, and other appropriate radionuclide and radiographic studies. CBC and platelet counts were performed weekly; electrocardiograms, chest x rays, physical examinations, and tumor measurements were done at 3-week intervals, and renal and hepatic function tests were repeated every 6 weeks.

Mitomycin C was administered every 6 weeks, and adriamycin was administered every 3 weeks. Both drugs were given by rapid intravenous injection. The cumulative adriamycin dose did not exceed 550 mg/m^2. The planned dose escalations for the phase I study are presented in Table II. Doses were not escalated within patients.

Complete response was defined as the complete disappearance of all measurable disease. Partial response was defined as a $\geqslant 50\%$ decrease in the sum of the products of measurable disease. No response was defined as a $\leqslant 50\%$ decrease in the sum of the products of measurable disease. Progressive disease was defined as a $\geqslant 25\%$ increase in measurable disease. Response duration was measured from the date a patient qualified as a responder to the date of disease progression. Survival was the time from initiation of therapy to death.

III.   RESULTS

Myelotoxicity

A total of six previously untreated patients received mitomycin C and adriamycin at the 10 mg/m^2 and 50 mg/m^2 dose, respectively (Group I). Four patients were treated in the initial phase I evaluation, and two patients were treated in the early phase II evaluation. The myelotoxicity encountered in Group I patients is presented in Table III. The acute myelotoxicity seen during the first course of therapy was mild. Four patients received five courses of therapy and one patient received six courses of treatment. Cumulative myelotoxicity occurred with repeated courses of therapy and was manifested primarily by platelet suppression during the first 21 days of treatment. No patient required a permanent dose reduction during therapy.

Thirteen previously untreated patients were treated with 12.5 mg/m^2 and 60

TABLE III. Myelotoxicity of MA (Group I): No Prior Therapy

Course	No. patients	Median WBC and Platelet Counts				Dose reductions/course
		0-21 days		21-42 days		
		$WBC \times 10^3$	$PLT \times 10^3$	$WBC \times 10^3$	$PLT \times 10^3$	
1	6	2.6 (2.0-9.5)	240 (88-795)	4.5 (1.6-6.0)	290 (145-10)	0
2	5	3.2 (2.0-6.8)	170 (49-10)	3.7 (2.9-7.6)	265 (175-345)	0
3	4	3.9 (2.5-6.5)	174 (130-200)	4.2 (2.4-5.0)	257 (225-400)	1
4	4	3.2 (1.2-3.8)	155 (115-176)	3.5 (3.2-4.3)	275 (1.85-500)	1
5	4	3.3 (0.8-3.9)	115 (59-300)	3.4 (3.5-3.7)	275 (59-300)	2
6	1	2.9	135	6.0	170	

mg/m^2 of mitomycin C and adriamycin, respectively (Group II). The myelotoxicity encountered with this dose level is presented in Table IV. Approximately half of the patients required adriamycin dose reductions during the first course of therapy. With subsequent courses of therapy most patients required permanent reductions of both the adriamycin and mitomycin C dose. As a result, the median blood counts presented in Table IV do not reflect the cumulative nature of the toxicity. It should be noted that platelet counts $< 50 \times 10^3$ were seen at all dose levels in Group II. Two of the five patients who received more than three courses of therapy developed protracted myelosuppression for 7 and 12 weeks, respectively.

Myelotoxicity tended to be more severe in patients who had received prior

TABLE IV. Myelotoxicity of MA (Group II): No Prior Therapy

Course	No. patients	Median WBC and Platelet Counts				Dose reductions/course
		0-21 days		21-42 days		
		$WBC \times 10^3$	$PLT \times 10^3$	$WBC \times 10^3$	$PLT \times 10^3$	
1	13	2.2 (0.3-5.7)	170 (18-517)	3.4 (1.3-6.2)	330 (94-479)	6
2	13	3.6 (0.8-8.1)	175 (38-386)	3.1 (0.5-5.2)	304 (130-455)	8
3	7	2.9 (1.5-5.0)	54 (15-144)	3.1 (2.2-42)	188 (50-352)	7
4	5	3.6 (2.6-4.9)	124 (45-295)	3.1 (2.8-3.4)	120 (60-138)	5
5	4	2.6 (2.3-3.9)	177 (24-138)	—	—	4

TABLE V.   Myelotoxicity of MA: Prior Therapy

Course	No. patients	Median WBC and Platelet Counts				Dose reductions/course
		0-21 days		21-42 days		
		Group I				
		WBC x 10^3	PLT x 10^3	WBC x 10^3	PLT x 10^3	
1	4	3.1 (1.3-5.0)	228 (150-320)	2.5 (1.6-3.1)	277 (142-410)	1
2	4	2.0 (1.2-4.5)	179 (36-320)	3.2 (2.3-3.4)	214 (87-435)	4
		Group II				
1	3	0.8 (0.5-0.9)	135 (18-230)	3.4 (2-5.3)	415 (265-514)	3

radiotherapy or chemotherapy (Table V). All patients treated with the Group I required dose reductions during the second course of therapy. Severe myelosuppression occurred during the first course of therapy in all the Group II patients.

Nonhematologic Toxicities (Table VI)

Gastrointestinal

Gastrointestinal toxicity occurred in one third of the patients. In general, the gastrointestinal side effects were mild. No patient developed gastrointestinal side effects severe enough to require dose reduction, interruption, or discontinuation of therapy.

Cardiac

Two patients developed apparent cardiotoxicity. The first patient was a 47-year-old white male with metastatic squamous cell lung cancer who had no prior history of heart disease. Acute congestive heart failure developed three weeks after having received the first dose of mitomycin C (10 mg/m^2) and adriamycin (50 mg/m^2). The congestive heart failure was controlled with appropriate medications, and the patient died 2 weeks later from progressive disease. The second patient was a 48-

TABLE VI.   Nonhematologic Toxicity

Gastrointestinal	9/27 (33%)	
Anorexia	1/27	(4%)
Nausea and vomiting	6/27	(22%)
Stomatitis	2/27	(7%)
Diarrhea	3/27	(11%)
Cardiac	2/27	(7%)

year-old white female without a previous history of heart disease. The patient presented with metastatic adenocarcinoma in the mediastinal lymph nodes. In addition, the mediastinal lymph nodes contained numerous noncaseating granulomata. The patient was treated with the Group I dose level and developed complete resolution of mediastinal adenopathy on chest x ray. After having received a cumulative adriamycin dose of 440 mg/m², the patient developed cardiomegaly and acute pulmonary edema. In addition she developed fibrous percardial and pleural effusions, with associated symptoms of pericarditis and pleuritis. The patient died from refractory heart failure. At autopsy, there was a diffuse interstitial nephritis and pneumonitis present along with an associated vasculitis. The heart showed severe myocardial degeneration consistent with adriamycin cardiomyopathy.

Objective Response

Two of four patients with gastric cancer who had measurable disease developed partial responses which lasted 11 and 3+ months. One patient with measurable disease died within 3 weeks of initiation of therapy. Three patients had complete surgical resection of advanced primary gastric cancer with involvement of multiple regional lymph nodes and/or adjacent local extension into visceral organs. One patient died at 5.5 months with progressive disease and two are alive and clinically disease free at 12+ months.

Four of eleven patients (36%) with adenocarcinoma of the lung developed partial responses. The response duration was brief, 4.25 ± .9 months. Survival in the patients who responded was 9.5 ± 1.3 months, whereas survival in the nonresponders was 4.5 ± .9 months. Two patients with adenocarcinoma of the lung had no measurable disease, and for one patient it is too early to evaluate response.

Additional responses were seen in two of six patients with other tumors, including one patient with metastatic breast cancer who had failed CMF adjuvant therapy and a second previously untreated patient with metastatic adenocarcinoma from an unknown primary source.

Six of the eight responding patients received mitomycin C and adriamycin at a dose of 10 mg/m² and 50 mg/m², respectively. The two additional responses were seen at the higher dose level.

CONCLUSIONS

Myelosuppression, as expected, was the dose-limiting toxicity of the combination of mitomycin C and adriamycin. At a dose of 10 mg/m² and 50 mg/m² of mitomycin C and adriamycin, respectively, mild cumulative toxicity was apparent after four courses of therapy. Significant dose reductions of adriamycin were generally not required during the combined treatment program at these dose levels.

Increasing the dose of mitomycin C and adriamycin to 12.5 mg/m² and 60

mg/m^2, respectively, yielded increased acute myelotoxicity during the first course of treatment as well as more severe cumulative toxicity during subsequent courses. This increase in myelotoxicity necessitated dose reductions of adriamycin in approximately one half of the patients during the first course of treatment and of both drugs in most patients by the third course of therapy. Protracted myelotoxicity was encountered at the higher dose of the combination, but not at the lower dose.

Prior chemotherapy or radiotherapy accentuated the myelotoxicity of both dose schedules, leading to significant dose reductions by the second course of therapy, even in patients administered the lower doses of mytomycin C and adriamycin. Therefore, it might be necessary to reduce the dose of both drugs even further in patients who have had extensive prior chemotherapy or radiotherapy.

Gastrointestinal toxicity was mild and not dose limiting in any patient. Cardiotoxicity was seen in two patients, at total doses of 90 and 440 mg/m^2, respectively. Acute cardiac decompensation after single doses of adriamycin has been reported, as well as cardiac toxicity at doses lower than the recommended maximal dose of 550 mg/m^2 (Von Hoff et al., 1978). Therefore, it is difficult to assess the role of mitomycin C in potentiating adriamycin cardiotoxicity, as has been recently reported (Buzdar et al., 1978).

Objective responses were observed in patients with both gastric cancer and adenocarcinoma of the lung. Responses occurred at both the lower and higher dose levels. Therefore, it appears that a dose of 10 mg/m^2 of mitomycin C q6 weeks and adriamycin, 50 mg/m^2 q3 weeks is well tolerated and has significant antitumor activity. A controlled study is in progress to compare the objective response rate and toxicities of the combination of mitomycin C and adriamycin (MA) to the FAM regimen in advanced gastric cancer.

REFERENCES

Ansfield, F., Klatz, J., Nealon, T., Rimaraz, G., Minton, J., Hill, G., Wilson, W., Davis, H. and Cornell, G. (1977). Cancer 39, 34-40.

Baker, L. H., Fzbicki, R. M., and Vaitkevicius, V. K. (1976). Med. and Pediatr. Oncol. 2, 207-213.

Blum R. H. and Carter, S. K. (1974). Ann. Intern. Med. 80, 249-259.

Buzdar, A. U., Legha, S. S., Tashima, C. K., Hortobagyi, H., Yap, H. Y., Krutchik, A. N., Luna, M. A., and Blumenschein, G. R. (1978). Cancer Treat. Rep. 62, 1005-1008.

Cortes, E. P., Holland, J. F., Wang, J. J., and Glidewell, O. (1975). Cancer Chemother. Rep. 6, 305-314.

Crooke, S. T., and Bradner, W. T. (1976). Cancer Treat. Rev. 3, 121-139.

Jones, E. (1959). Cancer Chemother. Rep. 55, 3-7.

Macdonald, J., Schein, P., Ueno, W., and Wooley, P. (1976). Proc. Am. Assoc. Clin. Oncol. 17, 264.

Macdonald, J., Butler, T., Smith, F., Smith, L., and Schein, P. (1977). Proc. Am. Assoc. Cancer Res. 19, 54.

Moertel, C. G. (1975). Cancer 36, 675-682.

Von Hoff, D. J., Layard, M., Basa, P., Davis, H. L., Rozencweig, M., and Muggia, F. M. (1978). Proc. Am. Assoc. Cancer Res. 19, 54.

Chapter 10

MITOMYCIN C IN BREAST CANCER

Thomas E. Godfrey

I. INTRODUCTION

It was reported by Hata *et al.* (1957) that mitomycin C had antitumor effect in animal tumor systems. Initial reports of human trials with mitomycin conducted in several different clinics in Japan indicated the drug to have activity against solid tumors, including breast cancer (Shiraha *et al.*, 1958). On the basis of these reports, clinical trials of mitomycin were initiated in the United States in 1959. The dosage schedules in these trials were such that the patients were receiving large amounts of the drug in a relatively short period of time, and this resulted in substantial hematologic toxicity. As a result, interest in the drug quickly waned.

In 1966 we obtained a supply of the drug and began using it as treatment for a wide variety of neoplasms resistant to the standard chemotherapeutic agents. The results of our experience were published in 1972 (Godfrey and Wilbur, 1972). Four of nine patients with advanced breast cancer responded to treatment. In 1976 we published our results using mitomycin in the treatment of advanced breast cancer; in that study the drug showed solid evidence of activity (Wise *et al.*, 1976). The present report reviews our experience with the drug as treatment for breast cancer from 1966 through June 30, 1978.

II. MATERIALS AND METHODS

A total of 129 patients with histologically proven advanced breast carcinoma received one or more injections of mitomycin. All patients were considered evaluable for response and all but 4 were evaluable for toxicity. There were 127 females and 2 males ranging in age from 31 to 82 years. Nearly all the patients had been treated earlier with alkylators and antimetabolites as single agents or, more recently, with combination cytoxan, methotrexate and fluorouracil (CMF) chemotherapy.

The patients were divided into two groups dealing upon patterns of metastatic spread. Group 1 included those patients with directly measurable tumor bulk involving soft tissues and viscera. Complete objective response was defined as total disappearance of all metastatic disease. Partial response was defined as a 50% or greater reduction in tumor mass for at least 1 month. Those patients in whom tumor bulk showed less than a 50% decrease in size were regarded as treatment failures and classified as nonresponders.

Group 2 consisted of patients with only bone metastasis. These patients were difficult to evaluate as objective responders since repair of metastatic bone lesions requires about 3 months to be seen on serial x rays and the response to treatment was frequently less than this. Therefore relief of bone pain was used as an indication of tumor response in these patients. Subjective response was defined as significant reduction in bone pain for at least 1 month.

Mitomycin C was initially obtained from Kyawa Hakko Kogyo Company Limited of Tokyo, Japan, later from the Clinical Drug Section, Cancer Therapy Evaluation Branch of the National Cancer Institute, and since August 1974 it has been purchased commercially. After reconstituting the 5 mg drug vials with 10 mg of saline, the drug is injected intravenously over a period of several minutes through a #23 Butterfly needle taking care to avoid extravasation.

Most patients received 30-45 mg of the drug initially, given in a divided dose over a 2-week period. Responsive patients received an additional 10 to 15 mg at monthly intervals. If there was a 25% reduction in the WBC or platelet count, the drug dosage was reduced by half; if there was a 50% or greater reduction in these concentrations, the dose was withheld until safe levels returned.

III. RESULTS

Table I summarizes our results of treatment. The overall response rate of the 90 patients in Group 1 with measurable tumors was 23%. Seven of the 21 responders experienced a complete response that lasted from 4 to 8 months. The duration of partial response ranged from 1 to 3 months. Responsive patients demonstrated a decrease in tumor size within 2 weeks of the start of therapy. Four of 10 patients with metastasis to the remaining breast responded to treatment. Eleven of 35 patients with skin and subcutaneous metastasis showed response. Patients with visceral metastasis (lung and liver) showed only a 10-15% response rate.

TABLE I. Mitomycin C Patients Treated from 1966 to 1978

	Group 1: with measurable tumor		Group 2: without measurable tumor (bone metastases)	
Number of patients	90		39	
Age in years				
range	31-82		40-79	
mean	57.6		58.8	
Principal site of metastases				
skin-subcutaneous	11/35[a]	(31%)		
lung	3/28	(10%)		
breast	4/10	(40%)		
liver	2/13	(15%)		
nodal	1/3			
peritoneal	0/1			
bone			13/39	
Total responders	21/90	(23%)	13/39	(33%)
Duration response (mo.)	2.9	(1-8)	3.4	(1½-10)

[a] Responders/total treated.

Thirteen of the 39 patients with only bone metastasis experienced a marked decrease in bone pain for an average of 3.4 months. The relief of bone pain began within 3 to 4 days of the onset of treatment and reached its maximum within 2 weeks. Because of the short duration of response, healing was usually not apparent on bone x rays. Improvement in the bone scan was reported in several responsive patients; and in the patient with a 10-month response, healing of lytic and blastic lesions was apparent on serial bone films.

Table II details the previous chemotherapy the patients received. The use of mitomycin was reserved for patients who were unresponsive or had become resistant to the standard alkylators and antimetabolites. Prior to 1975, single agents were used sequentially; since then, our initial chemotherapy has been CMF followed in some instances by adriamycin, before the mitomycin.

The response to prior chemotherapeutic agents in 57 patients treated since 1975

TABLE II. Prior Chemotherapy

	Single agents used sequentially
1966-1974	72 patients
Alkylators	93%
5-FU	93%
Methotrexate	18%

	Combination chemotherapy initially
1975-1978	57 patients
CMF[a]	89%
Adriamycin	26%

[a] Cytoxan, methotrexate, fluorouracil.

TABLE III.   Response of Patients Treated from 1975 to 1978

	Responders	Nonresponders
Mitomycin	12	45
Other chemotherapy		
Prior CMF	6/11[a] 54%	13/41 31%
Adriamycin		
Premitomycin	1/2	0/13
Postmitomycin	2/7	4/20
Hormonal manipulation		
Estrogens	0/3	3/23
Oophorectomy	0/1	0/3
Androgens	2/3	0/4
Adrenalectomy	–	2/2
Orchiectomy	–	2/2

[a] Responders/total treated.

is detailed in Table III. Mitomycin responders showed a higher response rate to prior CMF than nonresponders: 54% versus 31%. Twenty-eight percent of mitomycin responders also responded to adriamycin, whereas only 20% of the nonresponders benefited. Response to mitomycin appears to have little predictive value of response to hormonal manipulation.

The 57 patients treated from 1975 to 1978 are further analyzed in Table IV. The mean initial drug dosage was essentially the same in the responsive and nonresponsive groups, whereas the total dose was greater in the responsive patients re-

TABLE IV.   Comparative Data of Responsive and Nonresponsive Patients Treated from 1975 to 1978

	Responders	Nonresponders
Number of patients	12	45
Initial drug dose (mean)	22 mg	23 mg
Total dose (mean)	55.4 mg	37.8 mg
Ranges	20-85 mg	10-115 mg
Disease free interval		
(median)	27½ mo.	19 mo.
Menopausal status		
Pre	2	4
Post	10	39
Survival time[a]		
range	42-932[b]	28-1148[c]
median	436	224
mean	404	314

[a] Days from date of first mitomycin administration.
[b] 9 of 12 patients still alive.
[c] 16 patients alive.

TABLE V.   Estrogen Receptors[a]

	Positive	Negative
Chemotherapy		
mito C	0/4[b]	2/7
CMF	0/1	2/7

[a]Sucrose density gradient method (Jensen, 1975).
[b]Responders/total treated.

flecting maintenance therapy. The median disease-free interval was 27½ months in responsive patients and 19 months in nonresponders. Two of 6 premenopausal patients responded to mitomycin whereas 10 of 49 postmenopausal patients showed response. The median survival time after mitomycin was first administered was 436 days for responsive patients and 224 days for nonresponders. This suggests that the drug induced remissions and prolonged life.

Estrogen receptors were positive in 4 out of 11 patients checked (Table V). None of the 4 responded to chemotherapy. Two of 7 patients with negative receptors responded to mitomycin and 2 to CMF therapy.

IV. TOXICITY

Great care should be taken to avoid drug extravasation. Even small amounts of the drug outside the vein will result in redness and itching of overlying skin in 3 to 4 days and this will be followed by tissue necrosis that progresses over a period of several weeks. Necrosis may involve not only skin and subcutaneous tissue but also tendons if it occurs on the dorsum of the hand. While the necrosis is progressing the patient will experience intense pain at the site. I am unaware of any way of reducing the likelihood of tissue necrosis once drug spillage has occurred. The necrosed area must be surgically debrided and skin grafted 3 to 4 weeks after the extravasation.

Nausea and vomiting or lethargy and generalized weakness, or both, were seen in about 10% of the patients. The nausea and vomiting occurred 1-2 hours after the drug was given. The vomiting usually cleared within 3-4 hours, but the nausea often persisted for up to a week.

TABLE VI.   Hematologic Toxicity

	WBC (/mm^3)			Platelets (/mm^3)		
	<2000	2000-4000	>4000	<50,000	50,000-100,000	100,000
Total patients (125)	9	66	50	18	31	76
(%)	(7%)	(53%)	(40%)	(14%)	(25%)	(61%)
Objective responders (21)	2/21	10/21	9/21	1/21	4/21	16/21
(%)	(9%)	(48%)	(43%)	(5%)	(19%)	(76%)

One hundred and twenty-five patients were evaluated for hematologic toxicity (see Table VI). Thrombocytopenia was more common than leukopenia and tended to be more severe with repeated doses of the drug. Small drops in the hemoglobin concentration often occurred during therapy, but a drop of 2 gm of more was rarely seen. In 61% of the patients the platelet count remained above 100,000, in 25% it was reduced to between 50 and 100,000 and in 14% the platelets decreased below 50,000.

The white blood count remained above 4000 in 40% of the patients, in 53% it dropped to between 2000-4000, while in 7% it was reduced to less than 2000. There were no deaths attributed to drug toxicity. There appeared to be no significant correlation between drug dose and hematologic toxicity, and there was no correlation between the pretherapy WBC or platelet counts and subsequent toxicity. Responding patients did not experience any greater hematologic depression than nonresponders. The majority of patients experiencing severe hematologic toxicity were those with bone scan or x ray evidence of bone metastasis (and often a history of previous radiation therapy to areas of bony involvement). As expected, severely debilitated patients also tolerated the drug poorly.

While renal toxicity from mitomycin has been reported (Liu et al., 1971) in only one instance did we note elevation of the blood urea nitrogen and serum creatinine. This patient had a preexistent mild azotemia and hypertension prior to the mitomycin therapy; the deterioration of her renal function could have been explained solely on a renovascular basis.

V. DISCUSSION

Mitomycin has established itself as an effective single agent in the management of far-advanced breast cancer. Thirty-four of 129 patients (26%) we treated responded to the drug for an average of 3 months.

In a review of the literature in English, 39 of 124 patients (31%) with breast cancer treated with mitomycin responded to therapy (Table VII). All of these patients except those of Buzdar et al. (1978) were treated with the drug alone; Buzdar used mitomycin and the progestational agent megestrol acetate. Our patients, as well as those in the studies reported by Hum et al. (1974) and Buzdar, had received extensive prior chemotherapy and in some instances hormonal therapy. The response rate of breast cancer patients to mitomycin has been relatively constant with the exception of those in the studies of Saba et al. (1969) and Hum. In these studies the mitomycin schedule was 125 μg/kg body weight weekly which represents a lower drug dosage than reported in the other studies. It should be mentioned that while the average duration of response to mitomycin is approximately 3 months, Buzdar, when adding the progestational agent, reported a 7-month median duration of response.

Several investigators, including ourselves, have used a large loading dose of the drug followed by smaller maintenance injections at 4-week intervals. From our ex-

TABLE VII. Literature in English

	Objective responses[a]	Drug dosage	Definition and duration (where specified) response
Jones (1959)	4/7	Phase I study with initial dose of 10 μg/kg day	Measurable reduction in tumor size for 2-3 months
Manheimer (1966)	2/3	125 μg/kg twice weekly	↓ in tumor size lasting weeks or months
Moore (1968)	15/42	0.050 mg/kg body weight daily for 6 days, then every 2nd day until total dose of 50 mg delivered	Reduction in size of 1 or more lesions by 50% or more
Saba (1969)	0/3	125 μg/kg body weight weekly in post adrenalectomy cases	
Guerrero (1972)	5/9	125 μg/kg every 3 or 4 days for total of 50 to 60 mg. Maintenance doses were one half the induction dose	↓ in measurable lesion by at least 50%
Hum (1974)	0/12	0.25 mg/kg/wk later decreased to 0.125 mg/kg/wk because of excessive toxicity	Any subjective or objective evidence of improvement
Buzdar (1978)	13/48	20 mg/m^2 IV day 1 and repeated at 4-6 week intervals with megestrol acetate 40 mg p.o. q.i.d.	↓ reduction in the size of all measurable lesions for 1 month or longer

[a] Responders/number treated.

perience I would suggest that in good risk patients the initial dose of the drug should be 15 mg/m² followed by half that dose at monthly intervals when indicated. In poor risk patients (those with bone scan or x ray evidence of metastatic bone disease or patients with severe debility) half the recommended dose can probably be safely tolerated. The platelet count should be checked at 2-week intervals, and if at any time it drops below 100,000, the next dose of the drug should be reduced by 50%. This same dosage reduction should be applied if the white count drops below 2500. If the platelet or white blood counts remain below these levels, withhold chemotherapy until safer levels are achieved.

As with hormone therapy, our experience indicates that mitomycin is most effective in the treatment of soft tissue and bone metastasis and less effective where tumor extension to the liver and lung has occurred.

The results of a five-drug combination in the treatment of hormone resistant advanced breast cancer were presented by Cooper (1969). He combined cytoxan, methotrexate, 5-fluorouracil, vincristine, and prednisone and reported a 90% complete remission rate. Many subsequent studies (Carter, 1976) using combination chemotherapy have shown response rates ranging from 20 to 70% with a cumulative response rate of 47%. No study has reproduced the original 90% rate reported by Cooper, and in fact the abstract has never been followed by a full paper detailing the study.

With the improved management of advanced breast cancer apparent through the use of combination therapy, we began a phase I study combining mitomycin and adriamycin as treatment for these patients in 1975. The initial dosage of mitomycin was 10 mg/m² followed by one half that dose at 3-week intervals; the adriamycin dosage was 30 mg/m² every 3 weeks. The WBC and platelet counts were checked at weekly intervals. The dosage was tolerated quite well, though one patient developed a thrombopenia of 51,000 following the initial injections and then showed a persistent thrombopenia of less than 100,000 following the second injection of the drugs. In one of the four patients there was a 6-week partial response of her liver metastasis.

At the next dosage schedule mitomycin was administered at 15 mg/m² followed by half that dose at 3-week intervals, and the adriamycin was given at a dose of 45 mg/m² every 3 weeks. We encountered significant hematologic toxicity at this dose level, with the white blood count being reduced to 2000 in all 5 patients treated and with the platelet count at some time during the course of treatment decreasing to 40,000 in 3 of the 5. None of these patients showed evidence of tumor response.

It appears that the greatest potential for mitomycin in breast cancer lies in its incorporation into a combination of drugs. It is possible that the mitomycin-adriamycin combination might be more successful in tumor control at different drug dosages or schedules. A study utilizing the drug in combination with other alkylators and antimetabolites should also be considered.

REFERENCES

Buzdar, A., Tashima, C., Blumenschein, G., Gortobagyi, G., Yap, H., Kruchik, A., Bodey, G., and Livingston, R. (1978). *Cancer 41,* 392-395.

Carter, S. (1976). *Cancer Treatment Rev. 3,* 141-174.

Cooper, R. (1969). *Proc. Amer. Assoc. Cancer Res. 10 (abst.),* 15.

Crooke, S. T. and Bradner, W. (1976). *Cancer Treatment Rev. 3,* 121-139.

Godfrey, T. and Wilbur, D. (1972). *Cancer 29,* 1647-1652.

Guerrero, R. C., Abello, E., Custodio, D., and San Diego, E. (1972). *Philippine Med. Assoc. J. 48,* 559-564.

Hata, T., Shimada, N., and Ishy, Y. (1957). "Symposium on the Chemotherapy of Cancer of Univ. Internationalis Centra Cancerum and Cancer Chemotherapy Comm. of Japan," Tokyo, Oct. 24-28, pp. 21-23.

Hum, G., Bogdon, D., and Bateman, J. (1974). *Oncol. 30,* 236-243.

Irwin, L. W., Pugh, R., Sadoff, L., Hestorff, R., and Weiner, J. (1974). *Abst. of the 11th Internal. Cancer Cong.,* 597.

Jensen, E. (1975). *Cancer Res. 35,* 3362.

Jones, R., Jr. (1959). *Cancer Chemother. Rep. 2,* 3-7.

Liu, K., Mittleman, A., Sproul, E. E., and Elias, E. G. (1971). *Cancer 28,* 207-212.

Moore, G. E., Bross, I. E., Ausman, R., Nadler, S., Jones, Jr. R., Slack, N., and Rimm, A. (1968). *Cancer Chemother. Rep. 52,* 675-684.

Saba, Z., Hall, T. C., and Griffiths, C. T. (1969). *Cancer 23,* 1122-1125.

Shiraha, Y., Sakai, K., and Teranaku, T. (1958). *Sixth Ann. Symp. on Antibiot., No. 70.*

Wise, G., Kuhn, I., and Godfrey, T. (1976). *Med. and Ped. Oncol. 2,* 55-60.

Chapter 11

ADRIAMYCIN AND MITOMYCIN C IN ADVANCED BREAST CANCER

Lee Roy Morgan

I. INTRODUCTION

Since the initial demonstrations by Greenspan (1966) and subsequent ones by Cooper (1969) indicating that patients with metastatic breast carcinoma frequently respond better to combination cytoxic chemotherapy, such treatment has played a significant role in the management of these patients. The general trend is that those patients that respond the best survive longer. Many combination treatment programs have been studied. Most are not strictly comparable.

Adriamycin is the most effective single agent available for inducing responses in patients with metastatic carcinoma of the breast (Broder and Tormey, 1974). Attempts to improve the number of responses by combining adriamycin with other drugs have generated considerable interest. The interest, however, continues to be tempered by cardiotoxicity. As a result, most recent reports have documented experiences with combinations that contain lower doses of adriamycin with the hope of reducing cardiotoxicity and of increasing tumor response through combinations with other cytotoxic agents (Smalley *et al.,* 1978; Plesant *et al.,* 1977). Most of the combinations with adriamycin contain an alkylating agent. Cyclophosphamide is generally considered to have an overall response rate of about 35% in advanced breast cancer (Broder and Tormey, 1974). Combinations of adriamycin and cyclophosphamide have been effective in this disease with reproducible rates of approximately 50% being observed (Jones, 1975; Lokich, 1974).

Preliminary data suggest that mitomycin C is an active alkylating agent in breast cancer (Godfrey and Wilbur, 1972; Crooke and Bradner, 1976). The preliminary results of Comis and Abou-Mourad (1978) further support the possible usefulness of mitomycin C in combination therapies for advanced breast cancer, especially with those patients who have failed on CMF therapies. This report communicates our experience to date with an adriamycin-mitomycin C regimen in advanced breast cancer.

II. PATIENTS AND METHODS

A. Patients

Twenty-seven female patients with advanced breast cancer were selected to receive adriamycin and mitomycin C. The majority of the patients possessed multiple lesions and all patients had biopsy-proven breast cancer. Patients were excluded from the study if there was organ dysfunction unrelated to tumor, other previous cancers, if it had been less than 4 weeks since treatment with cobalt, hormone, or chemotherapy, if a Karnofsky performance index < 60. Informed consent was obtained from all patients.

When possible, tumor tissue from either cutaneous or other metastatic sites was selected for biopsy, and the remaining skin nodules and/or metastases were evaluated for response to drug therapy. Ages ranged from 32 to 76, and one third of the patients were black. All patients were evaluated for postmenopausal status.

The patients were stratified by dominant disease sites (visceral, osseous, soft tissue, or lymphatic), number of organ sites of involvement, and prior treatment responses.

B. Drug Regimen

Adriamycin (ADR) and mitomycin C (MMC) were administered on schedules as described in Table I. An excellent risk was a patient with a history of receiving no

TABLE I. Adriamycin Plus Mitomycin C Therapy in
Advanced Breast Cancer

Excellent risk	ADR	$50/m^2$
	MMC	$10/m^2$
Normal risk	ADR	$40/m^2$
	MMC	$7\frac{1}{2}/m^2$
Poor risk	ADR	$30/m^2$
	MMC	$5/m^2$

Schedule: Adriamycin: every 3 weeks
Mitomycin C: every 6 weeks

prior chemotherapy and only chest wall irradiation. A normal risk was a patient who received prior chemotherapy and cobalt therapy and had a pretreatment WBC between 3000 and 5000/mm^3; and a poor risk was a patient receiving extensive cobalt therapy ($>$ 2 sites and/or $>$ 2000 rads to more than 25% of the normal bone marrow) and chemotherapy. Adriamycin was given every 3 weeks and mitomycin C was given every 6 weeks.

Each course of therapy consisted of the intravenous administration of adriamycin in 50 ml 5% dextrose in water, followed by mitomycin C in 50 ml 5% dextrose in water. Each was slowly given over 15-20 min duration. The adriamycin was repeated in 3 weeks. After a patient receives ADR and MMC on day 1, the day 22 dose of the adriamycin should be adjusted (Table II) depending on the nadir counts. If no drug was given, weekly CBC and platelet counts were obtained and adriamycin was given when WBC 4.0 x 10^3/mm^3 and platelets 100 x 10^3/mm^3 were obtained.

If a patient had a platelet nadir $<$ 50,000 and/or a WBC nadir $<$ 2000, no drug was administered until counts were platelet $>$ 100,000 and WBC $>$ 4000. After recovery, the following modified dosage schedule was used to reduce the doses 75% of the planned schedule, that is, MMC 7.5 mg/m^2, ADR 37.5 mg/m^2. In patients with a serum bilirubin concentration greater than 2.0 mg/dl or a serum alkaline phosphatase concentration greater than 150 IU/liter due to hepatic disease, only 25% of the calculated adriamycin dose was administered.

Patients were evaluated prior to therapy by physical examination, history, electrocardiogram, complete blood cell counts, liver and renal function tests, chest and skeletal roentgenograms, and bone and liver scintiscans.

During therapy, weekly CBC and platelet counts and serum creatinine values were obtained. Prior to drug administration, a complete liver profile was obtained. EKG was obtained at 6-week intervals. Prior to initial therapy, after 220 mg/m^2 and after 440 mg/m^2 total doses of adriamycin, echocardiograms were also obtained. Patients were discontinued from the study when a total of 440 mg/m^2 of adriamycin was given.

TABLE II.   Dose Deescalation of Adriamycin

Nadir Counts x 10^3					Dose adjustment for adriamycin
Day 0-20			Day 21		Day 22
WBC		PLT	WBC	PLT	% of planned dose
$>$4.0		$>$100	$>$4.0	$>$100	100
$\geqslant$2.0-3.9	or	$\geqslant$75-99	$>$4.0	$>$100	100
$\geqslant$1.0-2.9	or	50-75	$>$4.0	$>$100	75
$\geqslant$1.0	or	$<$50	$>$4.0	$>$100	50
$\geqslant$2.0	or	75-100	3-3.9	$>$100	50
$<$2.0	or	$<$50	$<$3.0 or	$<$100	0

C. Criteria for Response

Patients were evaluable if they received one complete course (6 weeks) of therapy. Complete response was defined as disappearance of all objective evidence of disease or recalcification of osteolytic lesions in measured and unmeasured sites for 12 weeks. A partial response was a decrease by > 50% in the product of the two largest perpendicular diameters of measurable lesions and/or partial recalcification of osteolytic lesions (regression or no change in osteoblastic lesions). No change indicated regression of < 50% in measured areas which lasted for at least 3 months. Progression was an increase of > 20% of measured lesions and/or the occurrence of new lesions and/or progression of osteolytic lesions.

D. Estrogen Binding Protein (EBP) and Enzyme Assays

The method of handling specimens after biopsy, preparation of cytosol, and assays for EBP by the dextran-coated charcoal and the sucrose gradient techniques were previously reported by Leung *et al.* (1975), Wittliff *et al.* (1972), Morgan *et al.* (1976), and Lippman and Huff (1976). Specific estrogen-binding capacity was specified as femtomole (fmol) of ^{3}H-17β-estradiol bound per mg of cytoplasmic protein (Wittliff *et al.*, 1972). In this study, tumors were classified as positive for EBP if the cytoplasmic estrogen-binding capcity was > 10 fmols/mg of protein. Tissue lactate dehydrogenase (LDH) activities were determined according to previously described procedures (Savlov *et al.*, 1974). Values for LDH activities were described as international units per gram wet tumor tissue.

III. RESULTS

Twenty-seven patients were treated with adriamycin and mitomycin C for at least 6 weeks, and evaluated. The overall response rate was 48% (13 of 27 patients) which included complete and partial responders and no change in size of lesions. Table III describes the patients' responses. As indicated, all the patients were in the postmenopausal status. Table IV is an evaluation of the postmenopausal status and response to therapy. The patients who responded to the greatest extent were in the older age group and those with the greatest number of years postmenopausal.

Durations of response are listed in Table V. The present study has been in progress for only 13 months. The first patient treated is still responding after 13 months although she has been off therapy for 4 months. At present, the median duration of response is 6+ months for the patients in the study with 80% of the responders still in remission and alive. Two patients who have reached maximum accumulated dosage of adriamycin, one demonstrating a complete response and the other no change, are currently being maintained on methotrexate 30 mg/m^2 intramuscular every 2 weeks. Table VI analyzes response rate in relation to specific organ sites of evaluable disease. In our study, the predominant lesions were visceral

TABLE III.   Responders to ADR-MMC According to
Menstrual Status

Status	Number of patients (27)	CR	PR	NC	NR
Postmenopausal[a]					
0-5 yrs.	5	1	1		3
> 5 yrs.	22	1	8	2	11
	27	2	9	2	14
		13 (48%)			
		11 (40%)			

[a] Postmenopausal: ≥55 years old and/or >6 mos. post-
oöphorectomy.

metastasis. Seven of the thirteen responders had pulmonary lesions that responded to therapy. Cutaneous lesions were the next most frequent site in which responses were noted. In the present patients, the responders with visceral disease had only lung involvement.

The clinical toxicities observed with this drug combination are presented in Tables VII and VIII. The observed nonhematological toxicities are what have been reported for adriamycin and mitomycin C alone. There were no renal or pulmonary toxicities noted of the type that have been described for high doses of mitomycin C alone. Cardiac toxicity was monitored carefully as mentioned in the methods section.

Electrocardiograms were performed on a regular basis. Only two patients demonstrated a reduction in QRS voltage $\geq$ 30% at total doses of adriamycin of 318 and 412 mg/m^2. Echocardiograms in these two patients demonstrated hypo- and dyskinetic movements of their intraventricular septum. However, no clinical evidence of cardiomegaly or congestive heart failure was noted. Off adriamycin therapy, the echocardiograms and electrocardiograms of both patients improved.

All patients developed alopecia. The nausea and vomiting noted were controlled with barbiturates and phenothiazine-type tranquilizers.

No evidence of hypercalcemia was noted. No patients expired as a result of sep-

TABLE IV.   Years Menopausal and Response

Years postmenopausal	Number of patients	Number of responders[a]
<5	5	2
>5-10	3	1
11-15	7	3
>15	12	5

[a] CR + PR only.

TABLE V. Duration of Response[a]

Duration of response[a] (Months)	Number of patients
<3	5
3-6	4
7-12	4

[a] CR + PR + NC.

sis. One patient experienced some increase in bone pain which subsided after one week of therapy, and then went on to achieve a partial response. No uterine bleeding was noted.

In Table VIII, hematological changes noted are described. Not all patients demonstrated a decrease in their hematological profile. No correlation between response to therapy and toxicities was noted. Sixty-nine percent of the patients developed WBC $< 3500/mm^3$, and 41% of the patients developed a platelet count of $< 100,000/mm^3$. The median nadir for WBC was seen within the second to third week after adriamycin and had little correlation with mitomycin C administration. The median platelet count nadir was less predictable and appeared around the third week of the course.

Table IX correlates previous therapy with disease-free intervals and response to therapy. There was little correlation between response to ADR-MMC therapy, prior therapies, and disease-free intervals.

In Table X is described the response to therapy and the initial performance status. As would be expected, the patients that responded the best had the better initial performance status. Table XI compares time in hospital after initial therapy was started, response, and performance status. There was an overall significant difference between the time that the responders and nonresponders spent in the hospital. The nonresponders, independent of performance status, all spent the same amount of time in the hospital. Similarly, the responders, irrespective of performance status, spent less time in the hospital.

The median survival of all patients in this study was 163 days. The median survival of patients with complete or partial response was 188 days (range 60 to 390 days) with nine patients still alive. The two patients with objective improvement

TABLE VI. Organs Involved: Responders versus Nonresponders[a]

Patients	Bone	Viscera	Lymphatics	Cutaneous tissue
Responders (13)	3	7	1	4
Nonresponders (14)	5	10	0	2

[a] CR + NR + NC.

TABLE VII. Nonhematologic Side Effects

Side effects	Number of patients
Gastrointestinal (N/V)	23
Stomatitis	11
Mucositis	9
Hepatic	0
Edema	0
Skin rash	0
Infection	0
CNS	0
Renal	0
Alopecia	27
Cardiac (EKG changes)	2
Neurotoxicity	0
Virilization	0

and no change in lesions had a survival range of 250-278 days with one patient still alive. The nonresponding patients had a median survival of 74 days (range 35 to 340 days) with six patients still alive. These data are not significantly different at present (Table XII).

IV. DISCUSSION

Adriamycin is still the most effective single agent available for inducing remissions in patients with metastatic carcinoma of the breast (Broder and Tormey,

TABLE VIII. Hematologic Side Effects

Toxic effect	Incidence (% of 27 patients)	Day of nadir	
		Mean	Range
Leukopenia (cells/mm^3)			
Responders			
$<$3500 $\geqslant$2000	15	12	11-19
$<$2000	19	14	12-21
Nonresponders			
$<$3500 $\geqslant$2000	19	11	14-21
$<$2000	26	14	14-21
Thrombocytopenia (cells/mm^2)			
Responders			
$<$100,000 $\geqslant$50,000	15	27	21-36
$<$50,000	4	28	19-32
Nonresponders			
$<$100,000 $\geqslant$50,000	11	27	20-42
$<$50,000	11	31	21-56

TABLE IX.   Effect of Pretherapy Variables on the Response to ADR-MMC

Patients	Number	No prior therapy	Cobalt therapy	Hormone therapy (responded)	Chemotherapy (responded)
Responders	13				
Disease-free intervals:					
<2 years	6	1	2	2 (0%)	3 (0%)
≥2 years	7	–	6	6 (50%)	3 (33%)
Nonresponders	14				
Disease-free intervals:					
<2 years	7	1	4	6 (0%)	5 (0%)
≥2 years	7	–	7	7 (43%)	7 (57%)

1974). Attempts to improve the quantity and quality of responses by combining adriamycin with other anticancer agents have generated considerable interest. The use of adriamycin in combination therapy for breast cancer increased after Jones (1975), Muggia (1974), Horton (1970), and Lokich (1974) reported that there was an increased response when an alkylating agent such as cyclophosphamide was combined with adriamycin.

There have been attempts to combine adriamycin with from one to four other single agents also proving effective in breast cancer. These combinations have resulted in increases in number of responses, duration of responses, and a longer duration of disease control but no significant increase in survival. Subclassification of patients by site of dominant disease has indicated improved results with the adriamycin combinations for all; but statistically, superiority to date has been achieved only in the skin-bone dominant group. Often, these combinations have not been compared and have not increased survival. Morbidity associated with the adriamycin was significant, and patients often refused to continue on therapy despite their being in remission.

Adriamycin is a planar molecule that binds to double-stranded DNA probably by intercalating between complementary strands. It is thought that this results in DNA synthesis inhibition (DiMarco and Lenaz, 1974), and inhibition of certain types of RNA synthesis (Blum and Carter, 1974).

The antibiotic adriamycin inhibits DNA synthesis when given during any phase of the cell cycle; however, the most sensitive phase is late S (Drewinco, 1975).

The combination of adriamycin with an alkylating agent such as cyclophospha-

TABLE X.   Initial Performance Status and Response

Performance status	CR	PR	NC	NR
100	1			
90	1	4	1	1
80		1		2
70		2	1	5
60		2		6

TABLE XI. Time in Hospital after Initial Therapy,
Response[a] and Performance Status

Performance Status	Responder		Nonresponder	
	Patients (%)	Time in Hospital (days) (mean)	Patients (%)	Time in Hospital (days) (mean)
100	3	0	–	–
90	22	4	3	14
80	2	0	7	24
70	11	3	19	21
60	7	7	22	21

mide represents the use of a phase-specific and a non-phase-specific agent. However, in order for the classical alkylating agents to interact with the guanosine bases in DNA, the latter must be unprotected and vulnerable for attack, with few histones protecting the DNA, as in late G and early S phases. Despite these considerations, these agents are generally considered to be active throughout the entire cell cycle.

Cyclophosphamide has been reported to have an overall response rate of 35% in breast cancer (Broder and Tormey, 1974; Bayer and Howard-Flanders, 1960). However, it did potentiate the cardiac toxicity of adriamycin (Jones, 1975). Mitomycin C in preliminary studies may be an active alkylating agent in breast cancer (Crooke and Bradner, 1976).

Mitomycin C is an antibiotic that contains an aziridine ring and an amino quinone moiety. When activated through reduction of the quinone ring, mitomycin C is a bifunctional, or possibly a trifunctional, alkylating agent that alkylates the guanosine bases of DNA, cross-linking bases and inhibiting of DNA synthesis. The most sensitive phases of the cell cycle are also late G, or early S. G_2 is much less sensitive (Blumenschein, 1975). Therefore, combinations of adriamycin and mitomycin C would provide a regimen that acts at different times in the cell cycle, but probably needs actively replicating cells and would have little affect on resting cells or cells in the G_0 phase. Comis and Abou-Mourad (1978), have recently reported that adriamycin and mitomycin C will produce objective remissions in advanced gastric and lung adenocarcinomas. These reports encouraged our study of adriamycin and mitomycin C in breast carcinoma.

TABLE XII. Duration of Survival in Responders

Response of Patients (No.)		Survival (days)	
		Median	Range
CR + PR	(11)	188	60-390
NC	(2)	–	250-278
NR	(14)	74	35-340

In the present study, adriamycin and mitomycin C produced significant objective responses of good quality that are continuing in $> 80\%$ of the patients that responded.

Subclassification of patients by site of dominant disease indicated improved results with adriamycin combination for all, but statistical superiority to date has been achieved only in the cutaneous dominant group. The study is ongoing, and the inclusion of more patients in the less dominant group will indicate whether there is statistical superiority in these less responsive groups. In this study, only pulmonary lesions responded.

Many of our patients had prior hormone and adjunct CMF chemotherapy; however, response to prior therapy had little affect on responses to ADR-MMC therapy.

The present regimen was reasonably well tolerated, and we were impressed with the quality of life the patients demonstrated, especially those with good initial performance status. The older patients that were > 10 years postmenopausal had the better responses.

In the present study, only seven patients had enough tissue to be assayed for both EBP and enzymes at the time of starting therapy. The results in the present work confirm our previous findings that patients who respond to chemotherapy have elevated tumor tissue LDH activities and normal or slightly elevated EBP values (Morgan et al., 1975). Although only a few patients had sufficient tissue to evaluate, the five patients that responded (5/7) to therapy had elevated LDH activities (> 350 units/g tumor tissue); the two nonresponders had normal LDH activities (50-349 units/g tumor tissue). Only one patient (a responder) had an elevated EBP (35 fmoles/mg protein). The other six patients had EBP < 10 fmoles per mg proteins.

It is well established that most malignancies, especially the anaplastic, poorly differentiated forms, have elevated LDH activities (Savlov et al., 1974; Burke et al., 1978). This may be associated with increased anaerobic glycolysis, resulting in a reducing environment. Mitomycin C requires reduction for activation. Cells that demonstrate increased anaerobic glycolysis and elevated LDH activities might reduce and activate mitomycin C more effectively. The use of LDH activities as a tissue marker for mitomycin C sensitivity is in progress and merits more investigation. Adriamycin and mitomycin C is a useful, reasonably well-tolerated combination in advanced breast cancer.

New combinations utilizing adriamycin and mitomycin C in breast cancer must be devised that cause less morbidity and have less potential for cardiotoxicity. The addition of an antimetabolite to the above two-drug combination is in order.

REFERENCES

Bayer, R. P., and Howard-Flanders, P. (1960). A. Verebung, 95, 345-350.

Blum, R. H., and Carter, S. K. (1974). Ann. Int. Med. 80, 249-259.

Blumenschein, G. R. (1975). In "Cancer Chemotherapy, The M. D. Anderson Clinical Conference," pp. 403-417. Year Book Med. Publ., Chicago, Ill.

Broder, L. E., and Tormey, Q. D. (1974). *Cancer Treat. Rev. 1,* 183-203.

Burke, R. E., Harris, S. C., and McGuire, W. L. (1978). *Cancer Res. 38,* 2773-2776.

Comis, R. L., and Abou-Mourad, N. (1978). *Proc. Am. Soc. Clin. Oncol. 19,* 377.

Cooper, R. G. (1969). *Proc. Am. Assoc. Cancer Res. 10,* 15.

Crooke, S. T., and Bradner, W. T. (1976). Mitomycin C: A review. *Cancer Treat. Rev. 3,* 121-137.

DiMarco, A., and Lenaz, L. (1974). Daunomycin and adriamycin, *In* "Cancer Medicine" (J. P. Holland and E. Frei, eds.) pp. 826-834. Lea & Febiges, Philadelphia, Pa.

Drewinco, B. (1975). *In* "Cancer Chemotherapy, the M. D. Anderson Clinical Conference," pp. 79-93. Year Book Publ., Chicago, Ill.

Godfrey, R. E., and Wilber, D. W. (1972). *Cancer 29,* 1647-1652.

Greenspan, E. M. (1966). *J. Mt. Sinai Hosp. 33,* 1-27.

Horton, J. (1970). *Proc. Am. Soc. Clin. Oncol. 11,* 240.

Jones, S. E. (1975). *Cancer 36,6,* 90-97.

Leung, B. S., Moseley, H. S., Davenport, C. E., Krippachne, W. W., and Fletcher, W. L. *In* "Estrogen Receptors in Human Breast Cancer" (W. L. McGuire, P. P. Carbone, and E. P. Vollmer, eds.) pp. 107-114. Raven Press, New York.

Lippman, M., and Huff, K. (1976). *Cancer 38,* 868-874.

Lokich, J. (1974). *Abst. 11th Int. Cancer Congress, (Florence) 1,* 369-370.

Morgan, L. R., Hungerford, L. E., Gillen, L. E., Hagardorn, A. N., Carter, R. D., Krementz, E. T., Leung, B. S., and Fletcher, W. (1975). *Clin. Res. 23,* 173.

Morgan, L. R., Schein, P. S., Woolley, P. V., Hoth, D., Macdonald, J. Luppman, M., Posey, L. E., and Beazley, R. W. (1976). *Cancer Treat. Rep. 60,* 1437-1443.

Muggia, F. M. (1974). *Cancer Chemother. Rep. 58,* 919-926.

Plesant, C. A., Van Amburg, III, and Klair, C. (1977). *Cancer 40,* 987-993.

Savlov, E. D., Wittliff, J. L., Hilf, R., and Hall, T. C. (1974). *Cancer 33,* 303-309.

Smalley, R. V., Carpenter, J., Bartolucci, A., Vogel, C., and Krauss, S. (1978). *Cancer 40,* 987-993.

Wittliff, J. L., Hilf, Brooks, W. F., Jr., Savlov, E. D., Hall, T. C., and Orlando, R. A. (1972). *Cancer Res. 32,* 1983-1992.

Chapter 12

A NEW COMBINATION CHEMOTHERAPY CONTAINING MITOMYCIN C FOR METASTATIC BREAST CANCER

Michael A. Friedman

I. INTRODUCTION

Many single chemotherapeutic agents are effective in treating patients with disseminated breast cancer. More importantly, the use of these agents in combination has resulted in enhanced rates of response and survival (Broder and Tormey, 1974). Currently, several effective combination chemotherapies are widely employed. These therapies usually consist of an alkylating agent (often cytoxan), antimetabolites (5-fluorouracil [5-FU], methotrexate, or both), an anthracycline antibiotic (adriamycin), and a vinca alkaloid (oncovin [vincristine]). Virtually all possible permutations of the individual agents have been explored. Combinations of cytoxan plus methotrexate plus 5-FU (CMF), adriamycin plus cytoxan (AC), and cytoxan plus adriamycin plus 5-FU (CAF) have been most extensively used.

All these programs have proven beneficial; the objective response rate for each has been reported to be 60% ± 15%. Few complete responses have been noted, and the duration of all responses has averaged 8 months. Patients who respond usually survive 1 year (Broder and Tormey, 1974). Despite many manipulations of drugs and schedules, little improvement in clinical results has been demonstrated for patients with disseminated breast cancer.

Additionally, increasing numbers of patients are receiving adjuvant postmastectomy chemotherapy, which most frequently consists of single-agent phenyl-alanine mustard (L-PAM) or combination CMF. Although many premenopausal women benefit from this therapeutic approach, more women (especially those who are postmenopausal) have recurrent disease that requires a different program of chemotherapy.

Recognizing that our therapeutic effectiveness in disseminated breast cancer has reached a plateau, we are aware of the need for an effective, tolerable combination therapy that will address the need for:

1. A therapy that will benefit patients who, despite adjuvant CMF or L-PAM, have recurrent disease.
2. A therapy that will yield more responses (especially more complete regressions of disease) and longer duration of response (therefore, increased length of survival).

Of the active agents available for breast cancer patients, we elected to test a combination of 5-FU plus oncovin plus adriamycin plus mitomycin C (FOAM). The activity of each of these agents is shown in Table I. Mitomycin C is a potent antibiotic alkylator in which there has been renewed clinical interest. Intermittent schedules of this agent appear to be effective and more easily tolerated than the "loading course" therapy described previously (Wise *et al.*, 1976). Moreover, it is an effective agent in breast cancer (and is probably not cross-resistant with other alkylators). The combination of adriamycin plus oncovin has been widely and effectively employed in patients for whom previous therapy has failed (Brambilla *et al.*, 1976). Additional preclinical information has been reported indicating that mitomycin C plus oncovin and adriamycin plus oncovin are synergistic combinations (Pouillant *et al.*, 1974).

The inclusion of 5-FU in our FOAM protocol was based on its activity in breast cancer. Although patients who have not benefited from previous CMF therapy may be resistant to 5-FU, theoretically they may still respond to 5-FU used in a different manner (Ullman *et al.*, 1978). The simultaneous administration of methotrexate and 5-FU (as in CMF therapy) may be the least effective way to use these two agents (Cadman *et al.*, 1978).

Moreover, a considerable amount of information about toxicity was available

TABLE I.   The Activity of the Components of FOAM Therapy in Cumulative Studies of Breast Cancer[a]

Drug	No. of patients	No. of responders	%
5-Fluorouracil	1236	324	26
Oncovin	226	47	21
Adriamycin	221	81	37
Mitomycin C	75	26	35

[a] Broder and Tormey, (1974).

from a similar program, FAM, used for gastric cancer (Macdonald *et al.,* 1976). In this study the nadir white count and platelet count were acceptable. However, breast cancer patients may have more generalized marrow insufficiency because of previous radiation or drug therapy or tumor invasion. Therefore, we embarked upon a phase I-II study of FOAM in breast cancer patients as a Northern California Oncology Group (NCOG) pilot study.

II. MATERIALS AND METHODS

The criteria in Table II were established to determine the eligibility of patients for the study. Patients satisfying all requirements were entered into the study and given a combination of chemotherapy as shown in Table III.

The doses were modified according to the magnitude of hepatic and hematopoetic dysfunction present. Adriamycin was decreased by 50% if the patient's serum bilirubin concentration was between 1.5 and 3 mg%, and by 75% if the bilirubin was < 3 mg%. The doses of 5-FU, adriamycin, and mitomycin C were diminished according to the patient's blood count (see Table IV).

Since the initiation of this study, 23 patients with metastatic breast cancer have been treated. Fifteen of these patients have been followed for 8 weeks (one full treatment cycle) and will be reported on here. Some of the important characteristics of this group of patients are presented in Table V. Eight of the women were premenopausal. All had received some surgical therapy; most had received radiation (14/15) and chemotherapy (8/15 CMF, 1/15, L-PAM). The specific sites of disease are also summarized in Table V.

III. RESULTS

The efficacy of FOAM in the treatment of these 15 patients is summarized in Table VI. This summary indicates that the entry KPS scores of these patients were

TABLE II.   Eligibility Criteria

Eligible	Ineligible
1. Biopsy proven adenocarcinoma of the breast	1. Age > 72 years
2. Measurable disease	2. Karnofsky performance status (KPS) $< 50\%$
3. Estimated survival $\geqslant 8$ weeks	3. Previous therapy with mitomycin C, oncovin, or adriamycin
4. Blood Urea Nitrogen (BUN) $\leqslant 35$ mg%; Serum creatinine $\leqslant 1.5$ mg%	4. Intrinsic heart disease precluding use of adriamycin
5. White blood count (WBC) $\geqslant 4000/\text{mm}^3$	5. Concomitant radiation therapy to $> 20\%$ of bone marrow
6. Platelet count $\geqslant 100,000/\text{mm}^3$	6. Active secondary tumor
7. Signed informed consent	

TABLE III. Combination Chemotherapy Schedule

Drug	Dose (Repeated every 8 weeks)	Day			
		1	8	29	36
(F) 5-Fluorouacil	400 mg/m^2 IV	X	X	X	X
(O) Vincristine[a]	1 mg/m^2 IV	X		X	
(A) Adriamycin[b]	40 mg/m^2 IV	X		X	
(M) Mitomycin C	10 mg/m^2 IV	X			

[a] Maximum single dose = 2 mg.
[b] Maximum Total Dose = 550 mg/m^2.

moderately low (an average of 64) and no patient's score exceeded 80. Standard NCOG criteria for clinical response were used to classify patients as having a complete response, a partial response, stable disease, or progressive disease. The majority of patients in this pilot study benefited from treatment. Nine of 15 patients had objective responses (1/15 complete) and 7/9 are still receiving FOAM. Stable disease was noted in 4/15 patients and 3/4 are still receiving therapy. Regressions of metastatic tumor have been noted in soft tissues, lungs, and liver. Treatment failed for two patients who had progressive disease.

The duration of these responses and overall length of survival is not known at this time. To date, the most durable response has been > 12 months, the median duration of response has been > 3.5 months, and the mean as yet cannot be determined.

IV. TOXICITY

Blood count depression was the main toxic effect of this therapy. Table VII summarizes this toxicity in terms of nadir platelet and WBC counts and the percentage of the protocol-dictated drug doses actually administered that correlate with these nadirs. For the 15 patients receiving one complete cycle of therapy the median white cell and platelet counts were 3300 and 150,000/mm^3 respectively. The lowest WBC count was 600/mm^3 and the lowest platelet count was 25,000/mm^3, both in a patient who was receiving concurrent intrathecal methotrexate (this probably contributed to the toxicity). The number of patients treated decreased with subsequent cycles but no unexpected toxicity was evident. At this time, one patient has received 6 full cycles of therapy, and her most recent nadir WBC and

TABLE IV. Dose Modification of 5-FU, Adriamycin, and Mitomycin C

Platelet Count	WBC		
	>4000	3-4000	<3000
>100,000	100%	50%	0%
75-99,000	50%	50%	0%
<75,000	0%	0%	0%

TABLE V. Patient Characteristics

Patient	Age	Prior Rx	Site(s) of disease
1	40	CMF, RT, H	lung, soft tissue
2	44	CMF, I	lung
3	49	CMF, RT	soft tissue
4	36	CMF, RT	lung, soft tissue
5	68	L-PAM, RT, H	lung, bone, soft tissue
6	48	CMF, RT, H	pleura, soft tissue
7	58	CMF, RT	liver
8	58	CMF, RT	brain, bone, lung
9	57	CMF, RT	soft tissue
10	44	RT	meninges, soft tissue
11	54	RT, H	ascites, bone, soft tissue
12	71	RT, H	soft tissue, bone, pleura
13	45	RT	lung, pleura, bone
14	52	RT	bone
15	43	RT	soft tissue

RT = radiation therapy; H = hormonal therapy; I = immunotherapy.

platelet counts were 4500 and 108,000 respectively. The amount of chemotherapy administered was in excess of 80% of the doses designated by the protocol for the first 3 cycles.

Other toxic effects included alopecia in 15/15, nausea and vomiting in 9/15 patients (mild in 5, moderate to severe in 4), and mucositis in 4/15 patients (mod-

TABLE VI. Efficacy of FOAM Therapy

Patient	KPS	Response[a]	Site(s) of response	Duration of response (months)	Survival (months)
1	50	PROG	–	–	1.5*
2	50	CR	lung	12+	12+
3	80	PR	soft tissue	10+	10+
4	80	S	–	–	6.5+*
5	80	PR	lung soft tissue	6.5+	6.5+
6	80	PR	pleura	2	6+*
7	50	PR	liver	3.5+	3.5+
8	60	PR	lung	3.5+	3.5+
9	50	PROG	–	–	2+*
10	60	PR	soft tissue	2.5	5.5+*
11	80	PR	ascites soft tissue	3.5+	3.5+
12	70	S	–	–	2+
13	60	S	–	–	2+
14	70	S	–	–	2+
15	70	PR	soft tissue	1.5+	1.5+

[a] CR = complete response; PR = partial response; S = stable; PROG = progression
* = off study

TABLE VII. Hematotoxicity of FOAM Therapy

	Course			
	1	2	3	4
Number of patients treated	15	9	3[a]	3
Nadir platelet (x 1000/mm^3)				
Median	155	167	124.5	90
Range	25-269	57-270	5-174	66-322
Nadir WBC (x 1000/mm^3)				
Median	3.3	4.1	4.8	2.8
Range	0.6-5.8	2.0-5.0	2.7-6.9	2.2-6.4
Percentage of protocol-specified dose delivered				
5FU	82	71	83	73
Oncovin	97	89	102	102
Adriamycin	87	82	92	100
Mitomycin C	97	92	92	92

[a] Cycle 3 nadir counts not available for one patient.

erate in 3, severe in 1). Only one patient had severe leukopenia-associated infection. No renal, cardiac, or central nervous system toxicity was noted. In general, patients indicated that the side effects of this program were less severe than their previous CMF treatment.

V. DISCUSSION

This report summarizes our phase I-II study of patients with metastatic breast cancer treated with FOAM chemotherapy. These data are both preliminary and incomplete. More patients and longer periods of evaluation are necessary to reach definitive conclusions. Nevertheless, some preliminary assessments can be made:

1. This combination is reasonably well tolerated, even in patients previously treated with radiation therapy and chemotherapy. The primary toxicity of this chemotherapy is hematologic.
2. Objective regressions have been noted in patients with soft tissue, lung, and liver disease, and they have occurred even in those for whom previous CMF therapy has failed.

If these tentative conclusions are supported by further experience, we envision a phase III study in which the chemotherapies FOAM and CMF will be compared.

ACKNOWLEDGMENTS

The author acknowledges the assistance of Fred Marcus, Michael Cassidy, Robert Hammers, and Kenneth J. Resser in this study.

REFERENCES

Brambilla, C., DeLena, M., Rossi, A., Valagussa, P., and Bonadonna, G. (1976). *Brit. Med. J. 1,* 801-804.

Broder, L. E. and Tormey, D. C. (1974). *Cancer Treat. Rev. 1,* 183-203.

Cadman, E. C., Davis, L. K., and Heimer, R. (1978). *Clin. Res. 26,* 432A.

Macdonald, J., Schein, P., Uneno, W., and Wooley, P. (1976). *Proc. Amer. Assoc. Cancer Res. 17,* C-111.

Pouillant, P., Hoang, T., Brugerie, E., and Lheritier, J. (1974). *Biomed. 21,* 471.

Ullman, B. Lee, M., Martin, D. W., Jr., and Santi, D. V. (1978). *Proc. Nat. Acad. Sci. 75,* 980-983.

Wise, G. R., Kuhn, I. N., and Godfrey, T. E. (1976). *Med. Pediatr. Oncol. 2,* 55-60.

Chapter 13

CLINICAL STUDIES OF MITOMYCIN C IN ADVANCED ADENOCARCINOMA OF THE LUNG[1]

Michael K. Samson
Roberto J. Fraile
Lawrence P. Leichman
Laurence H. Baker

I. INTRODUCTION

Mitomycin C, an antitumor antibiotic isolated from *Streptomyces caespitosis,* has been used in clinical trials in the United States since 1958. Initial reports from Japanese investigators were encouraging, with an overall response rate of 37%, documented in a review by Frank and Osterberg (1960). Attempts to reproduce the Japanese experience in this country, following their daily dose schedule, led to serious, hematopoietic toxic side effects (Whittington and Close, 1970; Van Der Merwe *et al.,* 1971; and Hata *et al.,* 1961). Sokoloff *et al.* (1959) demonstrated in mice with Ehrlich ascites tumors a therapeutic advantage utilizing an intermittent schedule of mitomycin C. Since then, several studies in man utilizing the single-dose intermittent schedule have demonstrated therapeutic antitumor activity with apparently more predictable and managable hematopoietic toxicity (Baker *et al.,* 1974; Buroker *et al.,* 1978; and Baker *et al.,* 1976).

[1] Supported by a research grant from Bristol Laboratories, Syracuse, New York, and Contract NO 1-CM-67105 from the National Cancer Institute (NCI), NIH, DHEW.

Since 1976, two clinical studies employing mitomycin C alone and in combination with adriamycin and cyclophosphamide (MAC) have been completed, and form the substance of this report. The first effort was in collaboration with Dr. Robert Comis of the Upstate Medical Center, State University of New York, Syracuse, New York (Samson *et al.,* 1978) and the second with Dr. Robert Talley of Henry Ford Hospital, Detroit, Michigan.

II. MATERIALS AND METHODS

Eligibility requirements for both studies included histologic proof of adenocarcinoma of the lung confirmed by a referral pathologist, documented evidence of local incurability and/or the presence of metastatic disease. Other criteria for entry into these studies included the following: written consent as to the investigational nature of the study; a life expectancy of at least 8 weeks; no prior chemotherapy with mitomycin C, cyclophosphamide or adriamycin; measurable disease; and adequate hematopoietic reserve defined as $WBC > 4000/mm^3$, platelet count $> 100,000/mm^3$, a serum creatinine of $\leqslant 1.5$ mg/100ml, and BUN $\leqslant 25$ mg/100ml.

The following definitions were utilized in determining the effects of tumor therapy: Complete remission (CR) was defined as the disappearance of all clinical evidence of active tumor for a minimum of 4 weeks together with a disappearance of all tumor-related symptoms. Partial remission (PR) was defined as $> 50\%$ decrease in the sum of the products of the largest perpendicular diameters of all measured lesions lasting for at least 4 weeks in the absence of significant increase in any one lesion or the appearance of new lesions. Progressive disease was defined as unequivocal increase of any measured lesion or the appearance of new lesions.

III. RESULTS

A. Mitomycin as a Single Agent

Mitomycin C was given at an initial dose of 20 mg/m² by IV push into an established IV line and repeated in 6 weeks. Third and subsequent courses were reduced to 10 mg/m². Each treatment course was administered provided there was sufficient evidence of recovery from the nadir leukocyte and platelet counts observed with the previous course of therapy. Patients were evaluated while receiving therapy with serial CBCs, chest roentgenograms, liver and renal function tests, and tumor measurements.

Twenty evaluable patients (8 female and 12 male) whose median age was 56 (range 41-77 years) and median Karnofsky performance status was 60 (range 40-100) were entered in the study. There were five PRs for an overall response rate of 25%. Median survival for responders was 33 weeks, whereas survival for nonresponders was 9 weeks (Fig. 1). This difference was found to be statistically significant (p=0.02).

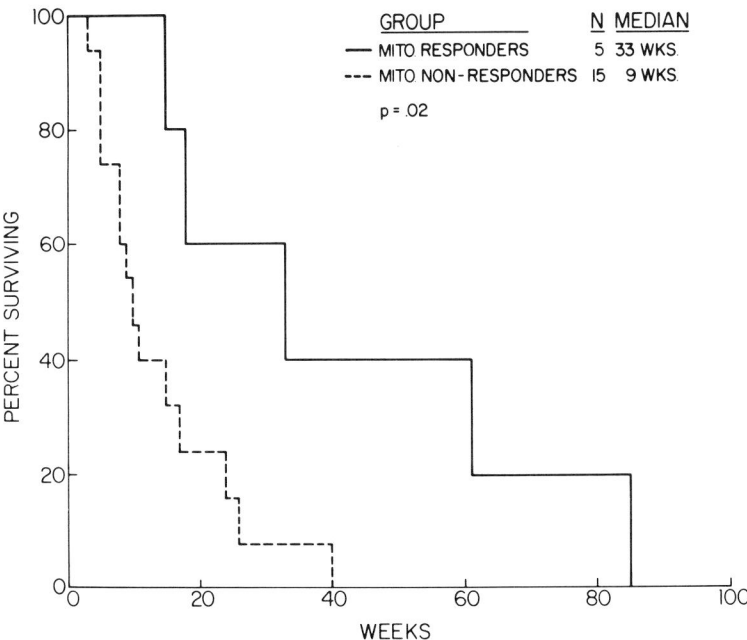

Fig. 1. Survival (weeks) of patients who received mitomycin C: responders versus nonresponders.

Nonhematologic toxicity could be evaluated in all 20 patients and consisted of nausea, vomiting, and diarrhea in 5% of patients. One patient developed alveolar fibrosis that may be attributed to mitomycin C since other etiologies were eliminated at postmortem examination. Renal toxicity was not observed.

Hematologic toxicity is outlined in Table I. Twenty-six percent of courses were associated with significant leukopenia (< 3000); 50% of courses had significant thrombocytopenia ($< 100,000$).

B. Mitomycin, Adriamycin and Cyclophosphamide (MAC) in Combination

In this study, mitomycin C was given at a dose of 7 mg/m^2 IV bolus and repeated every 6 weeks, constituting a course of therapy, while adriamycin and cyclophos-

TABLE I.   Hematologic Toxicity–Mitomycin C

Course	WBC Nadir (x 10^3 cells/mm^3)		Median Days To Nadir	Median Days To Recovery	Platelet Nadir (x 10^3 cells/mm^3)		Median Days To Nadir	Median Days To Recovery
1	Mean	4.6	16	29	Mean	122	16	28
	Median	4.3			Median	91		
	Range	(0.3-9.8)			Range	(14-257)		
2	Mean	4.5	19	21	Mean	120	14	28
	Median	4.9			Median	105		
	Range	(2.1-6.6)			Range	(29-255)		

phamide were administered IV bolus at doses of 40 mg/m^2 and 400 mg/m^2, respectively, and repeated every 3 weeks. Follow-up examinations were similar to the previously mentioned mitomycin study.

Twenty-eight evaluable patients (13 female and 15 male) with a median age of 60 (range 40-77 years) and a median Karnofsky performance of 75 (range 35-90) were entered into the study. Seven PRs were observed for an overall response rate of 25%. Median survival for responding patients was at least 39 weeks, while median survival for nonresponding patients was 17 weeks (Fig. 2). This difference was found to be statistically significant (p = 0.004).

Nonhematologic toxicity consisted of nausea and vomiting (45%) and stomatitis (3%). Alopecian was reported in 60% of patients. Renal, pulmonary, or cardiac toxicity were not noted in this group of patients.

Table II enumerates the hematologic toxicity observed through four courses of chemotherapy with MAC. No cumulative myelosuppression was noted, nor was there any significant delay in administering subsequent courses of therapy. Significant leukopenia ($<$ 3000) was observed in 18% of courses, but in contrast to the mitomycin study only in 3% of courses were platelets noted to fall below 100,000. This is clearly the result of the reduced dose of mitomycin in the three-drug combination.

Metastatic sites in responding patients in both studies included both soft tissue and visceral organs and are shown in Table III.

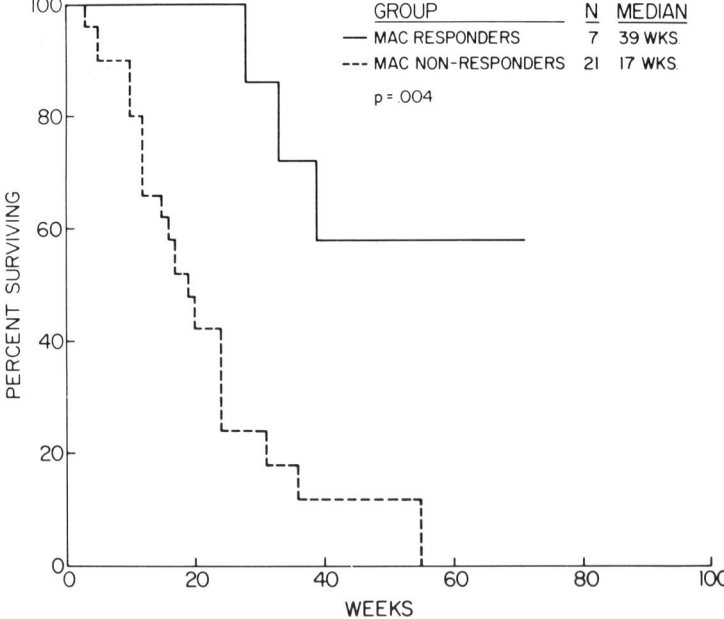

Fig. 2. Survival (weeks) of patients who received MAC: responders versus nonresponders.

TABLE II.   Hematologic Toxicity–MAC

Course	WBC Nadir (x 10 cells/mm)		Median Days To		Platelet Nadir (x 10 cells/mm)		Median Days To	
			Nadir	Recovery			Nadir	Recovery
1	Mean	4.7	14	23	Mean	275	20	22
	Median	4.0			Median	266		
	Range	(1.9-17.3)			Range	(87-436)		
2	Mean	6.2	15	23	Mean	295	–	–
	Median	4.9			Median	310		
	Range	(1.6-18.6)			Range	(115-550)		
3	Mean	7.0	13	, 23	Mean	213	–	–
	Median	4.6			Median	214		
	Range	(1.9-22.2)			Range	(95-406)		
4	Mean	4.5	8	18	Mean	220	14	21
	Median	3.9			Median	230		
	Range	(1.4-7.9)			Range	(82-333)		

IV. DISCUSSION

Although these two studies were conducted sequentially and not in a randomized prospective fashion, we attempted to evaluate the comparability of both patient populations in terms of several prognostic factors known to have significance in lung cancer. For sex, prior or concurrent radiation therapy, prior chemotherapy, disease-free interval, and age and performance status, no statistical differences were found. However, there were three significant differences in the two patient populations:

1. There were more nonwhite patients entered in the MAC study.
2. More patients on the MAC study had undergone "curative" lung resections, and
3. A higher percentage of patients on the mitomycin study had extra-pulmonary metastatic disease.

However, in spite of the aforementioned differences, we feel that these two treatment groups are comparable.

The mitomycin study demonstrates the activity of this drug in adenocarcinoma of the lung. However, as has been shown in previous studies with mitomycin C in solid tumors, the duration of response was brief. In addition, cumulative hematologic toxicity, although not a factor in our studies, clearly limits prolonged administration of the drug. Adriamycin and cyclophosphamide have both been shown

TABLE III.   Metastatic Sites in Responding Patients[a]

	Lymph Nodes	Lung	Bone	Liver	Skin
Mitomycin C	3	1	2	1	1
MAC	2	3	1	2	2

[a] Most patients had multiple sites of metastases.

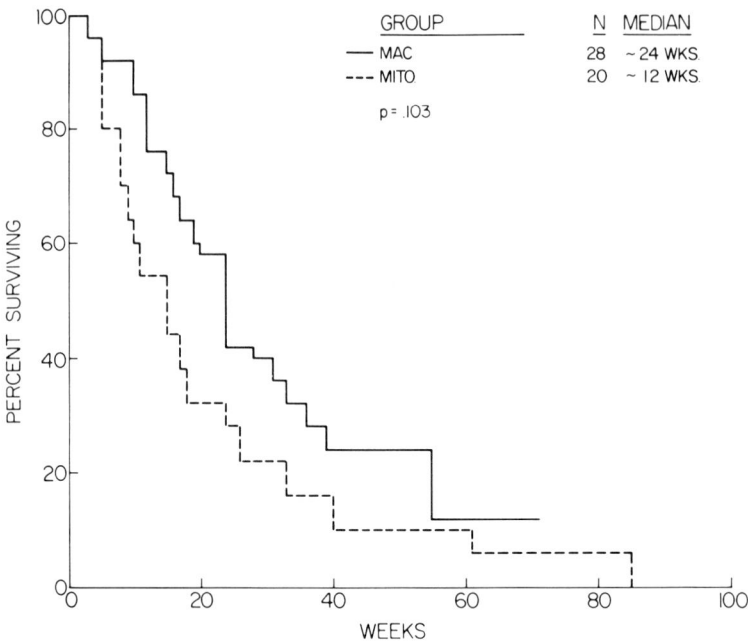

Fig. 3. Survival (weeks) of all patients who received MAC versus those who received mitomycin C.

to have activity in adenocarcinoma of the lung (Selawry, 1976). We had hoped that by combining these two agents with mitomycin C the response rate, response duration, and survival could be significantly enhanced. While the response rates for both studies were identical (25%), the median duration of response (6 weeks for mitomycin C, 14 weeks for MAC) and overall survival for responding patients (33 weeks for mitomycin C, 39 weeks for MAC) appear to favor the three-drug combination, but they fell short of reaching statistical significance. Both studies were able to show a significant survival advantage of responding patients over nonresponding patients; however, median survival of all patients did not differ (Fig. 3).

In the past, squamous cell carcinoma has been regarded as the more prevalent type of lung cancer in the United States (Cliffton and Luomanen, 1968). A recent study, however, has shown that the incidence of adenocarcinomas is rising, and if current trends continue this may become the predominant cell type (Vincent *et al.,* 1977). The therapeutic implications are obvious—new, active tumorcidal agents are urgently needed. Once these agents are found, they then can be incorporated into drug combination programs with other active agents, one of which is mitomycin C.

REFERENCES

Baker, L. H., Caoili, F. M., Izbicki, R. M., Opipari, M. I., and Vaitkevicius, V. K. (1974). *Proc. AACR and ASCO 15,* 182.

Baker, L. H., Izbicki, R. M., and Vaitkevicius, V. K. (1976). *Med. Pediatr. Oncol. 2,* 207-212.

Buroker, R. R., Kim, P. N., Baker, L. H., Ratanatharathorn, V., Woitaszak, B., and Vaitkevicius, V. K. (1978). *Med. Pediatr. Oncol. 4*, 35-42.

Cliffton, E. E., and Luomanen, K. J. (1968). *In* "Lung Cancer" (W. L. Watson, ed.), p. 376. C. V. Mosby, St. Louis, Mo.

Frank, W., and Osterberg, A. E. (1960). *Cancer Chemother. Rep. 9*, 114-119.

Hata, T., Hassenlopp, C., and Takita, H. (1961). *Cancer Chemother. Rep. 13*, 67-77.

Samson, M. K., Comis, R. L., Baker, L. H., Ginsberg, S., and Crooke, S. T. (1978). *Cancer Treat. Rep. 62*, 163-165.

Selawry, O. S. 1976). *Semin. Oncol. 1*, 259-272.

Sokoloff, B., Nakabayashi, K., Enomoto, K., Miller, T. R., Bicknell, A., Bird, L., Travner, W., Niswonger, J., Renningar, G. (1959). *Growth 23*, 1-27.

Van Der Merwe, A. M., Falkson, G., and Falkson, H. C. (1971). *Med. Proc. 17*, 90-92.

Vincent, R. G., Peckren, J. W., Lane, W. W., Bross, I., Takita, H., Houten, L., Gutierrez, A. C., and Rzepka, T. (1977). *Cancer 39*, 1647-1655.

Whittington, R. M., and Close, H. P. (1970). *Cancer Chemother. Rep. 54*, 195-198.

Chapter 14

MITOMYCIN C IN GASTRIC CANCER

Robert L. Comis

I. INTRODUCTION

Mitomycin C was first noted to have antitumor activity against gastric cancer in early Japanese clinical trials (Frank and Osterberg, 1960). During the 20 years of evaluation in the United States, the activity of mitomycin C against gastric cancer has been confirmed. Mitomycin C has been the second most commonly employed single agent in American clinical trials. Clinical evaluations in over 100 patients have shown a 25% objective response rate (29/116) when mitomycin C was employed as a single agent (Comis and Carter, 1974). The data from several studies spanning the two decades of evaluation indicate a consistent 20-30% response rate in patients with metastatic gastric cancer (Table I, Table II). Although mitomycin has consistently induced objective tumor regressions, the durations of remission have been uniformly short. The average remission duration ranges from 1 to 3 months.

Initial enthusiasm for mitomycin C waned because of the severe, cumulative myelotoxicity encountered when the drug was administered on a daily or every other day schedule until myelotoxicity developed. After the cumulative nature of the myelotoxicity was appreciated, manipulation of the schedule of drug administration led to more manageable toxicity without attenuation of antitumor effects (Baker *et al.*, 1976).

Only four chemotherapeutic agents, or classes of agents, have been adequately evaluated in metastatic gastric cancer. In addition to mitomycin C, these drugs

TABLE I. Mitomycin C in Gastric Cancer: Historical Perspective

Year of report	Investigators	No. patients	Objective response (%)
1959	Frank and Osterberg (1960)	113	35
1966	Manheimer and Vitale (1966)	14	21
1968	Moore et al. (1968)	16	31
1974	Moertel (1974)	12	27
1978	Buroker et al. (1978)	18	28

include 5-fluorouracil, adriamycin, and the nitrosoureas. Of the latter class of compounds 1, 3-bis-(2-chloroethyl-1-nitroso) urea (BCNU) appears to be most active. Each agent yields about a 20-25% objective response rate. As with mitomycin C, the duration of response to these other agents is relatively short, ranging from 3 to 4 months.

Prior to the disease-oriented execution and analysis of clinical trials, it was not generally appreciated that gastric cancer was a potentially chemotherapy-responsive disease. Drugs that were found to be inactive in colonic cancer, the disease most frequently represented in drug-oriented studies in gastrointestinal cancer, were assumed to be inactive in gastric cancer. A good illustration of the confusion caused by combining chemotherapy data on all gastrointestinal cancers is available from a randomized prospective trial of single-agent versus combination chemotherapy in gastrointestinal cancer performed by Reitemeier et al. (1970). The data presented in Table III are an adaptation of those presented in the study.

II. MATERIALS AND METHODS

Patients were randomly assigned to treatment with either 5-fluorouracil, mitomycin C, BCNU, or two- and three-drug combinations including the single agents. When all gastrointestinal cancers were considered, the objective response rates to the single agents versus the combinations showed no evidence that combination chemotherapy was superior to single-agent treatment. When the data were analyzed for single-agent versus combination chemotherapy response in the three major gastrointestinal cancers, there was some indication that gastric cancer was more re-

TABLE II. Objective Response Rates for Various Single Agents

Drug	Reference	Response rate (%)
5-fluorouracil	Comis and Carter (1974)	23
Mitomycin C	Comis and Carter (1974)	25
Adriamycin	Moertel (1975)	26
BCNU	Comis and Carter (1974)	18
CCNU	Comis and Carter (1974)	3
MeCCNU	Comis and Carter (1974); Moertel et al. (1976)	7

TABLE III.   Studies with 5-FU, Mitomycin, BCNU:
Alone or in Combination

	Gastrointestinal Cancer	
	No. treated	% Response
Single agents	88	19-23
Combinations	126	13-20
	Gastric Cancer	
Single agents	10	20
Combinations	16	50

sponsive to combination chemotherapy than it was to single-agent treatment. The possible advantage of combination chemotherapy was not evident for pancreatic or colon carcinomas. Fortunately, the data were analyzed for the major subtypes of gastrointestinal malignancy in this report leading to subsequent controlled evaluations of combination chemotherapy in metastatic gastric cancer.

III.   RESULTS

Subsequently, controlled evaluations have shown a superiority for combination chemotherapy over single-agent chemotherapy in gastric cancer. Kovach *et al.* (1974) showed that the objective response rate for the combination of 5-fluorouracil and BCNU was superior to that obtained with 5-fluorouracil used as a single agent, 41% versus 29%, respectively. More importantly, there was a significant increase in 18-month survival for the combination compared to single-agent treatment, 25% versus 7%, respectively. In an Eastern Cooperative Oncology Group study, Moertel *et al.* (1976) showed a statistically significant increase in objective response rate for the combination of methyl-CCNU and 5-fluorouracil over methyl-CCNU *alone.* Buroker *et al.* (1978) reported a controlled evaluation of single-agent mitomycin C versus the combination of mitomycin C and 5-fluorouracil. The objective response rate for the combination was 48% versus 28% for the single agent, but no statistically significant difference in survival or response duration was reported. In addition, a recent combined modality study has indicated that combination chemotherapy was superior to combined modality therapy including chemotherapy plus radiation in patients with locally advanced unresectable gastric cancer having measurable and nonmeasurable disease (Schein and Childs, 1978). Thus it appears from most studies that combination chemotherapy has a definite role in the treatment of gastric cancer. Furthermore, mitomycin C is an integral part of the more recent FAM combination which has been reported to yield a greater than 50% objective response rate in patients with metastatic gastric cancer (Macdonald *et al.*, 1976). The FAM regimen is currently being intensively evaluated in controlled clinical trials.

IV. DISCUSSION

In summary, mitomycin C is an effective agent in inducing objective response in metastatic gastric cancer. The usefulness of the drug employed as a single agent is limited because of the short duration or remissions and cumulative bone marrow toxicity. Its more important role appears to be in the development of effective combination chemotherapy programs.

REFERENCES

Baker, L. H., Izbicki, R. M. and Vaikevicius, V. K. (1976). *Med. Pediatr. Oncol. 2,* 207-213.

Buroker, T. R., Kim, P. N., Baker, L. H., Ratanatharathorn, V., Wajtaszak, B., and Vaitkevicius, V. K. (1978). *Med. Pediatr. Oncol. 4,* 35-42.

Comis, R. L., and Carter, S. K. (1974). *Cancer 34,* 1576-1586.

Frank, W., and Osterberg, A. E. (1960). *Cancer Chemother. Rep. 9,* 114-119.

Kovach, J. S., Moertel, C. G., Schutt, A. J., Hahn, R. G., and Reitemeier, R. J. (1974). *Cancer 33,* 563-567.

Macdonald, J., Schein, P., Uneo, W., and Wooley, P. (1976). *Proc. Amer. Soc. Clin. Oncol. 17,* 264.

Manheimer, L. H. and Vitale, J. (1966). *Cancer 19,* 207-212.

Moertel, C. G. (1974). *JAMA 228,* 1290-1291.

Moertel, C. G. (1975). *Cancer 36,* 675-682.

Moertel, C. G., Mittleman, J. A. Bakemeier, R. F., Engstrom, R., and Hanley, J. (1976). *Cancer 38,* 678-682.

Moore, G. E., Bross, L. D., Ausman, R., Nadler, S., Jones, R., Slack, N., and Rimm, A. A. (1968). *Cancer Chemother. Rep. 52,* 675-684.

Reitemeier, R. J., Moertel, C. G., and Hahn, R. G. (1970). *Cancer Res. 30,* 1425-1428.

Schein, P. S. and Childs, D. (1978). *Proc. Amer. Soc. Clin. Oncol. 19,* 329.

Chapter 15

THE FAM (5-FLUOROURACIL, ADRIAMYCIN, MITOMYCIN C) AND SMF (STREPTOZOTOCIN, MITOMYCIN C, 5-FLUOROURACIL) CHEMOTHERAPY REGIMENS[1]

Philip S. Schein
Jack S. Macdonald
Daniel F. Hoth
Paul V. Woolley

I. INTRODUCTION

Since 1974 a series of phase II trials of new combination chemotherapy regimens have been conducted at the Vincent T. Lombardi Cancer Research Center, with specific emphasis on adenocarcinomas of the upper gastrointestinal tract and lung. The chemotherapy programs were developed using anticancer agents that have undergone an adequate clinical trial as single agents and have demonstrated reproducible activity in patients with advanced measurable disease. The principal regimens tested, the FAM and SMF combinations, were specifically developed for patients with advanced gastric and pancreatic cancer, respectively. A major consideration in the design of these regimens was patient tolerance. They were to be used as outpatient treatment, while preserving the patient's overall quality of life. In 1974 the combinations incorporated several innovations in therapy: (*a*) mitomycin C was

[1] Supported by NIH-NCI NO1-CM 67110.

administered in a single-dose schedule every 2 months in recognition of the delayed onset of myelosuppression produced by this agent. Baker and co-workers had described activity in upper gastrointestinal cancer, with acceptable hematologic toxicity, using a similar regimen of 20 mg/m² every 6-8 weeks (Baker *et al.*, 1974); (*b*) adriamycin was employed in the FAM combination after it became apparent in early phase II trials that this drug had important antitumor activity in gastric cancer. Adriamycin has since been demonstrated to produce objective responses in patients with advanced measurable pancreatic cancer (Gastrointestinal Tumor Study Group, 1978); (*c*) streptozotocin, an agent that has been used extensively in the management of pancreatic islet cell carcinoma, has also been reported to have activity for adenocarcinoma of the same organ (Ratanatharathorn *et al.*, 1977). This drug was employed in the SMF regimen for pancreatic cancer.

II. MATERIALS AND METHODS

The FAM regimen was administered in 8-week cycles (Table I) (Macdonald *et al.*, in press). 5-FU was administered at a dose of 600 mg/m² intravenously on days 1, 8, 29, and 36. Adriamycin was administered intravenously at a dose of 30 mg/m² on days 1 and 29; and mitomycin C, 10 mg/m², was administered on day 1 only of each course. Drug dosage was modified for subsequent courses according to the degree of hematologic toxicity as measured by white blood cell and platelet counts (Table II). Blood counts were obtained weekly during the first cycle of chemotherapy and in subsequent courses immediately prior to each treatment. Since the nadir of hematologic toxicity produced by mitomycin C occurs 4-5 weeks after administration, blood counts measured at this time period were used to adjust the dosage of this agent for the subsequent cycle.

SMF was administered in 8-week cycles (Table III) (Wiggans *et al.*, 1978). Streptozotocin was administered at a dosage of 1 gm/m² IV on week 1 only. The cycle was repeated on week 9. Streptozotocin was discontinued for the following conditions: protein-urea > 1 gm/24 hr, renal glycosuria, renal tubular acidosis, Fanconi's syndrome, elevation of serum creatinine above 2 mg/100 ml, or decrease in creatinine clearance to less than 70 ml/min. Streptozotocin was resumed at a dosage of 0.5 gm/m² per treatment only if there was a complete return of renal function to pretreatment values. Dosage modifications of 5-FU and mitomycin C were based on nadir WBC and platelet counts (Table III).

TABLE I.   The FAM Combination Chemotherapy Regimen

Drug	Dose	Time (weeks)								
		1	2	3	4	5	6	7	8	9
5-fluorouracil	600 mg/m² IV	X	X			X	X			X
Adriamycin	30 mg/m² IV	X				X				X
Mitomycin C	10 mg/m² IV	X								X

TABLE II. Dose Attentuation Schedule for Bone Marrow
Depression Based upon Nadir WBC and Platelet Counts

Drug/dose (%)	WBC/mm^3	Platelets/mm^3
100	3500	100,000
75	2500-3499	75,000-99,999
50	1500-2500	25,000-75,000

All patients had biopsy-proven adenocarcinoma, and unless otherwise specified, none had previously been treated with chemotherapy or radiation therapy. The performance status of each case was assessed at the time of entry into this study using the Eastern Cooperative Oncology Group system. To be eligible for this program the patient must have had a lesion measurable by palpation and x ray or radionuclide scan in order to assess the effectiveness of therapy. Liver scans were employed provided that they demonstrated a clearly defined perfusion defect of > 3 cm. Malignant hepatomegaly was used as an indicator lesion if the liver contained proven metastases and was enlarged to at least 5 cm below the xyphoid or costal margins.

Patients were evaluated for response using the following system: A partial response (PR) was defined as a 50% or greater decrease in the products of the two largest perpendicular diameters of the most clearly measurable lesion, without increase in the size of other known areas of malignant disease. This result must have been observed at a minimum of 4 weeks after initiation of treatment. If hepatomegaly was followed, there must have been a decrease of at least 30% in the sum of measurements below the xyphoid process and both costal margins at the midclavicular line, with improvement or stability of pretreatment liver function tests. If, at the end of an 8-week cycle, patients demonstrated disease progression they were defined as nonresponders (NR), and alternate therapy was initiated. Duration of response and survival were measured from the start of therapy. The data was analyzed by the life table method (Hill, 1961) and survival times were compared using the Mann-Whitley U Test (Zar, 1974).

III. RESULTS

A. FAM Chemotherapy for Advanced Gastric Cancer
(Macdonald et al., in press)

Thirty-six consecutive patients with advanced gastric cancer were admitted to this study between September 1974 and September 1977. The ages ranged from 49

TABLE III. The SMF Combination Chemotherapy Regimen

Drug	Dose	Time (weeks)								
		1	2	3	4	5	6	7	8	9
Streptozotocin	1 gm/m^2 IV	X	X			X	X			Repeat
Mitomycin C	10 mg/m^2 IV	X								cycle at
5-fluorouracil	600 mg/m^2 IV	X	X			X	X			ninth week

to 62 years. Fourteen of the 36 patients (39%) were fully ambulatory, and 11 were bedridden for greater than 50% of the time. The following sites constituted the measurable lesions for the 36 patients: liver, 17/36 (47%); abdominal mass, 15/36 (42%); osseous metastases, 1/36 (3%); and malignant lymph node masses 3/36 (8%). In 5/17 patients with followable liver disease, radionuclide scan was used as the measurable parameter; in the remaining 12 patients, measurable hepatomegaly was followed. A single pathologist who had no prior knowledge of clinical response reviewed the grade of differentiation in 31 cases. The majority of cases (18) were poorly differentiated, and only 3 patients had well-differentiated neoplasms.

Eighteen of 36 patients (50%) achieved a partial remission. The median duration of response was 9.5 months (range 2-19.5 months). The median duration of survival in responding patients was 13.5 months; 2 patients remain alive and in remission at 14.5 and 26 months after initiation of therapy. All responding patients except for one were treated until there was evidence of progression of disease on chemotherapy. The remaining case was noted to have significant resolution of an unresectable gastric mass after 9 months of treatment, and subsequently underwent an abdominal exploration. At that time, there was marked reduction in the size of the primary gastric tumor, and a subtotal gastric resection was performed with removal of all visible disease. Of the 18 patients who did not respond to FAM, all are dead, and their median survival is 3.0 months (range 0.5-6.0 months) from the initiation of therapy. The difference in survival time between the responding and nonresponding patients is statistically significant ($p = 0.001$) and is presented in Fig. 1.

An analysis of possible prognostic variables including initial performance status, resectability of the primary gastric tumor, and histologic differentiation of the neoplasm failed to account for the observed differences in patient response and survival. The activity of the FAM regimen for advanced gastric cancer has now been confirmed in many centers, including studies conducted by Prof. Lagarde of the Fondation Bergonie, Bordeaux, and Prof. Boiron of the Hospital St. Louis, Paris, under the auspices of the French-American Agreement on Cancer Research. A similar regimen, FAM, developed by the Gastrointestinal Tumor Study Group, has produced a survival significantly better than 5-FU plus methyl-CCNU, in a randomized controlled trial.

B. FAM Chemotherapy for Advanced Colorectal Cancer
(Macdonald *et al.*, 1976)

Thirty-five consecutive patients with histologically proven colorectal adenocarcinoma were entered into this study. The clinical data for these patients are as follows: The patients ranged in age from 39 to 76 years (median 58 years) and all were ambulatory with a median ECOG performance status of 1 (range 0-3). Fifteen of these patients had failed prior chemotherapy or radiotherapy regimens. Fourteen had been treated with 5-FU, methyl-CCNU, and vincristine and one

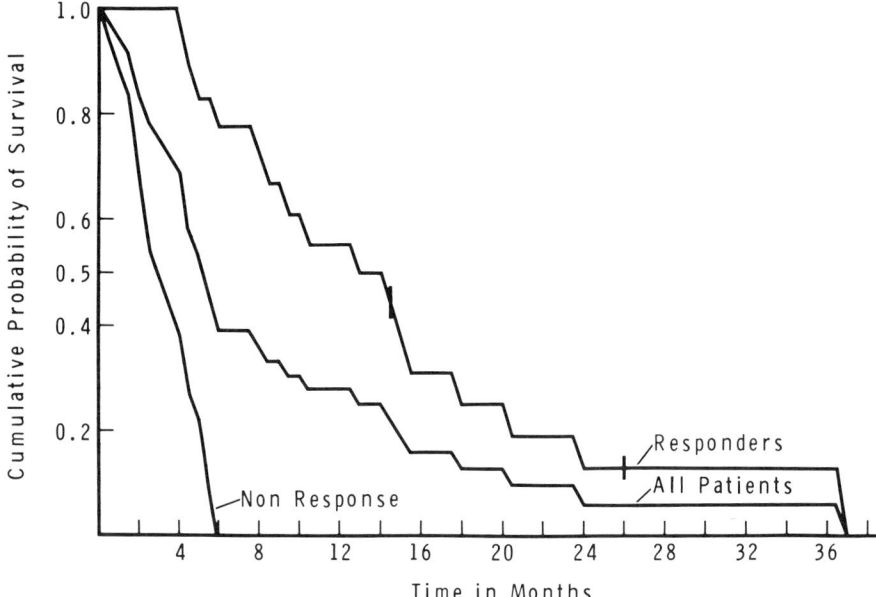

Fig. 1. Life-table analysis of survival for patients with advanced gastric cancer treated with the FAM regimen.

with weekly 5-FU. Two additional patients had received radiation therapy to mass lesions in the abdomen. All patients had disease that was readily measured by physical examination and x rays or radionuclide scans prior to beginning therapy.

Partial responses were observed in 6 of 35 patients (17%) treated with FAM chemotherapy, including 2 patients who had failed prior chemotherapy. Regression of hepatic lesions was documented in two patients by the use of radioisotope scans, computerized tomography, and ultrasonography. Two patients demonstrated responses in abdominal masses, whereas pulmonary nodules and malignant hepatomegaly were the followable lesions in two remaining patients. The median duration of response was 4.5+ months (range 3+-12+ months). The median survival for the responding group was 5.5+ months (range 3+-13+ months), and 4 patients are alive in continued response.

Seven patients (20%) demonstrated stabilization of disease with a duration of 7 months (range 3-9 months). The median survival for this group was 9+ months (range 4+-14 months) with 4 patients alive. The median survival for the 22 nonresponding patients is 6.5+ months but will not be greater than 8 months. Performance status did no significantly effect the likelihood of response since 16 of 22 nonresponding patients had performance scores of 0 or 1. It is obvious that FAM combination chemotherapy did not significantly improve survival in responding patients, nor was it more effective than 5-FU alone in achieving objective regression of disease.

C. SMF Chemotherapy for Advanced Pancreatic Cancer

Ten of 23 patients (43%) have achieved a CR (one case) or a PR. The median duration of response is in excess of 6 months, with 4 patients alive and in remission at 7+, 7.5+, 15+, and 23+ months. Of the nonresponders, there is one patient alive 4+ months from diagnosis. The median survival of all cases from time of diagnosis is 6 months. Those patients who showed an objective response have a median survival in excess of 7.5 months (range 3-23 months), (Fig. 2) as compared to 3 months (range 1-6.5 months) for those with disease progression ($p < 0.01$). Five of 23 patients (22%) showed disease stabilization. The median duration of this stabilization was 5 months (range 3-6 months) and the median survival for this subgroup was 9 months (range 5.5-15 months).

No significant differences were demonstrated when the responders and nonresponders were compared with respect to initial performance status and site of disease. Two of the 3 patients with an initial status of 3 or 4 responded, and the median of the responding group was 1 as compared to 1.5 for those with progressive disease. Patients with metastatic liver disease demonstrated a higher response rate (4/6, 67%) than patients in whom an abdominal mass was the followable parameter (6/17, 35%). The survival results of the SMF program are similar to those of Kovach, *et al.* (1974), a 6-month median. While the patient populations in the present SMF study and in the study by Kovach *et al.* are composed of advanced metastatic cases, these two series differ in an important respect. In the latter study, 40% of cases were presumptively diagnosed as pancreatic in origin based on histology and negative barium contrast studies, whereas all but one patient of the SMF series were confirmed at surgery. Although the objective response rate with SMF is higher than that reported for 5-FU + BCNU, 33%, it is apparent that SMF has not made any appreciable impact on survival for the majority of patients. Nevertheless, the results clearly demonstrate that clinically useful and durable remissions can be achieved for a small subgroup treated with a well-tolerated form of chemotherapy. The SMF regimen using loading course and weekly administration of 5-FU is now being tested by the Gastrointestinal Tumor Study Group.

D. FAM Chemotherapy for Advanced Pancreatic Cancer

Following the demonstration that adriamycin had activity for advanced pancreatic cancer when used as a single agent, this drug was substituted for streptozotocin. This program has been active at the Lombardi Center for only the past 15 months. Twenty-five patients with advanced measurable disease have been treated; ten (40%) have achieved a partial response. In addition, 2 cases evidenced an apparent stabilization of their disease. The median duration of response is 8 months, with a range of 3+ to 13 months. The median survival of the responding group is in excess of 9 months (3+ to 14+), in contrast to a 3-month median for nonresponders ($p < 0.01$).

Based upon these early results this program has now been accepted for further

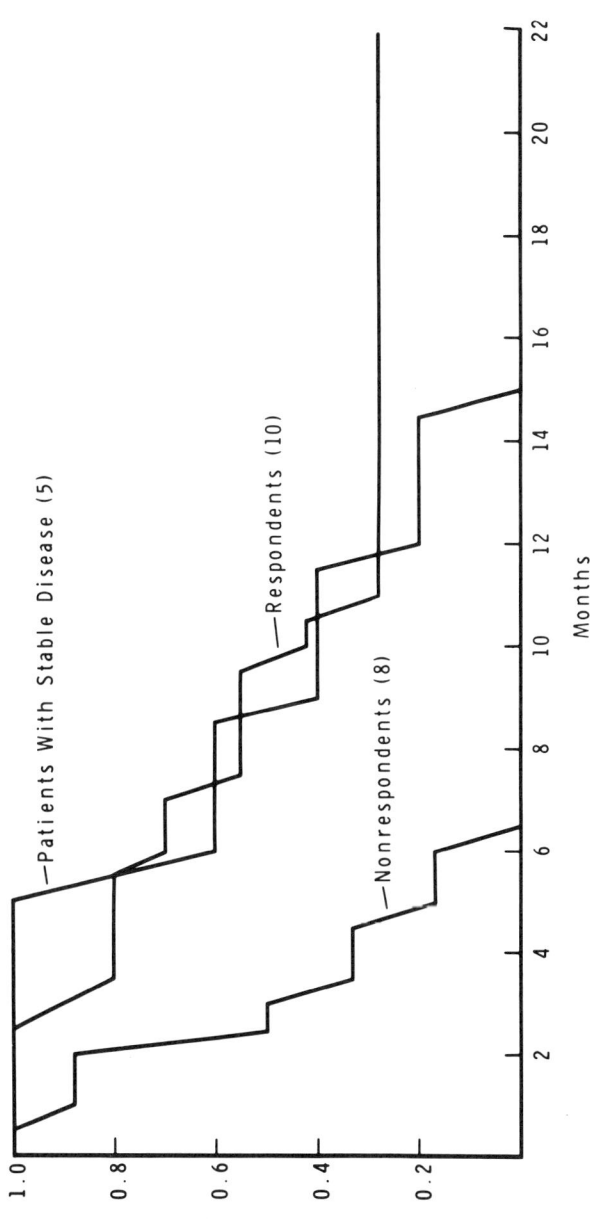

Fig. 2. Life-table analysis of survival for patients with advanced pancreatic cancer treated with the SMF regimen.

clinical trial by the Gastrointestinal Tumor Study Group and the Cancer and Acute Leukemia Group B.

E. FAM Chemotherapy for Adenocarcinoma of the Lung

Between October 1975 and April 1977, 25 patients (14 men and 11 women) with histologically confirmed unresectable and measurable adenocarcinoma of the lung were entered in the phase III protocol. All patients were ambulatory with performance 0-3. No patients had received prior chemotherapy. Four patients had undergone surgery for their original tumor and were to receive chemotherapy for recurrent tumor. Six patients had received radiation therapy to unresectable pulmonary tumors prior to chemotherapy, and three others began radiation therapy concomitantly with the institution of chemotherapy. Irradiated areas were not regarded as evaluable for response.

Nine of 25 patients (36%) treated with FAM had an objective response (one CR, 8 PR) with a median response duration of 7.0 months.

The one CR remains disease-free at 23.5 months, and 4 PRs remain alive (2 in remission, 2 with progressive disease) 5.5-13 months after initiation of therapy. Four patients (16%) had stabilization of disease, and 3 of the 4 remain alive at 10,18.5, and 23 months after the initiation of therapy. Twelve of 25 patients (48%) evidenced progressive disease and had a median survival of 2.5 months; no patient lived longer than 7 months. Survival curves are shown in Fig. 3. Median survival for the entire series is 6.5 months, whereas the projected median survival for responders is 11.5 months. Survival is significantly longer for objective responders (CR + PR) than for patients with progressive disease (PD), $p < 0.001$. Four patients died of progressive cancer before receiving their first full course of FAM and are included in the PD group (Butler *et al.*, in press).

F. Clinical Toxicity

A major consideration in the design of the FAM regimen was patient tolerance. Many patients with advanced stages of gastrointestinal cancer are already debilitated by the cachexia syndrome that is frequently associated with malignant disease. In contrast to nitrosourea-containing drug regimens, there was little acute gastrointestinal toxicity with the FAM regimen, and when observed it was readily controlled with phenothiazine antiemetics in almost all instances. The use of streptozotocin in SMF did result in nausea and/or vomiting in the majority of patients. While there were no instances of renal toxicity associated with FAM, the SMF regimen did produce definite nephrotoxocity in 30% of cases. Streptozotocin is a known nephrotoxin (Schein *et al.*, 1974), and mitomycin C at higher doses (20-40 mg/m^2 intravenously every 4-8 weeks) than employed in the SMF regimen has been reported to cause glomerular damage with proteinuria and azotemia in 3 of 32 patients (Liu *et al.*, 1971). In all three cases renal insufficiency progressed after

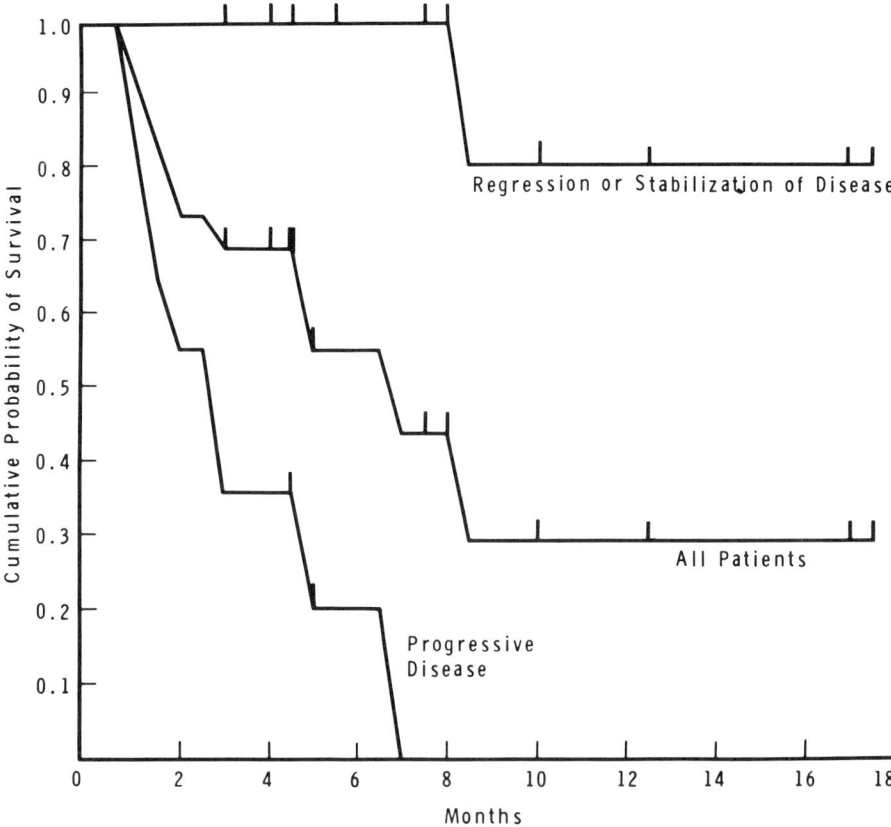

Fig. 3. Life-table analysis of survival for patients with adenocarcinoma of the lung treated with the FAM regimen.

mitomycin C was discontinued. Mitomycin C nephrotoxicity has been evaluated by Ratanatharathorn *et al.* (1977). When mitomycin C was administered at a dosage of 20 mg/m^2 intravenously every 6-8 weeks, no significant clinical nephrotoxicity was observed. Seven of 23 patients treated with SMF developed 1+ or greater proteinuria, which quantitatively did not exceed 1.25 gm in 24 hr. One additional patient, not a diabetic, developed glucosuria with a blood glucose of 200 mg% after a total dose of 24 gm of streptozotocin. Two of 23 cases (9%) developed renal impairment with BUN concentrations of 25 and 48 mg/ml, and serum creatinines of 2.7 and 4.8 mg/ 100 ml. The total doses of streptozotocin in these cases were 24 and 17 gm respectively. In both instances of azotemic nephrotoxicity no other etiology was documented, and renal function stabilized at the reduced level of function after streptozotocin alone was omitted from the regimen. It was because of these instances of streptozotocin gastrointestinal and renal toxicity that adriamycin has been substituted for patients with pancreatic cancer, following the demonstration that the latter agent was active in this disease.

There have been no serious treatment-associated complications resulting from hematologic toxicity with the FAM regimen. The use of an intermittent schedule of mitomycin C has largely avoided the past problem of cumulative bone marrow depression, and has allowed for continued treatment at 70-80% of projected doses after 1 year of therapy. This is an important feature of any drug combination developed for patients with advanced gastrointestinal or pulmonary tumors, since effective remission maintenance therapy must be continued for an indefinite period. All too often, an initially tolerated intensive regimen leaves the patient with little bone marrow reserve. The data obtained from the treatment of patients with advanced gastric cancer are representative of the hematologic toxicity of the FAM combination. The median WBC nadir in the group was $2600/mm^3$, and median platelet nadir was greater than $100,000/mm^3$, with a range of 13,000-825,000. The nadirs of white blood cell and platelet depression occurred during the fifth week of each treatment cycle in 90% of patients. There were no instances of leukopenia-related sepsis or thrombocytopenia hemorrhage. After 12 months of treatment, patients continued to tolerate 11% of the originally projected drug doses based upon body surface area. It should also be noted that the dose of adriamycin employed with each 8-week course of FAM is 60 mg/m^2, with a total dose of 360 mg/m^2 after 1 year of therapy. Therefore, it should be exceedingly uncommon to encounter cardiac toxicity related to this agent unless the patient received prior mediastinal irradiation.

IV. DISCUSSION

We are encouraged with the initial results achieved in these phase II trials of FAM chemotherapy in gastric and pancreatic cancer and adenocarcinoma of the lung, as well as with the low order of toxicity. In particular, the 50% response rate and the 9.5 month duration of remission observed in patients with advanced measurable stomach cancer are equivalent to previously reported phase II results for effective combination chemotherapy of advanced breast cancer. Although our data also suggest that objective response is associated with prolongation of survival, it is important to emphasize that the only appropriate manner in which to evaluate potential survival benefits for chemotherapy regimens is through prospectively randomized phase III trials, which are now being conducted in cooperative group studies. Surgical adjuvant trials for resected gastric cancer are being planned. In our current studies, we are incorporating a new nitrosourea, chlorozotocin, into the FAM combination in an attempt to improve the efficacy of this regimen.

REFERENCES

Baker, L. H., Caoili, E. M., Izbicki, R. M., Opipari, M. I., and Vaitkevicius, V. K. (1974). *Proc. Am. Soc. Clin. Oncol. 15,* 182.

Butler, T. P., Macdonald, J. S., Smith, E. P., Smith, L. F., Woolley, P. V., and Schein, P. S. (in press). *Cancer.*

Gastrointestinal Tumor Study Group (1978). *Cancer 42,* 19-22.

Hill, A. B. (1961). "Principles of Medical Statistics." Oxford University Press, New York.

Kovach, J. S., Moertel, C. G., Schutt, A. J., Hahn, R. G., and Reitemeier, R. J. (1974). *Cancer 33,* 563-567.

Liu, K., Mittelman, A., Sproul, E. E., and Elias, E. G. (1971). *Cancer 28,* 1314-1320.

Lokich, J., Chawke, P. L., Brooks, J., and Frei, E. (1974). *Ann. Surg. 179,* 450-453.

Macdonald, J. S., Kisner, D. F., Symthe, T., Woolley, P. V., Smith, L., and Schein, P. S. (1976). *Cancer Treat. Rep. 60,* 1597-1600.

Macdonald, J., Woolley, P. V., Smythe, T., Ueno, W., Hoth, D., and Schein, P. S. (in press). *Cancer.*

Ratanatharathorn, V., Cadnopaphorndai, P., Rosenberg, B., Baker, L. H., Taber, S., Ruffer, B. W., Mcdonald, F. D., Vaitkevicius, V. K. (1977). *Proc. Am. Soc. Clin. Oncol. 18,* 293.

Schein, P. S., O'Connell, M. J., Blom, J., Hubbard, S., Magrath, I. T., Bergevin, P., Wiernik, P. H., Ziegler, J. L., and DeVita, V. T. (1974). *Cancer 34,* 993-1000.

Stolkinsky, D. C., Sadoff, L., Braunwald, J. and Bateman, J. R. (1972). *Cancer 30,* 61-69.

Wiggans, R. G., Woolley, P. V., Macdonald, J. S., Smythe, T., Ueno, W., and Schein, P. S. (1978). *Cancer 41,* 387-391.

Zar, J. H. (1974). *In* "Biostatistical Analysis," p. 109. Prentice Hall, New York.

Chapter 16

EXPERIENCES WITH TWO TREATMENT SCHEDULES IN THE COMBINATION CHEMOTHERAPY OF ADVANCED GASTRIC CARCINOMA[1]

Frank J. Panettiere
Lance Heilbrun

I. INTRODUCTION

Although in the past, adenocarcinomas throughout the gastrointestinal tract were treated with essentially the same chemotherapy regimens irrespective of site of origin, recent data have indicated variations in tumor responsiveness depending upon the primary site of origin. The first clue to this came from the drug adriamycin. Although it is well recognized that it has only very meager effectiveness in colorectal carcinoma, it has a very significant effect in the management of gastric adenocarcinoma (Moertel, 1975). Although 5-FU is well known to have antitumor effect in the large bowel, this particular drug also has some degree of effectiveness more proximally in the gastrointestinal tract (Moore, 1968). Like 5-FU, mitomycin C is also somewhat effective in gastrointestinal malignancies of various primary sites.

For the treatment of gastric carcinoma, each of these drugs has been shown to have definite effectiveness individually. Moertel (1975) reported the response rate to adriamycin to be 36%. Moore (1968) in a large series reported a 24% response

[1] Supported by SWOG grants, DHEW 03096 and 12014.

rate to 5-FU. In another large study, 24% of patients with gastric carcinoma responded to mitomycin C (Comis and Carter, 1974).

Because these three particular drugs seem to be the most effective single agents today to manage disseminated gastric adenocarcinoma, it seemed very reasonable to test them in combination. The effects of one such combination of the three drugs was reported at the American Society for Clinical Oncology Meetings of 1976 by Macdonald *et al.* (1976). Although their published abstract reported that 9 of 18 gastric adenocarcinoma patients had attained partial regressions, in the verbal presentation at the meeting they stated that 10 of 21 (48%) experienced regressions of tumor with a median duration in excess of 9 months. In accordance with their particular program, adriamycin, mitomycin C, and 5-FU were given simultaneously, except that 5-FU was repeated 1 week later and mitomycin C was given only every other time the adriamycin was administered.

We questioned whether this was the optimal schedule to utilize these three drugs. Among our considerations was the fact that mitomycin C functions as a biological alkylating agent (Carter, 1968) and therefore is a cell-cycle-nonspecific drug. In addition adriamycin and mitomycin C bind to DNA (Zunio *et al.*, 1972). Although adriamycin's function seems to be accomplished by intercalation with the DNA molecule, both adriamycin and mitomycin C are cell-cycle-nonspecific agents, and both specifically affect cellular DNA. We felt that if both drugs are given simultaneously, many of the same tumor cells may actually be "killed twice." This could result in excessive toxicity without much gain in therapeutic efficacy. Therefore, rather than give the two drugs simultaneously, we felt that it might be more advantageous if their administration were separated by some time. We hoped that before sublethally damaged cells fully repair the damage of the first drug, the second drug might have an enhanced opportunity to destroy the still metabolically weakened cells.

Characteristically, one sustains, and recovers from, adriamycin myelosuppression earlier than from that of mitomycin C. Therefore, in order to preclude overlapping toxicity, we felt that adriamycin should be given first. Existing data demonstrate that adriamycin disassociates the chromatin from the cellular nuclear membrane. It appears that adriamycin alters surface properties of the cell and therefore promotes disassociation of DNA-membrane complexes (Murphee *et al.*, 1976). Theoretically, therefore, such an adriamycin effect on membrane permeability might permit subsequently administered mitomycin C to reach cellular DNA in higher concentrations than would have been the case otherwise.

5-FU is well recognized to be a S-phase-specific agent. Because adriamycin causes cell cycle progression delay (Valeriote, 1975), if 5-FU were administered simultaneously with, or soon after, adriamycin, one would expect that its effectiveness might be diminished by the decreased number of cells actively passing through the S phase of the cell cycle at that particular time. Therefore we reasoned that the 5-FU should be administered at a time significantly after adriamycin, when cycle progression delay is no longer in effect. Adriamycin pharmacokinetic studies indicate that this agent has a rather prolonged plasma decay curve (Benjamin *et al.*,

1973; Benjamin, 1975; Creasey et al., 1976; Chan et al., 1976). Thus, a multiple-day interval between adriamycin and 5-FU seems to be indicated. However, if 5-FU is given 1 or 2 weeks after adriamycin, there can be difficulties with overlapping bone marrow toxicity. We therefore decided to administer 5-FU 4 weeks after adriamycin, at a time after the usual recovery from adriamycin myelosuppression. We also expected that the subsequent myelosuppression from the 5-FU would occur after the expected recovery from the myelosuppression from the previously administered mitomycin C.

We felt that there was an additional theoretic advantage from the administration of such a cell-cycle-specific drug after the previous administration of the cycle-nonspecific agents. This was based on a rationale proposed by Schabel (1969). In accordance with his concept, when a previous agent (such as this particular combination's adriamycin and mitomycin C) destroys proliferating clonogenic cells, and when a cell-cycle-specific agent (such as 5-FU) is administered subsequently, at that particular time previously nonproliferating but still clonogenic cells would have been recruited into the cell cycle and so would be susceptible to the 5-FU to which they would have been resistant previously.

Based on these various multiple considerations, we designed a new program which we called a sequential regimen. Adriamycin is given on the first day of each 8-week course. Forty-eight hours later, mitomycin C is given. Four weeks after the initial dose of adriamycin, depending on marrow toxicity, up to four daily doses of 5-FU are administered. (We did not choose to use continuous infusion 5-FU because of the kinetic basis of the regimen. Doses of 5-FU can to some extent be "self-defeating" because 5-FU has been shown to cause cell-cycle progression delay by impairing the cells' entrance into the S phase of the cell cycle where 5-FU is optimally effective. We felt that daily IV bolus injections of 5-FU would allow time for cells to reenter the cell cycle and therefore allow them again to be susceptible to the next day's dose of 5-FU). As in the original simultaneous regimen of Macdonald et al. (1976), repeat courses were planned every 8 weeks.

Although the sequential regimen offers detailed *theoretic* justification as perhaps a better way of utilizing these three drugs to treat gastric carcinoma, the simultaneous utilization of the drugs as reported by the Georgetown group (Macdonald et al., 1976) was *proven* to offer approximately a 50% response rate. Therefore, we decided that it would be most rational to compare their original simultaneous regimen against our theoretically superior but unproven sequential regimen.

An important additional feature of this comparative study includes two specific areas of stratification. First patients who had previously received 5-FU or ftorafur or other similiar fluorinated pyrimidines would be eligible for the study but analyzed separately. We wanted to see if previous exposure to that standard therapy would have a deleterious effect on the subsequent utilization of such multiple-drug combination chemotherapy.

In addition, we allowed entry in two clinical categories: those patients with measurable disease, and those patients with nonmeasurable disease. We did this because so very often patients with gastric carcinoma have tumors that are quite difficult to measure such as vague, difficult to palpate abdominal masses or lesions that are poorly and indirectly seen at endoscopy or at upper gastrointestinal radiographs. With such weak parameters to judge response, often what is reported as tumor shrinkage may be wishful thinking more than objective tumor regression. We hoped that by allowing entry of patients both with and without definitely measurable lesions there would be a greater likelihood that those categorized as having measurable disease would have relatively accurately measured tumor masses. Those patients registered with measurable disease would be analyzed for tumor regression as well as for duration of survival. Those patients registered without objectively measurable disease could not, of course, be analyzed for responsiveness, but they could be analyzed for survival.

II. MATERIALS AND METHODS

This treatment program is outlined in Fig. 1. It was opened as Southwest Oncology Group Study Number 7639 in February 1977. When this current analysis was made, 1½ years later, nearly 200 patients from 23 different Southwest Oncology Group institutions had been included on the study. The biggest contributors were Wayne State University in Detroit, University of Texas Medical Branch in Galveston, the University of Hawaii in Honolulu, and the University of Utah in Salt Lake City (Table I).

For many of the patients more recently entered on the study, the data are far too immature at this time to include in the preliminary analysis. Currently, there are enough data for reasonable analysis from 110 patients known to be eligible and at least partly evaluable. Sixty-two currently known to be evaluable were randomized to the sequential limb and 48 to the simultaneous program. Of the 110, 79 were

TABLE I.   SWOG 7639: Case Entry by Member Institution

Wayne State University, Detroit	39
University of Texas Medical Branch, Galveston	15
University of Hawaii, Honolulu	11
University of Utah, Salt Lake City	11
Henry Ford Hospital, Detroit	10
Baylor College of Medicine, Houston	9
Cleveland Clinic, Cleveland	9
Ohio State University, Columbus	9
University of Mississippi, Jackson	8
Allegheny General Hospital, Pittsburgh	7
Oklahoma Medical Research Foundation, Oklahoma City	7
Tulane University, New Orleans	7
University of New Mexico, Albuquerque	6
University of Oregon, Portland	6

Nine other institutions entered between one and four patients. Twenty-three different SWOG institutions have participated to date.

SWOG 7639

Simultaneous Regimen

		Total Per Course
Adriamycin	30 mg/m^2/dose	day 1– – – –day 29– – – –	60
Mitomycin C	10 mg/m^2/dose	day 1– – – – – – – – – –	10
5-Fluorouracil	600 mg/m^2/dose	day 1 day 8 day 29 day 36	2400

Sequential Regimen

Adriamycin	50 mg/m^2/dose	day 1– – – – – – – –	50
Mitomycin C	10 mg/m^2/dose	– – – –day 3– – – – –	10
5-Fluorouracil	600 mg/m^2/dose	– – – –days 29, 30, 31, 32	2400

Fig. 1. Treatment program for SWOG Study 7639.

TABLE II. SWOG Toxicity Grading Criteria

Type	None	Mild	Moderate	Severe	Life threatening
Leukopenia	at least 4000	3000-3999	2000-2999	1000-1999	under 1000
Thrombocytopenia	at least 100,000	75,000-99,999	50,000-74,999	25,000-49,999	onder 25,000
Mucositis	normal	erythema	ulcers, can eat	unable to eat due to ulcerations	

registered as having measurable disease and 31 as nonmeasurable.

Standard criteria were used for response. For patients with objectively measurable tumors, we recorded each tumor's greatest diameter and its perpendicular. To judge for possible response, serial changes in the sums of the products of these bidimensional measurements were assessed. For a *complete regression,* total disappearance of all objectively measurable disease must last for at least 1 month. To qualify as a *partial response,* 50-99% regression of all measurable tumor was required and must have lasted for at least 1 month without the growth of any individual lesion. *Stable disease* was a category used only for those who were entered with known measurable disease. To be placed in this category, over at least a 1-month period there must be no tumor growth, and if any shrinkage were to be recorded, it must not meet the criterion of a partial response. *Increasing disease* categorized those whose measurable tumors grew progressively so that none of the other response categories were ever attained. Patients registered without preexisting measurable disease were not eligible for any of these 4 categories. Those with nonmeasurable disease (and those with measurable disease) were studied as to survival duration.

We utilized the survival curve estimation method of Kaplan and Meier (1958). Comparisons of survival curves between groups of patients were made using the generalized Wilcoxon test of Gehan (1965). Two-sided tests of significance were applied in making survival comparisons, except those involving response status. Those comparisons employed one-sided significance tests, since there were obviously *a priori* assumptions of directional differences in those cases (i.e., responders should survive longer than nonresponders).

Standard SWOG toxicity criteria were used. Table II defines our criteria for assessing severity of white blood cell, platelet, and gastrointestinal mucosal toxicity.

III. RESULTS

As implied previously, we feel that response is a very difficult parameter to ascertain in gastric carcinoma because of the very common difficulty in measuring objective tumor size. With that strong reservation as to the objective meaningfulness of the data, current response determinations are displayed in Table III.

A comparison of the survival of all eligible patients, measurable or not, is displayed by the treatment arm in Fig. 2. The survival of patients receiving the simultaneous regimen (median = 25 weeks) is not significantly different (two-sided $p = 0.227$) from that achieved by patients receiving sequential combination (median = 19 weeks).

In Fig. 3 is shown the survival of eligible patients by disease-measurability status. The survival of patients with measurable disease (median 21 weeks) is not significantly different (two-sided $p = 0.260$) from that of nonmeasurable patients (median = 16 weeks).

Survival of the eligible patients who were either fully or partially response-evaluable has been compared by response status in two ways. In Fig. 4, the survival

TABLE III. SWOG 7639: Responses of Patients with Measurable Disease

	Sequential	Simultaneous
Complete	0	0
Partial	4	8
Stable	15	9
Increasing	7	3
Not evaluable[a]	36	28
Total	62	48
CR + PR/Evaluable	4/26 = 11%	8/20 = 40%
CR + PR/Total	4/62 = 6%	8/48 = 17%

[a] Too early to evaluate; early death due to tumor, not toxicity; early loss to follow-up, etc.

of the 12 (partial) responders is compared to that of 34 nonresponders (stable disease plus increasing disease categories). The survival of the responders (median = 31 weeks) is slightly significantly longer (one-sided p = 0.065) than that achieved by the nonresponding patients (median = 21 weeks).

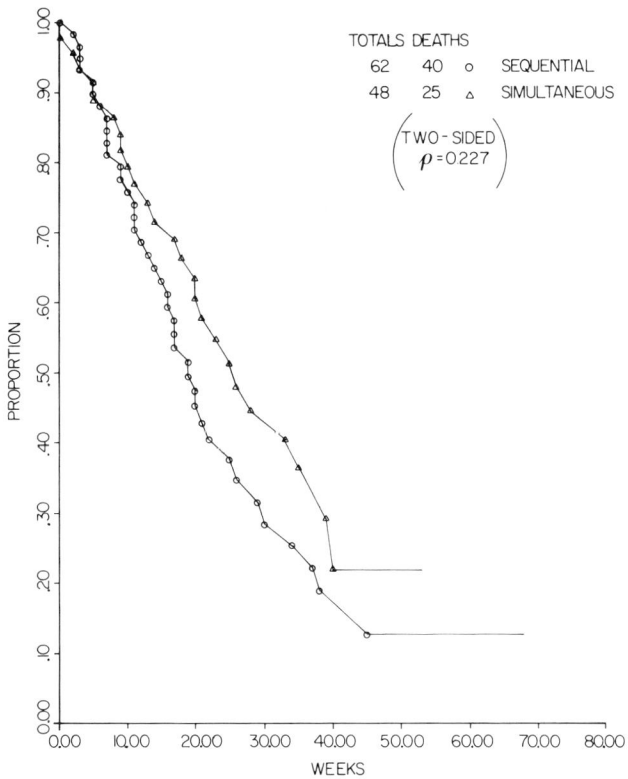

TOTALS DEATHS
62   40   o   SEQUENTIAL
48   25   △   SIMULTANEOUS

$$\left(\begin{array}{c} \text{TWO - SIDED} \\ p = 0.227 \end{array}\right)$$

Fig. 2. Survival of all eligible patients.

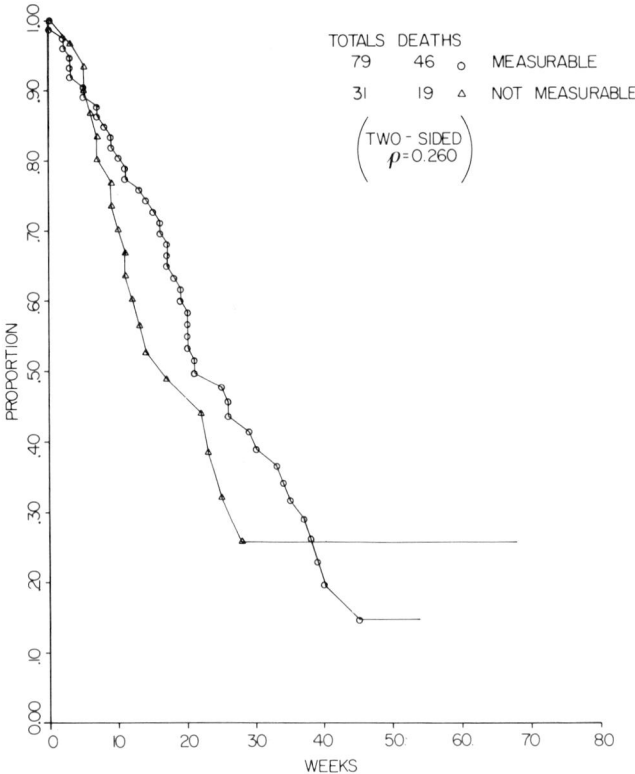

Fig. 3. Survival of patients with measurable disease versus patients with nonmeasurable disease.

Another way of examining survival by response status if presented in Fig. 5. Here 36 patients with nonincreasing disease (partial responders plus stable disease) are compared with the 10 patients who had observed increasing disease. The survival of the nonincreasing disease patients (median = 34 weeks) was highly significantly longer (one-sided $p = 0.001$) than that achieved by the patients with definite increasing disease (median = 18 weeks).

Sample size does not permit separate comparisons of survival by response status for the two treatment arms of this study at the present time. The survival data presented here are preliminary in terms of the total number of patients available for comparison of the different subgroups. However, these data are reasonably mature for those patients evaluated to date with respect to censoring rates (proportion of patients still alive and under follow-up). When censoring rates are high (e.g., 60-80% or more), the analyses can only be regarded as very preliminary due to insufficient follow-up time. In all survival comparisons made here, the censoring rates were only 20-50%; most were 35-45%. However, the median follow-up time for patients included in Figs. 1 and 2 is only 17 weeks; for Figs. 3 and 4 it is 22 weeks. Obviously, reanalysis at a later data is needed, and is planned.

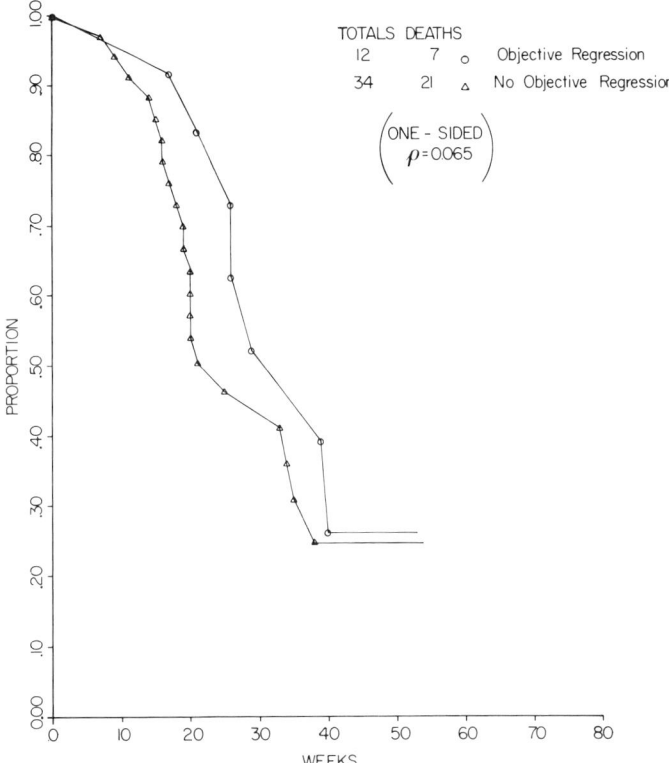

Fig. 4. Survival of responders and nonresponders.

The major toxicities are displayed according to severity in Table IV. In addition, alopecia, nausea, and vomiting were essentially equal in both limbs. Three patients on the sequential limb (and none on the simultaneous regimen) experienced skin necrosis, apparently due to drug infiltration. In addition, one patient on the sequential regimen was thought to have cardiac toxicity, and one patient on the simultaneous regimen is felt to have had drug-induced diarrhea with his drug courses.

The worst degree of toxicity of any type that each individual patient had is displayed in Table V. This includes in the denominators only the 51 sequential patients and 39 simultaneous patients who currently have had sufficient trial to be meaningfully at significant risk to experience toxicity.

IV. DISCUSSION

When this protocol was designed, we had strong question as to the meaningfulness of what are categorized as objective responses in diseases so characteristically difficult to measure as gastrointestinal carcinomas and, *a fortiori*, gastric carcinomas.

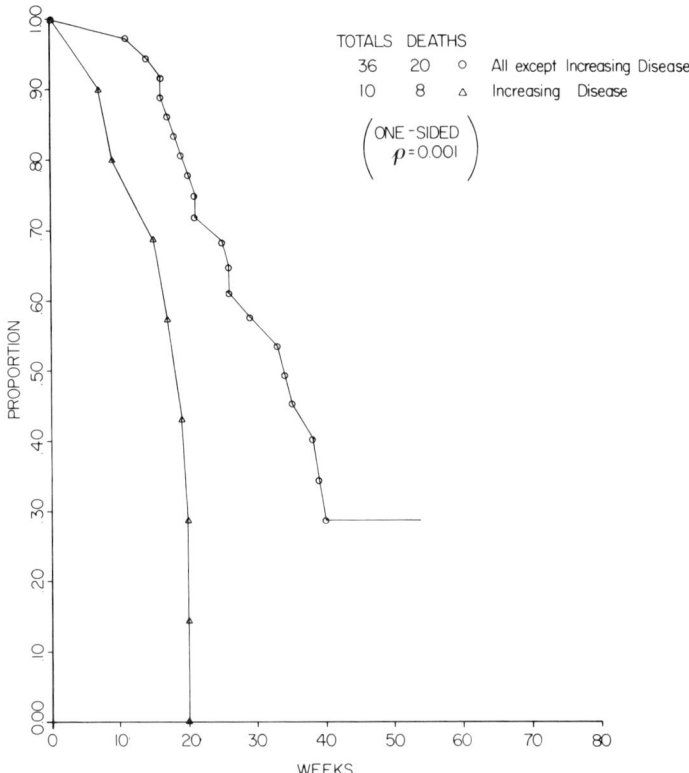

Fig. 5. Survival of patients with and without increasing disease.

It is certainly too early to confirm or deny this hypothesis on the basis of existing data, but it might serve to explain the apparent discrepancy between the apparent tendency toward response rate differences (Table III) and the apparent lack of survival differences (Fig. 2) of the two regimens. In the assessment of response, whether one uses as the denominator only evaluable patients or all entered patients, the

TABLE IV. SWOG 7639: Toxicity Type and Degree (51 Sequential and 39 Simultaneous)

	None	Mild	Moderate	Severe	Life threatening
Leukopenia					
Sequential	17	5	10	14	5
Simultaneous	12	6	12	7	2
Thrombocytopenia					
Sequential	41	3	4	1	2
Simultaneous	25	9	1	2	2
Mucositis					
Sequential	48	1	1	1	0
Simultaneous	33	3	2	1	0

TABLE V. SWOG 7639: Worst Degree of Toxicity

Degree of Toxicity	Sequential		Simultaneous	
None or mild	16	(31%)	14	(36%)
Moderate	13	(25%)	11	(28%)
Severe	16	(31%)	10	(26%)
Life threatening	6	(12%)	4	(10%)
Fatal	0	(0%)	0	(0%)
Totals	51	(100%)	39	(100%)

simultaneous regimen appears superior, with response rate differences of 40% versus 11% (evaluable only) or 17% versus 6% (all entered). However, if we use survival as a more objective, and definite, end point, we see no real evidence for a difference. The data on the graph in Fig. 2 indicate that 75% survive at 10 weeks in the sequential limb and at 12 weeks in the simultaneous limb. The 50th percentile is reached at 19 and 25 weeks respectively, and the 25th percentile at 34 and 40 weeks. The two-sided p value here is 0.227. It is not what one would expect if the apparent difference is response rates between the two limbs were clinically meaningful.

The data displayed in Fig. 2 also suggest that measurability, or the lack thereof, is not a meaningful parameter with reference to survival. One might have suspected a priori that those categorized as having measurable disease would have larger and more advanced tumors to allow measurability and that this, therefore, would result in a briefer survival. Certainly, there is no significant difference between the two curves (the two-sided p is 0.260). Surprisingly, however, those judged to have objectively measurable disease do not even tend to do more poorly. The 75th, 50th, and 25th percentiles for those with measurable disease are at 14, 21, and 38 weeks compared to 9, 16, and 28+ for those entered with nonmeasurable disease.

But despite this, at this early time in this ongoing study, all one can really say is that there is no clinically meaningful difference between those categorized as having measurable disease and those not so categorized. This might serve as further evidence that measurability is not a clinically meaningful parameter in this tumor type.

At the present time, no meaningful analysis can be made as to the possible effect of prior exposure to flourinated pyrimidines. Nine measurable disease patients had had such prior exposure and two are recorded as having developed partial regressions (one on each limb). To date, only seven nonmeasurable disease patients had previous exposure to fluorinated pyrimidines. Until larger numbers are accrued, their survival curve data will not be ready for calculations.

It would appear from Tables IV and V that the sequential limb and the simultaneous limb offer equal degrees of toxicity to the patient. Because toxicity cost seems to be quite comparable, the relative therapeutic effectiveness of the two regimens should be easier to judge. Based on the kinetic rationale of the sequential regimen, one would have expected it to offer an enhanced risk for toxicity as well as an expected greater therapeutic effect. However, the data thus far show neither greater toxicity nor greater antitumor benefit. Thus far, the only evident benefit from the sequential regimen appears to be that, for equal toxic effect as well as for apparently equal therapeutic effect, there might be a slight financial benefit to the patient. As Fig. 1 indicates, the per-course dosage of the rather expensive adriamycin is 50 mg/m^2 on the sequential regimen and 60 mg/m^2 for those on the simultaneous regimen.

But all of our data are quite preliminary. Although currently nearly 200 patients have been entered on this ongoing study, for no more than 110 do we have data for this current analysis. We anticipate that this study will remain open and continue to accrue patients until late 1979 or early 1980. The subsequent final analysis should give us far more definite conclusions than the preliminary ones we can make at this time.

V. CONCLUSIONS

Current preliminary data on this ongoing study indicate that both regimens are effective but not overwhelmingly so.

Although we have calculated response rates utilizing standard criteria, we see strong reasons to doubt the meaningfulness of what is categorized as a response when one is considering this particular tumor type.

The theoretic kinetic rationale that led to the design of the sequential regimen has not to date been reflected in an advantage in survival or in response rate. The new regimen's toxicity cost has thus far proven equal to that of the original simultaneous program as designed by the Georgetown group (Macdonald *et al.*, 1976).

All conclusions must be considered very preliminary at this time as they are based on only about 1/3 of the total number of patients whom we anticipate will eventually be entered on this multiinstitutional Southwest Oncology Group study.

ACKNOWLEDGMENTS

The authors wish to acknowledge the very valuable assistance of Mr. Tom Connor (programmer) and Ms. Sue Wimberly (data manager).

REFERENCES

Benjamin, R. S., Riggs, C. E., and Bachur, N. R. (1973). *Clin. Pharm. Ther. 14,* 592-600.
Benjamin, R. S., (1975). *Cancer Chemother. Rep. 6,* (part 3), 183-185.
Carter, S. K. (1968). *Cancer Chemother. Rep. 1,* (part 3), 99-114.
Chan, K. K., Cohen, J. L., Fross, J. F., Marlis, A. S., Bateman, Lee Y. T., and Marshall, J. G. (1976). *Proc. Amerc. Assoc. Cancer Res. 17,* abstract 757, 190.
Comis, R. L., Carter, S. K. (1974). *Cancer 34,* 1576-1586.
Creasy, W. A., McIntosh, L. S., Brescian, T., Odujirin, O., Aspines, G. T., and Murray, E. (1976). *Cancer Res. 36,* 216-221.

Gehan, E. A. (1965). *Biometrika 52,* 203-223.

Kaplan, E. L., Meier, P. (1958). *J. Amer. Stat. Assoc. 53,* 457-481.

Macdonald, J., Schein, P., Ueno, W., and Wooley, R. (1976). *Proc. Amer. Soc. Clin. Oncol. 17,* (abstract C-111), 264.

Moertel, C. G. (1975). *Cancer 36,* 675-682.

Moore, G. J. (1968). *Cancer Chemother Rep., part 1 52,* 641-653.

Murphee, S. A., Cunningham, L. S., Hwang, K. M., and Sartorelli, A. C. (1976). *Proc. Amer. Assoc. Cancer Res. 17,* abstract 164, 41.

Schabel, F. M. (1969). *Cancer Res. 29,* 2384-2389.

Schein, P. S., Macdonald, J. S. Hoth, D., and Wooley, P. V. (1978). *Cancer Chemother. Pharmacol. 1,* 73-75.

Valeroite, F. A. (1975). *In* "The Cell Cycle in Malignancy and Immunity: Proceedings of the 13th Annual Henford Biology Symposium," pp. 387-427. U. S. Energy Research and Development Administration.

Zunino, F., Gambetta, R., d.Marco, A., and Zaccara, A. (1972). *Biochem. Biophys. Acta 277,* 489-498.

Chapter 17

STUDY OF MITOMYCIN IN CERVICAL CANCER IN THE UNITED STATES

Laurence H. Baker

I. INTRODUCTION

In a 1977 review Wasserman and Carter were able to identify only 12 agents with evidence of clinical activity against disseminated cervical carcinoma. Seven of these drugs had alkylation as a predominant mechanism of action (two were mitomycin C and its N-methyl derivative porfiromycin). A review of data published (Manheimer, 1966; Moore, 1968; Godfrey and Wilbur, 1972; Izbicki et al., 1972; Panettiere et al., 1976) within the United States, in which criteria of response was stated to be 50% or more reduction in tumor volume, identified only 21 patients treated with mitomycin C alone (Table I). Responses were reported in 5 of these 21 patients, with the overwhelming majority coming from one single study.

Our interests in mitomycin C in cervical cancer actually began as a result of our studies with the N-methyl derivative porfiromycin. Previously, Izbicki et al. (1972) reported responses in 15 patients treated with cervical cancer by porfiromycin. When we decided that little significant difference existed (Baker et al., 1976a) between porfiromycin and mitomycin, our attention turned to the use of mitomycin in the treatment of cervical cancer. However, we no longer thought it necessary to confirm single-agent activity, but rather to study the use of combination chemotherapy.

In 1976, the final results of a study of mitomycin C, vincristine, and bleomycin

TABLE I. Mitomycin C Alone: Objective Response

Author	Responders/total
Manheimer (1966)	0/2
Moore (1968)	4/18
Godfrey (1972)	1/1
Izbicki et al. (1972)*	5/15
Panettiere et al. (1976)*	9/34

*N-Methyl, mitomycin C (porfiromycin).

in the treatment of advanced squamous cell carcinoma of the uterine cervix reported 13 partial responses in 27 fully evaluable patients treated (Baker et al., 1976b).

II. MATERIALS AND METHODS

In that study, as well as all future studies of mitomycin combinations, patient eligibility included: (a) patients with incurable squamous cell carcinoma of the uterine cervix who were no longer candidates for surgery or radiotherapy, (b) life expectancy of six weeks or longer; (c) no uncontrolled active or potentially active site of infection; (d) microscopic proof of malignancy and documented evidence of dissemination or recurrence; (e) at least one measurable lesion; (f) signed informed consent approved by our Human Experimentation Committee; (g) no evidence of renal impairment (creatinine less than 1.7 mg %); (h) no prior treatment with any of the drugs used.

As a result of what we interpreted to be initial success with this three-drug combination, we turned to the Southwest Oncology Group for confirmation in a larger number of patients. Within the Southwest Oncology Group, 130 patients who had far-advanced squamous cell carcinomas of the cervix were treated with mitomycin C, vincristine, and bleomycin. The results (Baker et al., 1978) of this three-drug combination are shown in Table II.

TABLE II. Mitomycin C Combinations

	Patients entered	Patients evaluable	Responders	Frequency of response
M(OB) 2 x weekly (1976)	30	27	13	
(1978)	58	50	30	
	88	77	43	
M(OB) 1 x weekly (1978)	25	24	6	
M(OB) infusion (1978)	47	41	16	
	160	142	65 (15 CR)	40% (46%)
Mito/Bleo[a]	12	10	2	

[a] Study still in progress.

All 160 patients received an identical dose of mitomycin C; namely, 20 mg/m²
IV bolus dose every 6-8 weeks for 2 doses, then 10 mg/m² every 6-8 weeks thereafter. In addition to the mitomycin, 88 patients received vincristine 0.5 mg/m²
twice weekly for 12 weeks and bleomycin 6 units/m² IM or IV 6 hr following the
vincristine administration for 12 weeks. Twenty-five patients were scheduled to receive vincristine 0.5 mg/m² once weekly for 24 weeks, and bleomycin 6 units/m²
IM or IV 6 hr following vincristine administration. The remaining 47 patients received vincristine 0.5 mg/m² IV on days 1 and 4 at 2 cycles and bleomycin 30
units/day as a continuous 96-hr infusion for 2 cycles (total dose = 240 units).

III. RESULTS

If we then combine patients from both series, 160 patients have been treated
with this three-drug combination in varying dose schedules, and 65 patients have
enjoyed clinical remission. Fifteen of these 65 were reported to be complete clinical responses, the combined activity of this three-drug combination appears to be
at least 40%. Miyamoto *et al.* (1978) reported on the effects of a combination of
bleomycin and mitomycin given sequentially, raising the question as to the need of
the vincristine in our previous studies. Currently, we are studying patients with
cervical cancer utilizing Miyamoto's dose schedule: bleomycin 5 mg IV continuous
infusion days 1-7, 6-22, 31-37, 46-52, and 61-67 and mitomycin C 10 mg on days
8, 23, 38, 53, 68 and every 6-8 weeks thereafter. Conclusions about this current
study are premature, but thus far we have been disappointed to have observed only
2 responses in 12 evaluable patients treated.

IV. DISCUSSION

It thus appears clear that the American experience with mitomycin C in disseminated squamous cell carcinoma of the uterine cervix has demonstrated activity
of this agent against this disease. Perhaps the biggest impact of this observation in
the United States is a resurgence of clinical trials in this disease category.

REFERENCES

Baker, L. H., Izbicki, R. M., and Vaitkevicius, V. K. (1976a). *Med. Pediatr. Oncol. 2,* 207-213.
Baker, L. H., Opipari, M. I., and Izbicki, R. M. (1976b). *Cancer 38,* 2222-2224.
Baker, L. H., Opipari, M. I., Wilson, H., Bottomley, R., and Coltman, C. A., Jr. (1978). *Obstet. Gynecol. 52,* 146-150.
Godfrey, T. E., and Wilbur, D. W. (1972). *Cancer 29,* 1647.
Izbicki, R., Al-Sarraf, M., Reed, M. L., Vaughn, C. B., and Vaitkevicius, V. K. (1972). *Cancer Chemother. Rep. 56,* (part 1), 615-624.

Manheimer, L. H. and Vital, J. (1966). *Cacner 19,* 207.

Miyamoto, T., Takabe, Y., Watanabe, M., and Terasima, T. (1978). *Cancer 41,* 403-414.

Moore, G. E., Bross, I. D. J., Ausman, R., Nadler, S., Jones, R., Jr., Slack, N., and Rimm, A. A. (1968). *Cancer Chemother. Rep. 52,* 675-684.

Panettiere, F. J., Talley, R. W., Torres, J., and Lane, M. (1976). *Cancer Chemother Rep. 60,* 907-911.

Wasserman, T. H., and Carter, S. K. (1977). *Cancer Treatment Rev. 4,* 25-46.

Chapter 18

RECENT RESULTS IN THE TREATMENT OF A METASTATIC CERVICAL CANCER WITH A SEQUENTIAL COMBINATION OF BLEOMYCIN AND MITOMYCIN C

Tadaaki Miyamoto

I. INTRODUCTION

Since Hata (1956) discovered mitomycin C (MMC), the drug has been widely used in Japan. A few papers refer to the objective response of cervical cancer to systemic MMC. It was found in Shinagawa's (1973) report that the shrinkage of primary tumor was observed in 16 of 41 (43%) operable patients by administering 40 mg MMC before operations.

After 10 years of clinical trials with MMC, the drug proved to be most effective when administered at a higher intermittent dose. Furthermore, two ways were found to overcome the limitations of MMC when used as a single agent. One method was combination therapy using other anticancer drugs with MMC. Ota *et al.* (1974) reported that 15 of 43 (35%) patients with metastatic lung cancer from the cervix responded to MMC combination therapy, as shown in Table I. The second method was to combine fibrinolytic agents which are thought to potentiate the effects of anticancer drugs with MMC. Niitani (1973) and Kurihara *et al.* (1974) reported that 26 of 45 (64%) patients with metastatic lung cancer from the cervix responded to MMC at a dose of 10 mg.

Miyamoto *et al.* (1978) reported that 14 of 15 (93%) patients with metastatic

TABLE I.   Effect of Mitomycin C on Cervical Cancer

	Objective response	Report
MMC alone	43% (16/41)	Shinagawa (1963)
METT[a], MFC[b]	35% (15/43)	Ota et al. (1974)
MMC + LL[c]	63% (26/45)	Niitani (1973)
		Kurihara et al. (1974)
MMC + BLM	93% (14/15)	Miyamoto (1978)

[a] METT: Mitomycin C, endoxan (cytoxin), tespamine, toyomycin.

[b] MFC: Mitomycin C, 5-FU, cytosine arsbinoside.

[c] LL: dextran sulfate + urokinase.

Total dose of MMC given: over 30-40 mg/body.

cervical cancer responded to the sequential combination of bleomycin and mito-mycin C which was devised on the basis of the information on cell kinetic inter-action between both agents.

In this paper, the results obtained by using a bleomycin-mitomycin combination in the treatment of metastatic cervical cancer will be reported.

II. MATERIALS AND METHODS

From July 1974 to June 1978, 30 patients with advanced cervical cancer were treated with a bleomycin (BLM) and mitomycin C (MMC) combination at the Hospital, National Institute of Radiological Sciences (HNIRS). All primary tumors, which histologically were squamous cell carcinomas, had received radical irradiation but no chemotherapy. At the time of chemotherapy, they had metastases in lung, bone, liver, skin, lymphatic node, and other sites.

The regimen of BLM and MMC combination is shown in Fig. 1. BLM at a daily dose of 5 mg was given for 7 consecutive days by drip infusion over 3 to 4 hr, followed by an intravenous push of MMC at a dose of 10 mg on day 8. This is one course of BLM and MMC combination, or B-M therapy, which is repeated two to five times with 1-week rest intervals depending on the response.

Complete remission (CR) was defined as the disappearance of all clinical evi-

Schedule of B-M Therapy

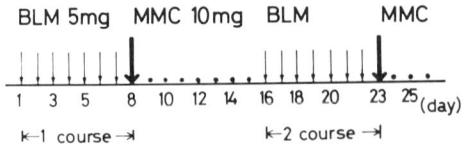

Fig. 1.   Protocol of bleomycin and mitomycin C (B-M) therapy.

TABLE II. Response Rate (%) of Metastatic Cervical Cancer by B-M Therapy (HNIRS)

		CR	PR	NR
All	(30)	86.6% (26/30)		13.3% (4/30)
Objective evaluated	(26)	65.3% (17/26)	23.0% (6/26)	11.5% (3/26)
		88.3% (23/26)		
B-M alone	(19)	57.8% (11/19)	31.5% (6/19)	10.5% (2/19)
		89.3% (17/19)		
B-M + radiotherapy	(7)	71.4% (5/7)	14.2% (1/7)	14.2% (1/7)
		85.6% (6/7)		

CR: complete remission; PR: partial remission; NR: no remission.

dence of tumor. Partial remission (PR) was defined as a 50% or greater decrease in tumor size. Other responses were classified as no remission (NR).

III. RESULTS

All patients at HNIRS received over two courses of B-M therapy. As shown in Table II, 26 of 30 (86.6%) patients responded in either subjective or objective evaluation. Objectively, 17 (65.3%) had CR and 6 (23%) had PR, respectively. In addition to the chemotherapy, seven patients were irradiated pre- and post-treatment for metastatic tumors. As a result, the CR rate was enhanced by approximately 5%.

Table III shows the respective response rates of metastatic tumor in lung, bone, liver, skin, and lymphatic node, obtained by using the chemotherapy alone. CR rate was approximately 60% in these organs, among which the rate did not differ significantly. The number of the patients with liver and skin metastases was too small to evaluate correctly. These results suggest that a sensitivity of the tumor to B-M therapy was not dependent upon metastatic sites.

As shown in Table IV, dose-limiting toxicities during remission induction were

TABLE III. Response Rate (%) of Metastatic Cervical Cancer In Various Sites by B-M Therapy

	CR	PR	NR
Lung (16)	62.5% (10/16)	25.0% (4/16)	12.5% (2/16)
Bone (9)	77.7% (7/9)	22.3% (2/9)	(0/9)
Liver (4)	50.0% (2/4)	25.0% (1/4)	(1/4)
Skin (2)	(2/2)	(0/2)	(0/2)
Lymph node (13)	61.5% (8/13)	30.7% (4/13)	7.8% (1/13)
Others (7)	57.1% (4/7)	28.1% (2/7)	6.8% (1/7)

CR: complete response; PR: partial response; NR: no response.

TABLE IV.   B-M Toxicity

Toxicity	Incidence (%)
Leukopenia (= 2,000/mm^3) or Thrombocytopenia (= 7.5 x 10^4/mm^3)	26.6% (8/30)
Lung fibrosis	6.6% (2/30)

studied in 30 patients. An average dose of BLM and MMC given during this period was 100 and 35 mg respectively. The percentage of our patients showing either leukopenia under 2000/mm^3 or thrombocytopenia under 7.5 x 10^4/mm^3 was 26.6%. This value is not significantly higher than the value seen with the use of MMC at the same dose. Frequency of lung fibrosis was 6.6%, which was even slightly higher than that with the use of BLM at the same dose. Other BLM-related toxicities such as alopecia, hyperpigmentation, and keratosis of the skin were frequently found, while other MMC-related toxicites such as renal failure were rarely seen.

The recurrence rate (Table V) was obtained for 15 out of 17 complete responders. Two excluded patients died within 3 months after receiving B-M therapy. As shown in Table V, the patients without a maintenance therapy had definite recurrence. An average remission duration was 4.5 months. An introduction of the maintenance therapy mentioned successfully reduced the recurrence rate from 100% to 12.5%.

To prevent the inevitable relapse in advance, an oral administration of Carboquon (carbazilquinon: CQ), a derivative compound of MMC, at a daily dose of 0.5 mg as a maintenance therapy was instituted. Thereafter, the average dose of CQ amounted to 52 mg for complete responders and 14 mg for partial responders, respectively. As a result, the recurrence rate of the patients receiving the maintenance remarkably decreased. Against such favorable results, unexpected adverse effects appeared as shown in Table VI. Some effects were fatal such as mycotic pneumonia, severe anemia, unknown causes of bloody stool, and malnutrition. Judging from the experience that no patients receiving CQ at a total dose of over 30 mg had recurrence, it seem evident that the dose of the drug administered actually was excessive.

The causes of death in 12 complete responders are listed in Table VII, in the order of the length of survival time. They may be subdivided into three groups. The first group consisted of two patients killed by perforation subsequent to radiation ulcer at the intestinal canal, which may be recalled by B-M therapy, and one patient

TABLE V.   Recurrence Rate (%) of
Complete Responders

Responders	Incidence (%)
Overall	53% (8/15)
Without maintenance	100% (7/7)
With maintenance	12.5% (1/8)

TABLE VI.   Maintenance Therapy (CQ: 0.5 mg/day) and Toxicity

Responder	Average total dose of CQ
Complete	52 mg (about 100 days)
Partial	14 mg (about 30 days)
	Adverse effects (13)
Sever anemia $(= 200 \times 10^4/mm^3)$	6
Infection	5
Cholecystitis	(1)
Pneumonia	(1)
Appendicitis	(1)
Herpes zoster	(2)
Bloody stool	1

who died of lung fibrosis. The second group consisted of five patients who died of recurrent tumor. The last group consisted of four patients who had received the maintenance therapy. It may have controlled the recurrence successfully, but it resulted in some fatal side effects.

In 24 patients, a 50% survival time of 10 months was observed from the onset of therapy. Five (20%) are still alive over 2 years without disease, however. This is a very hopeful result because other therapy in the past could not induce survival over 2 years (Arai *et al.*, 1976) (Fig. 2).

IV. DISCUSSION

Table VIII suggests that one B-M course was highly potent in patients who experienced complete responses. Would the effect of B-M therapy on cervical cancer be superior to that of simple addition of BLM and MMC? As shown in Table IX,

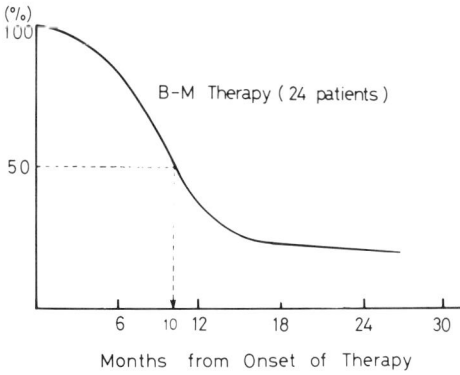

Fig. 2.   The survival of 24 patients after B-M therapy.

TABLE VII. Cause of Death of 12 Complete Responders

No. of patients	Survival time (mos.)	Maintenance	Cause of death
1	2.0	−	Perforation (ileum)
2	3.5	−	Perforation (esophagus)
3	4.0	−	Lung fibrosis
4	6.0	−	Relapse
5	8.0	−	Relapse
6	9.0	+	Relapse
7	9.0	−	Malnutrition
8	10.0	−	Relapse
9	10.0	+	Malnutrition
10	13.0	+	Diarrhea, anemia
11	18.0	+	Mycotic pneumonia
12	24.0	+	Unidentified

Suzuki *et al.* (1976) reported that the response rate of cervical cancer at stage IV, or relapse, to BLM was 35%, including 4% of excellent cases showing tumor shrinkage over 50% in diameter. Niitani (1973) (Table X) reported that metastatic lung cancer from the cervix responded to MMC at a 75% response rate including 17.8% of strongly effective cases showing tumor shrinkage over 90% in diameter. Assuming either excellent or strongly effective response identical with CR, the combination of both drugs would produce the additive (complete remission) rate of 21% shown in Table XI, which is inferior to CR rate (65.2%) (Table XI) found in B-M therapy by about 40% (Clarysse *et al.,* 1977). It is evident that the potentiation of CR rate must be attributed to the unique combination schedule of B-M therapy.

In order to clarify the effect of B-M therapy in further detail, the duration of complete remission was obtained for seven patients who had recurrence without the maintenance therapy. Figure 3 shows their remission duration against the number of B-M courses. As indicated by the dotted circle, the length seems to be roughly dependent upon the number of courses.

The volume change of the tumor of four complete responders was obtained as a function of the treatment time to estimate the therapeutic efficacy of the B-M course in a quantitative manner. As shown schematically in Fig. 4, a tumor at Vt decreased during three B-M courses and ultimately disappeared. After a certain

TABLE VIII. Potency of One B-M Course
in Complete Responders

Patient	Reduced relative tumor volume
A. N. (lung)	1.0×10^{-1}
S. O. (lung)	2.0×10^{-1}
E. K. (lung)	0.9×10^{-1}
T. N. (skin)	0.5×10^{-1}
Average	1.1×10^{-1}

TABLE IX.   Effect of Bleomycin on Cervical Cancer[a]

	Excellent[b]	Good or fair	Both
Stage IV recurrence	4% (1/22)	32% (7/22)	36% (8/22)

Suzuki *et al.* (1976).
[a] Total dose of bleomycin: over 120 mg/body.
[b] Over 50% reduction in tumor diameter.

TABLE X.   Effect of Mitomycin C on Metastatic Lung Cancer (Cervix)

	Strongly effective[a]	Effective	Both
MMC alone[b]	12.5% (1/8)	12.5% (1/8)	25% (2/8)
MMC + LL[c]	17.8% (5/28)	57.1% (16/28)	75% (21/28)

Niitani (1973).
[a] Over 90% reduction in tumor diameter including CR.
[b] MMC: 10 mg/body IV, once or twice a week.
[c] LL: dextran sulfate + urokinase.

	CR	PR	CR + PR
MMC + BLM	62.5% (10/16)	25.0% (4/16)	87.5% (14/16)

Miyamoto (1978).
MMC: 35 mg/body in average total dose.
BLM: 100 mg/body in average total dose.

period it reappeared and grew exponentially. Extrapolating the logarithmic portion of the regrowth curve back to zero time when the treatment started, V_o was obtained. Consequently, V_o/V_t means the net reduction of tumor by the therapy. The therapuetic potency per one course of B-M therapy was calculated by dividing V_t/V_o by the number of courses given. Table VIII shows the actual value for each patient thus estimated. It clearly indicates that one B-M course has the capability of reducing tumor size to slightly over one-tenth. Assuming the value to correlate with that of inactivated clonogenic cells in the tumor (Miyamoto *et al.*, 1976), five B-M

Remission Duration and No. of B-M Course

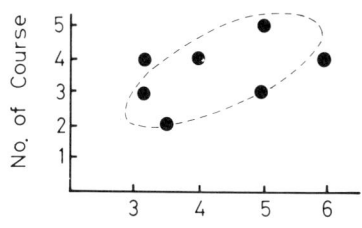

Fig. 3.   Each closed circle indicates a patient who had received a number of B-M courses and achieved CR, which lasted at least 1 month.

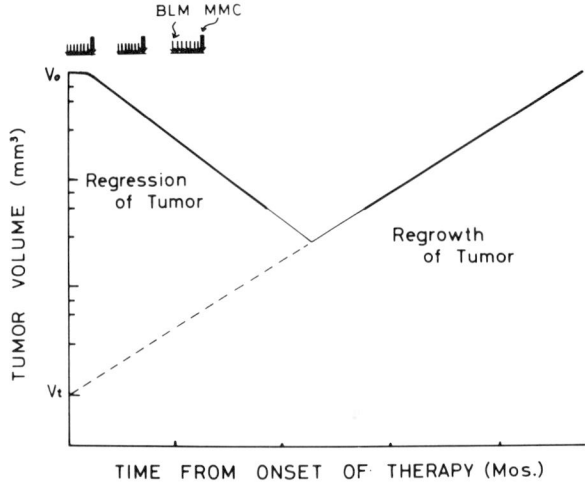

TIME FROM ONSET OF THERAPY (Mos.)

Fig. 4.   Shown schematically is the procedure to calculate the reduced tumor volume by the B-M courses given from the regrowth curve of a recurrent tumor. A tumor (Vo) begins to decrease in size as soon as the therapy starts and at last disappears clinically (fine lines). However, when approximately 4.5 months elapse after the initiation of therapy, the tumor reappears and continues to increase exponentially. The regrowth curve of the recurrent tumor obtained is then extrapolated to zero time when the therapy started (Vt). Consequently, three B-M courses decrease the tumor size by Vt/Vo.

courses can reduce 10^{12} tumor cells to 10^{7}, of which the remaining cells are thought to be sufficient to produce recurrent tumor.

Generally MMC is said to be about one-half of CQ in potency (Okada and Arakawa, 1976). However, the effect of CQ in oral administration is under one-half of that in intravenous administration. We may assume that the effect of MMC is almost the same as that of CQ in oral administration. Knowing that the patients receiving CQ at a total dose of 30 mg as a maintenance had no recurrence, the effective minimum dose of MMC as a maintenance drug is thought to be 30 mg. Theoretically, the addition of 30 mg MMC could not reduce 10^{7} remaining cells to 10^{4} even if the drug acts most effectively. Considering patients without disease surviving over 2 years, it is natural to infer that some other unknown factor such as immunity would be active on the remaining tumors.

TABLE XI.   Potentiation of B-M Therapy

Bleomycin (Table IX)	4% (CR)
Mitomycin (Table X)	17.8% (CR)

The additive combination of BLM + MMC should theoretically result in

$$17.8 + 4 (100-17.8/100) = 21\%$$

CR rate of B-M therapy (Table X) = 62.5%

It is very important to prevent the fatal side effects induced during remission induction and maintenance in advance in order for the patients with CR to survive over 2 years. New bleomycins such as pepleomycin, which produces lung fibrosis to a lesser degree, should be developed rather than the present BLM. The patients who received excessive doses of irradiation to the gut should be excluded to prevent the radiation ulcer induced by B-M therapy.

ACKNOWLEDGMENTS

The author thanks the doctors at the Hospital, National Institute of Radiological Sciences for helping him to take care of the patients, and Drs. Nakagima, Tanabe, Muto, and Terasima for their useful advice.

REFERENCES

Arai, T., Morita, S., and Kurisu, A. (1976). *Jap. J. Cancer Clin. 22,* 258-263.

Clarysse, A., Kenis, Y., and Mathe, G., Eds. (1976). *Cancer Chemotherapy.* 123. Springer Verlag, New York.

Hata, T. (1956). *J. Antibiot. 9.* 141-146.

Kurihara, M., Higuchi, K., and Nakatzu, T. (1974). *Gan To Kagakuryoho (Cancer Chemother.) 2,* 417-414.

Miyamoto, T., Takabe, Y., Watanabe, M., and Terasima, T. (1976). *Gan To Kagakuryoho (Cancer Chemother.) 3,* 1225-1236.

Miyamoto, T., Takabe, Y., Takabe, M., Watanabe, M., and Terasima, T. (1978). *Cancer 41,* 403-414.

Miyamoto, T. (1978). *Cancer Chemother. and Pharmacol.,* in press.

Niitani, H. (1973). *Saishinigagu 28,* 912.

Okada, N., and Arakawa, M. (1976). *GANN 67,* 805-812.

Ota, K., Murakami, M. and Sugiura, T. (1974). *Gan To Kagakuryoho (Cancer Chemother. 1,* 331-338.

Shinagawa, S. (1963). *J. Jap. Obstet. Gyn. Soc. (English) 10,* 152-160.

Suzuki, M., Watanabe, M. and Sato, A. (1976). *GANN Monograph on Cancer Research 19,* 221-230.

Chapter 19

MITOMYCIN TREATMENT FOR HEAD AND NECK CANCER IN JAPAN

Yukio Inuyama

I. INTRODUCTION

Since 1963, we have used chemotherapy as an adjunct to surgery and irradiation. Cancer chemotherapeutic agents used so far include cyclophosphamide, chromomycin A_3, mitomycin C, 5-fluorouracil, bleomycin, and adriamycin. These drugs, administered by intraarterial infusion, contributed greatly to improvement of the remote results of treatment of head and neck cancer.

Of the aforesaid drugs, MMC will be discussed here in respect to its primary effect, its histopathological effect, and the remote results of its use and its side effects, observed chiefly in patients treated by intraarterial infusion, as well as the clinical results obtained by the other researchers in Japan. In view of a growing tendency to correlate chemotherapy with cell kinetics, I would like to describe the clinical effect of B-M therapy, proposed by Miyamoto (1977), on cancer of the head and neck.

II. MATERIALS AND METHODS

MMC was used on 37 cases of malignant tumor of the head and neck from 1963 to 1966. The site of tumor was the nose and paranasal sinus in 22 cases, nasopharynx in 6 cases, mesopharynx and oral cavity each in 4 cases, and larynx in 1 case. The histologic type was squamous cell carcinoma in 32 cases, reticulum cell sarcoma in

TABLE I.   Mode of Treatment

Treatment	No. of cases
IA → surgery	14
IA + radiation	8
IA alone	7
IV + radiation	1
Polychemotherapy	7
Total	37

3 cases, and myogenic sarcoma in 2 cases. MMC was administered through the intra-arterial route in 29 cases and intravenous route in 8 cases. In 7 of 8 cases of intra-venous injection, MMC was used as one of the polychemotherapeutic agents. Dosage by intraarterial infusion was 2 mg/day daily or 6 mg/day twice a week. The total quantity of MMC administered by intraarterial infusion was 33.7 mg on the average. Dosage by intravenous injection was 2 mg/day daily, or in polychemo-therapy, 2-4 mg/day twice a week. The total quantity of MMC administered by intravenous injection was 30 mg on the average. The treatment consisted of intra-arterial infusion of MMC followed by surgery in 14 cases, which formed the largest group, as Table I shows; intraarterial infusion of MMC plus radiation in 8 cases; and intraarterial infusion of MMC alone in 7 cases. The effect was evaluated as excellent if the tumor shrank by over 90%, good if it shrank by 50-90%, and unchanged if the degree of shrinkage was under 50%.

Table II shows the effects of intraarterial infusion of MMC observed in our de-partment. In the 25 cases previously untreated, the effect was excellent in 4 cases (16%) and good in 13 cases (52%), from which the overall response rate was calculated as 68%. In the previously treated 4 cases, no favorable effect was observed. Kondo (1965) reported that he had obtained very good results in 25 cases, which consisted of total regression in 8 cases (32%), partial regression in 15 cases (60%), and overall response rate of 92% (Table III). Mohri (1969) treated maxillary carcinoma in 15 cases by intraarterial infusion of MMC and obtained excellent results in 8 cases (53%), good results in 4 cases (27%) and an overall response rate of 80% (Table IV).

In 25 cases where MMC treatment was combined with surgery or radiation, 5-year survival was achieved in 7 cases (28%). To be precise, the 5-year survival rate was 5/15 (33.3%) in cancer of the nose and paranasal sinus and 2/4 (50%) in naso-pharyngeal cancer, whereas none of the patients with cancer of the mesopharynx or oral cavity survived 5 years (Table V). Examination of the relationship between dose and prognosis disclosed that from 20-60 mg MMC had been administered with

TABLE II.   Effect of MMC by Intraarterial Infusion in 29 cases

Effect	Previously untreated	Response rate (%)	Previously treated	Response rate (%)
Excellent	4	16 ⎫ 68	0	0
Good	13	52 ⎬	0	0
Unchanged	8		4	

TABLE III. Effect of MMC by Intraarterial Infusion[a]

Effect	No. of cases	Response rate (%)
Total regression	8	32 ⎱
Partial regression	15	60 ⎰ 92
No response	2	
Total	25[b]	

[a] Kondo (1965).
[b] Of 25 cases, 12 were administered cyclophosphamide simultaneously.

TABLE IV. Effect of MMC by Intraarterial Infusion in Maxillary Carcinoma[a]

Effect	No. of cases	Response rate (%)
Excellent	8	53 ⎱
Good	4	27 ⎰ 80
Unchanged	3	
Total	15	

[a] Mohri (1969).

TABLE V. Survival Rates by MMC Treatment Combined with Radiation or Surgery

Site	Five-year survival	
	No.	%
Nose and paranasal sinus	5/15	33.3
Nasopharynx	2/4	50.0
Mesopharynx	0/2	0
Oral cavity	0/3	0
Total	7/25	28.0

excellent or good results in all the cases of over 5 years' survival (Fig. 1).

Table VI shows the histological changes in 36 cases of maxillary cancer treated preoperatively by intraarterial infusion of chemotherapeutic agent. The effect was evaluated on the basis of Shimosato's (1971) classification. In 13 cases where MMC was given by intraarterial infusion, III resulted in 1 case, IIb in 2 cases, IIa in 4 cases, and I in 5 cases. In 12 cases of the BLM intraarterial infusion group, III resulted in 2 cases, IIb in 4 cases, IIa in 5 cases, and I in 1 case, results which compare favorably with the findings in the MMC group. Compared with the above two drugs, chromomycin A_3 was far less effective, producing I in 5 cases, and 0 in 6 cases. Mohri (1969) performed surgery after intraaterial infusion of MMC for maxillary cancer in 15 cases and evaluated the histopathological effect of the treatment. His results were, according to Hayes' classification (1964), stage III in 1 case, stage II in

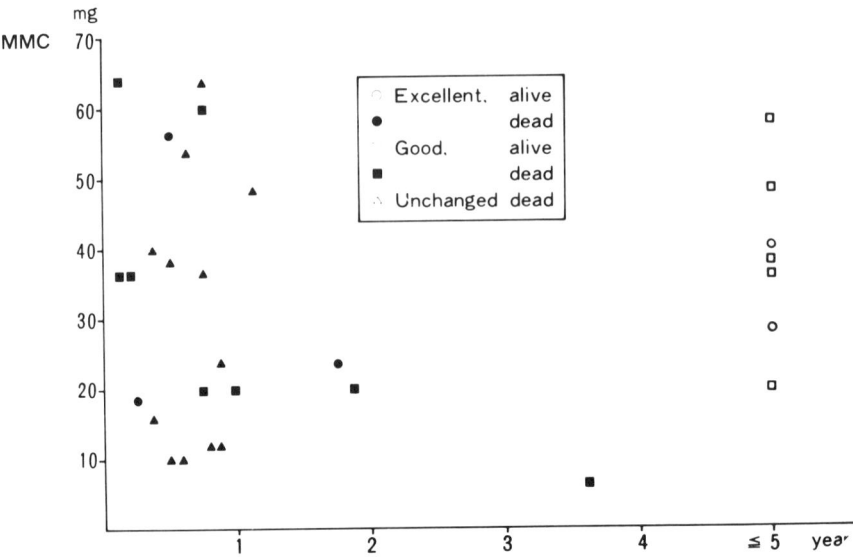

Fig. 1. Dose, clinical effect, and prognosis of 20-60 mg MMC.

8 cases, and stage I in 6 cases (Table VII).

In 31 cases, leukopenia occurred in the largest proportion (17 cases, 54.8%), and anemia in the second largest proportion (8 cases 25.8%). Alopecia was seen in 6 cases (19.3%) and stomatitis in 6 cases (19.3%) (Table VIII). Of 17 patients who presented leukopenia, 3 subsequently developed sepsis and died. Figure 2 shows the

TABLE VI. Histological Changes after Cancer Chemotherapy
by Intraarterial Infusion

	Shimosato's classification	MMC 13 cases	BLM 12 cases	CHR. A_3 11 cases
IV	Complete arrest of tumor proliferation			
III	Low probability of recurrence of tumor proliferation	1	2	
IIb	Moderate probability of recurrence of tumor proliferation	2	4	
IIa	High probability of recurrence of tumor proliferation	4	5	
I		5	1	5
0				6

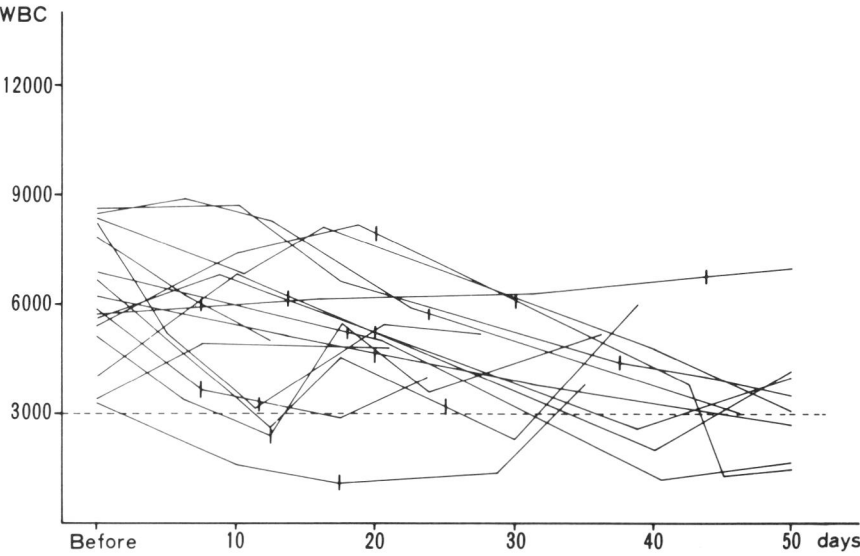

Fig. 2. Time-course change in WBC due to MMC treatment.

TABLE VII. Histological Changes after MMC Treatment by Intraarterial Infusion in Maxillary Carcinoma

Stage	Hayes' classification	No. of cases
I	Intercellular bridges and cytoplasmic vacuolization	6
II	Marked cytoplasmic vacuolization accompanied by contrasting nuclei	8
III	Extensive coagulation necrosis of the tumor	1

TABLE VIII. Toxic Effects of MMC[a]

Toxicity	No. of cases	Incidence (%)
Leukopenia	17	54.8
Anemia	8	25.8
Alpecia	6	19.8
Stomatitis	6	19.3
Thrombocytopenia	1	3.2
Nausea	1	3.2
Anorexia	1	3.2

[a] In evaluable 31 patients; total doses 32.3 mg on the average.

time-course change in white blood cell count that accompanied MMC treatment. WBC began to decrease about 1 week after the initiation of the treatment and continued to decrease almost linearly thereafter in some cases. Withdrawal of MMC was sometimes followed by rapid recovery; however, some patients did not recover until 30 days after treatment.

Kondo (1965) reported the incidence of leukopenia as 48%, and Mohri (1969) as 80%. An experiment with rabbits was performed to evaluate the method of MMC administration. MMC concentration was determined by Miyamura's method (1961) with the use of *Escherichia coli* B. In Fig. 3, 0.5 mg/kg MMC was infused by bolus injection into the femoral artery. The full line shows MMC concentration of blood in the ipsilateral femoral vein, and the dotted line MMC concentration in the ipsilateral femoral muscle. Whereas MMC concentration of blood in the femoral vein fell to ¼ the level observed immediately after infusion when 10 min elapsed, that in the femoral muscle was 7 μg/ml immediately after infusion and approx. 0.7 μg/ml even 30 min after that. Figure 4 shows MMC level in blood and the femoral muscle after its continuous infusion into the femoral artery and bolus injection into the auricular vein. Compared with MMC levels after one-shot intraarterial infusion, the latter levels were extremely low. From the above results as well as the action mode of MMC and the results of its clinical trials, one-shot intraarterial infusion was considered to be the best method for administration of MMC. Meanwhile, the therapeutic effects and the state of side effects suggest that the total quantity of MMC should preferably be in the range of 20 mg to 60 mg.

B-M therapy was performed on 37 cases of cancer of the head and neck in 2 years between October 1976 and September 1978 in our department. The site of tumor was the oral cavity in 11 cases, which formed the largest group; nose and paranasal sinus in 10 cases, the next largest group; nasopharynx in 6 cases; mesopharynx in 4 cases; and others in 7 cases. Of the said 37 patients, 29 (all with recurrence or metastasis) had been previously treated, and 8 untreated. In the majority of the untreated cases, only a single course was used prior to radiation therapy (Table IX).

A single course of therapy consisted of 5 mg/day BLM injected IM daily for 1 week and 10 mg MMC dissolved in 20 ml of 20% dextrose solution injected IV the

TABLE IX.   Sites of Tumor

Site	Previously treated	Previously untreated	Total
Oral cavity	8	3	11
Nose and paranasal sinus	8	2	10
Nasopharynx	5	1	6
Mesopharynx	4	0	4
Larynx	3	0	3
Hypopharynx	1	1	2
Ear	0	1	1
Total	29	8	37

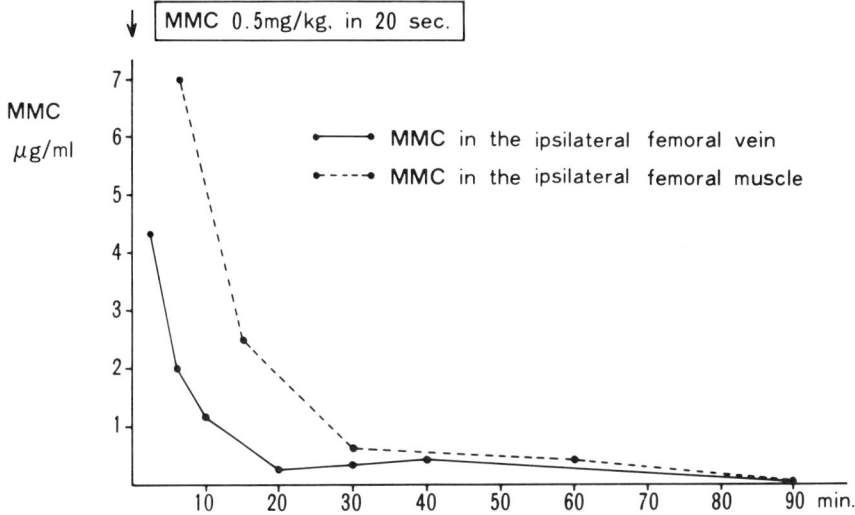

Fig. 3. MMC concentrations in the femoral vein and femoral muscle after bolus injection into the femoral artery.

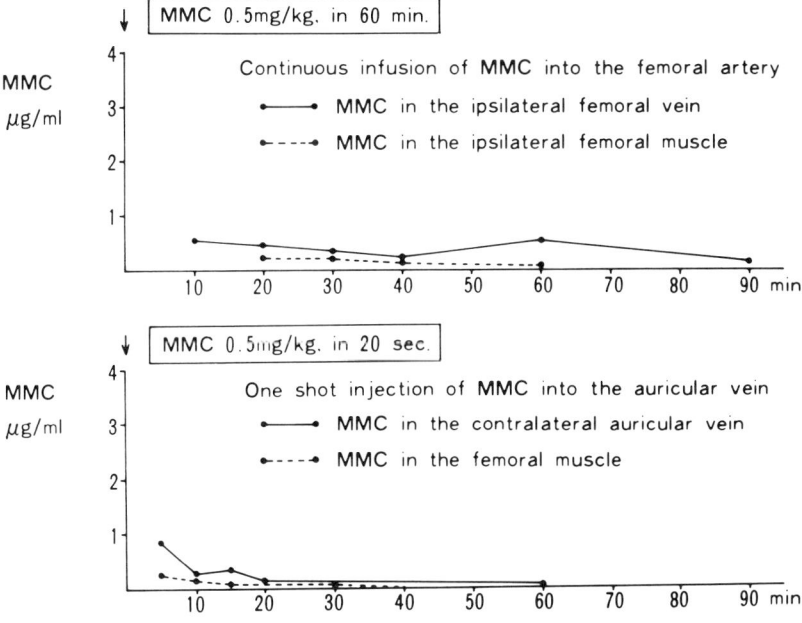

Fig. 4. Level of MMC in blood and femoral muscle after continuous infusion into the femoral artery and bolus injection into the auricular vein.

TABLE X. Effect of B-M Therapy

Effect	Previously untreated	Previously treated	Response rate (%)
Excellent		8	22
Good	2	2	10 32
Unchanged	6	19	
Total	8	29	

next day. Up to 6 courses were used. In 2 of 37 cases, B-M therapy was conducted by intraarterial infusion. In another 2 cases, an ordinary course of B-M therapy was given at first, then an additional therapy was performed with 10 mg MMC once a week until the total quantity of MMC reached 20-30 mg.

III. RESULTS

Among the said 37 cases, the responses were excellent in 8 cases (22%) and good in 4 cases, from which the overall response rate was calculated as 32%. The excellent response was not elicited in the untreated group, since, as stated above, only a single course was given before the initiation of radiation therapy in 7 of 8 such cases (Table X). The pattern of tumor regression due to B-M therapy had 3 varieties, as Fig. 5 shows. In the E (excellent) group, the tumor shrank by 50-60% in response to the first course, and disappeared or shrank by over 90% by the time 3 courses

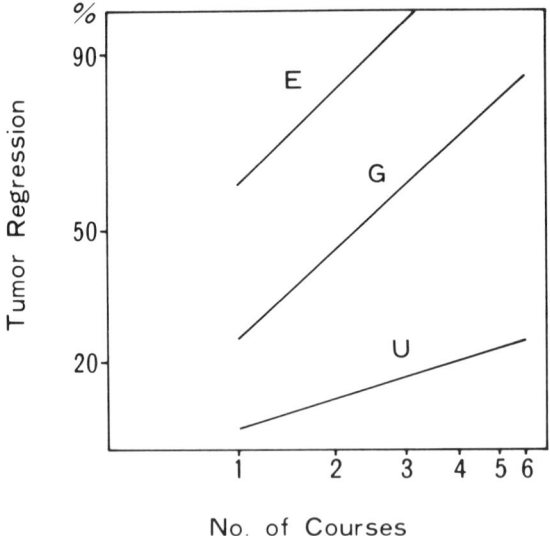

Fig. 5.   Three categories of tumor reaction to B-M therapy. E: excellent; G: good; U: unchanged.

were completed. In the G (good) group, on the contrary, the tumor shrank only by 20-30% at of the end of the first course, and over 90% shrinkage was not achieved even after application of 4-5 courses. In the U (unchanged) group, shrinkage of the tumor was scarcely observed after the first course, and subsequent application of the second and third course, failed to produce any effect. The aforesaid findings suggest that the response to the first course of B-M therapy roughly shows whether or not the tumor is sensitive to the therapy.

In cases where B-M therapy elicited the excellent response, maintenance therapy was conducted by IM injection of immunostimulative OK-432 (picibanil) combined with oral administration of futraful.

The cancer in case 1 was squamous cell carcinoma which had developed in the buccal mucosa; it had been treated by radiation and then recurred. When one course of B-M therapy was performed, and was followed by administration of 10 mg MMC twice, the tumor disappeared macroscopically. Picibanil was subsequently administered IM for 15 months until its quantity in total reached 235 KE. Recurrence or metastasis has not been observed so far. In case 5, on the other hand, marked shrinkage of the tumor was accompanied by hemorrhage from the lingual artery and pulmonary fibrosis, which led to death. In case 8, marked shrinkage of the neck tumor was accompanied by rupture of the carotid artery, which caused death (Fig. 6).

Of the side effects of B-M therapy, the most serious is pulmonary fibrosis. Pulmonary fibrosis developed in 5 of 37 cases, 13.5%. This incidence is higher than that of pulmonary disorder in the treatment with BLM alone, which is said to be

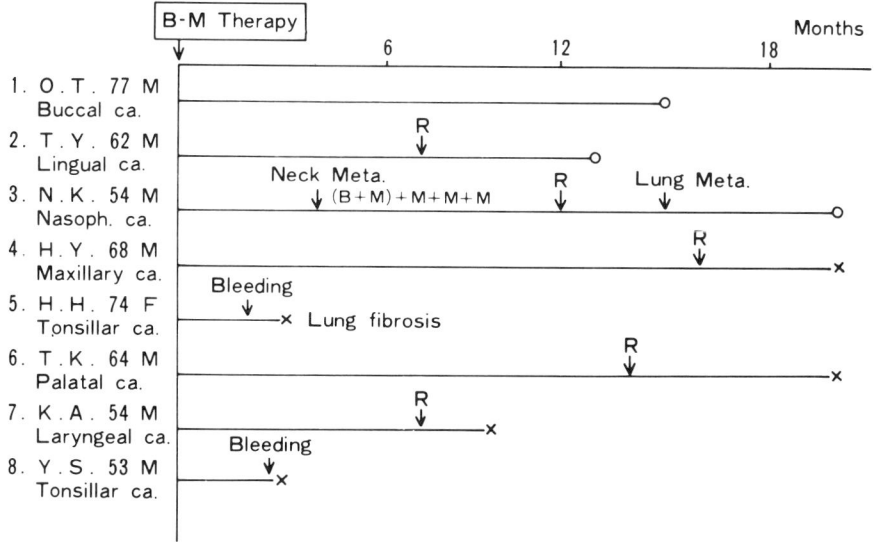

Fig. 6. Follow-up on 8 cases with excellent tumor response to B-M therapy.

TABLE XI.   Toxic Effect of B-M Therapy[a]

Toxicity	No. of cases	Incidence (%)
Lung fibrosis	5	13.5
Leucopenia	4	10.8
Thickening of the skin	2	5.4
Malaise	2	5.4
Fever	1	2.7
Alopecia	1	2.7

[a] In 37 evaluable patients.

1.5-7.7%. Utmost caution is therefore necessary, particularly with the aged. The high incidence of pulmonary fibrosis may partly be attributed to the fact that many of the patients with recurrent cancer had previously been administered BLM. As for bone marrow depression, WBC fell below 4000 in 4 cases, or 10.8% (Table XI).

IV.   DISCUSSION

Like BLM, MMC is quite effective against cancer of the head and neck. Because its effect is dependent on its concentration, the most suitable method for MMC administration is intraarterial infusion. MMC will also be most useful in the type of chemotherapy correlated to cell kinetics, such as B-M therapy proposed by Miyamoto (1977). Because MMC may cause bone marrow suppression, the utmost caution should be exercised in its administration.

REFERENCES

Hayes, M. D. (1964). *Arch. Surg. 88,* 1970-1976.
Kondo, H. (1965). *Otologia (Fukuoka) 11,* Suppl. 3, 109-132. (in Japanese).
Miyamoto, T. (1977). *Cancer and Chemother. 4,* 273-291. (in Japanese).
Miyamura, S. (1961). *Antibiotics, Ser. B14,* 251 (in Japanese).
Mohri, M. (1969). *Pract. Otol. Kyoto 62,* 1513-1532 (in Japanese).
Shimosato, Y. (1971). *Japan J. Clin. Oncol. 1,* 19.

Chapter 20

MITOMYCIN C, 5-FLUOROURACIL, AND RADIATION THERAPY IN SQUAMOUS (EPIDERMOID) CELL CARCINOMA OF THE ANAL CANAL

Thomas Buroker
Norman Nigro
Basil Considine
Vainutis K. Vaitkevicius

I. INTRODUCTION

Although squamous cell carcinomas only represent approximately 4% of tumors of the distal 18 cm of the large intestine, they account for approximately one-third of the neoplasms of the distal 2 cm of the rectum. Confusion regarding nomenclature, anatomy, site of origin, and therapy is greater with squamous cell carcinomas of the anal canal then perhaps with any other gastrointestinal tumor. Eponyms that have been applied to squamous cell carcinoma and its variants include: cloacogenic carcinoma, basaloid carcinoma, and transitional cell cloacogenic carcinoma. It is the authors', as well as others, opinion that although histological differences may exist between the classical squamous cell carcinoma of the anal canal and its variants, from the practical point of therapy, they may be considered to be identical tumors. Thus, in this paper these lesions will be described collectively as squamous (epidermoid) carcinomas (Quan, 1977).

The differential diagnosis of squamous carcinomas of the anal canal include three nonkeratinizing tumors: basal cell carcinoma, Bowen's disease, and Paget's extramammary disease.

Basal cell carcinomas of the perianal area have in the past been regarded as rare lesions. However, Turell (1966) has reported that the occurrence of this tumor may be more frequent than has been described. This tumor occurs twice as frequently in men as women, appears as a small skin nodule in hair-bearing areas near the anal margin, and usually ulcerates as it enlarges. In general, basal cell carcinomas of the perianal tissue resemble in appearance those seen elsewhere in the skin (Sawyer, 1977).

Bowen's disease is a chronic intraepidermal squamous cell cancer of the skin. It usually occurs after the fifth decade and is seen with equal frequency in men and women. The lesions are often large, erythematous, and spreading plaque-like with an eczematous crusting and weeping surface. This tumor obligates close follow-up of patients since most reports describe a significant number of these individuals will develop future cutaneous or systemic malignancies (Sawyer, 1977; Graham and Helwig, 1961).

The perianal lesion of extramammary Paget's disease is also usually elevated with an erythematous to whitish-gray scaly appearance. Microscopically an intraepithelial mucous adenocarcinoma is seen along with pale ovoid Paget cells with vesicular nuclei. The diagnosis of extramammary Paget's disease is facilitated by specific histochemical stains. Most cells in this tumor will stain strongly for mucicarmine, as well as demonstrate a positive aldehyde-fuchsin test (Sawyer, 1977; Wood and Culling, 1975). Here again, a careful search must be present for an underlying occult carcinoma which is frequently present (Kavlic, 1971).

Squamous cell carcinomas of the anal canal occur more frequently in women than men, have a propensity for patients in the fifth and sixth decades, and not infrequently are associated with antecedent benign anorectal disease, that is, chronic fistulae, hidradenitis suppurativa, and condylomata accuminata (Quan, 1977; Hickey et al., 1972; Sawyer, 1972).

The normal histology of the anal canal potentially lends itself to the development of different pathological entities. This may be simplified if one divides the normal epithelium of this area into two types: the distal squamous epithelia which give rise to squamous cell carcinomas; and the transitional epithelia present in the area of the dentate line which give rise to the so-called transitional cell of cloacogenic carcinomas. As was mentioned earlier, both these lesions will be termed squamous (epidermoid) carcinomas (Hickey et al., 1972).

In the past the therapy of choice for squamous cell carcinoma of the anal canal has been surgery. Small noninvasive lesions (musculature not penetrated) have done extremely well with local excision. Unfortunately, at the time of diagnosis most patients have invasive tumors and will require abdominal perineal resections to remove all evidence of malignancy. This latter group will still have a 5-year survival of only approximately 55% (Stearns and Quan, 1970).

Epidermoid carcinomas are radiosensitive and can be successfully treated with radiation therapy. Reluctance to use radiotherapy as a single modality developed because of the potential radionecrosis and fibrosis of the anal canal that may occur when optimal high dosages are employed (Kunkler and Das, 1968). This complication may be so disabling as to require subsequent radical surgery.

Nigro *et al.* (1974) in an attempt to use moderate dosages of radiotherapy to decrease the incidence of serious local radiotherapy complications, combined external irradiation with 5-fluorouracil and mitomycin C. Their success in a small series led to a prospective trial of preoperative combined modalities in squamous cell carcinoma of the anal canal.

II. MATERIALS AND METHODS

Eight women and six men, ranging in age from 49 to 65 years, with biopsy-proven squamous cell carcinoma of the anal canal were entered into the study. No patient had clinical evidence of inguinal lymph node metastases. In all patients, routine noninvasive metastatic work-up including chest x ray, liver scan, and IVP failed to demonstrated disseminated disease; and all were judged medically to be candidates for an abdominoperineal resection.

Preoperative combined chemo-radiation therapy was administered as illustrated in Table I. Chemotherapy and radiation therapy were begun jointly on day 1 of the therapy. 5-fluorouracil was given via a central venous catheter in a dosage of 1000 mg/m^2/24 hr for 4 days as a continuous infusion. This 96-hour infusion was repeated in 1 month even in the presence of bone marrow depression since 5-FU infusions have been shown to be nonmyelosuppressive (Seifert *et al.*, 1975). Mitomycin C was given as a bolus intravenous injection at a dosage of 15 mg/m^2. External irradiation was also begun on day 1 of therapy to the portal depicted in Fig. 1. Radiation therapy was given as 3000 rads, calculated at the midplane of the pelvis, at 1000 rads per week. The radiation portal measured 15 x 15 cm with its center on the patients midline. The lower edge of the beam included the ischial tuberosities. An abdominal perineal resection was performed 4 to 6 weeks following completion of the radiation therapy. Leukocyte and platelet counts were obtained weekly until the time of surgery.

TABLE I. Preoperative Therapy for Squamous Cell Carcinoma
of the Anal Canal

1.	*External irradiation* 3000 rads to rectum and local nodal areas. Day 1 to day 21. (200 rads/day/15 days)
2.	*Systemic chemotherapy*
a.	5-FU: 100 mg/m^2/24 hr as a continuous infusion for 4 days. Start on day 1.
b.	Mitomycin C: 15 mg/m^2 IV bolus on day 1.
c.	5-FU: Repeated day 20 to 31.

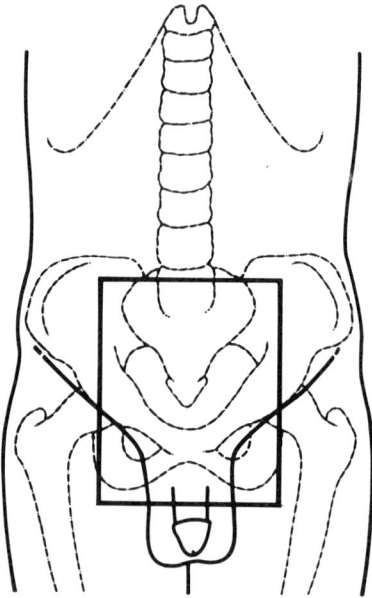

Fig. 1.   Radiation portal utilized for combined therapies for anal cancer.

III. RESULTS

All 14 patients were evaluable for the effect of the combined therapy on their preoperative lesion. In 10 patients the tumor was judged clinically to have disappeared completely. Even in the 4 patients in which tumor was clinically still present, a minimum of 50% reduction in tumor size was noted.

Ten of the 14 patients who received preoperative chemotherapy in conjunction with irradiation underwent an abdominal perineal resection. In 6 patients surgical specimens contained no residual neoplasm, whereas in the remaining 4 patients, 3 were histologically Duke B's and one individual was found to have biopsy-confirmed liver metastases at exploration. The 6 patients whose AP specimen contained no tumor were all felt to have no demonstrable clinical disease preoperatively after the combined therapy. The 4 patients who had residual disease were judged to have palpable tumor prior to surgery.

Four patients had tumors that clinically completely regressed preoperatively, and they subsequently refused an abdominal perineal resection. However, all consented to an excisional biopsy from the area where the tumor had arisen. None of the biopsies of these patients contained tumor. The clinical and pathological findings of all patients treated are shown in Table II.

It is noteworthy that of the ten patients in whom the tumor had disappeared clinically, as well as in the surgical or excisional biopsy specimen, all had lesions

TABLE II. Effect of Combined Preoperative Therapy on
Squamous Cell Carcinoma of the Anal Canal

No. of patients	Preop. tumor status after therapy	Surgery	Pathology
10	no disease	6 AP resections	no tumor
		4 local excision	no tumor
4	decrease by greater than 50%	4 AP resections	3 Duke B's 1 disseminated disease

prior to therapy that did not exceed 4 cm in diameter. Those patients whose disease remained after the combined therapy had larger lesions with diameters exceeding 6 cm.

Hematological toxicity was experienced but was tolerable. No patient experienced a nadir leukocyte or platelet count less than $1500\ cm^3$ or $50,000\ cm^3$, respectively. Radiation therapy was not interrupted in any patients. Additonal toxicities encountered included diarrhea, perianal proctitis, dysuria, and nausea. These side affects were all reversible and readily controlled.

The abdominal perineal operations varied in that some patients underwent the synchronous combined techniques whereas others had the abdominal and perineal phases done separately. No technical difficulties at surgery or postoperative healing problems were observed.

In the ten patients who had no residual tumor at the time of surgery, median follow-up is in excess of 30 months (range 6+ to 60+ months) with no evidence of recurrent disease.

IV. DISCUSSION

The authors believe this small pilot study demonstrates the feasibility of administering 5-FU-mitomycin C in conjunction with external irradiation preoperatively in patients with squamous cell carcinoma of the anal canal. It appears that a select group of patients may not require radical surgery for this disease but may be treated with an alternate approach.

It would also seem feasible that two additional groups of patients might benefit from this combined preoperative approach. First would be those patients who present with locally advanced disease that is so extensive that surgery can not be performed. Perhaps such patients could have their large tumor mass reduced to a resectable status. Secondly, in the unfortunate patient who presents with dissemnated disease palliative surgery for the primary lesion could be avoided if the combined chemotherapy-radiotherapy approach were to sterilize the disease in the anal canal.

To confirm the preliminary results obtained in our small series, a larger prospective cooperative study appears warranted.

REFERENCES

Graham, J., and Helwig, E. (1961). *Arch. Dermatol 83,* 738.

Hickey, R. C., Martin, R. G., Kheir, S., MacKay, B., and Gallager, H. S. (1972). *Surg. Clin. of North America 52, 4,* 943-950.

Kavlie, H., Stevenson, J. K., and Gould, V. E. (1971). *Am. Surg. 37,* 485.

Kunkler, P., and Das, R. (1968). *Proc. Roy. Soc. Med. 61,* 628-629.

Nigro, N., Vaitkevicius, V. K., and Considine, B. J. (1974). *Dis. Col. and Rectum 17, 3,* 354-356.

Quan, S. (1977). *N. Y. State J. Med.* 2056-2057.

Sawyer, J. (1972). *Surg. Clin. of North America 52, 4,* 935-940.

Sawyer, J. (1977). *Am. Surg.* 424-429.

Seifert, P., Baker, L. H., Reed, M. L., and Vaitkevicius, V. K. (1975). *Cancer 36,* 123-128.

Stearns, M., and Quan, S. (1970). *Surg. Gynecol. Obstet. 131,* 953.

Turell, R. (1966). *Am. J. Surg. 112,* 897.

Wood W., and Culling, C. (1975). *Arch. Pathol. 99,* 442-445.

Chapter 21

MITOMYCIN C IN EPIDERMOID CANCER OF THE LUNG

Lawrence S. Koons
Robert B. Catalano
David T. Harris

I. INTRODUCTION

An analysis of previous experience with mitomycin C in epidermoid cancer of the lung demonstrated antitumor activity when given by bronchial artery infusion (Neyazaki *et al.,* 1969; Neyazaki *et al.,* 1975), but no significant activity when given in low daily doses or frequent intermittent schedules (Selawry, 1973). Therefore, a study was designed to give mitomycin C in large intravenous doses at 4- to 6-week intervals to patients with advanced disease.

II. MATERIALS AND METHODS

Mitomycin C was given at a dose of 20 mg/m^2/IV over a 5-10 min interval. Induction therapy consisted of two doses separated by a 4-week interval. Evaluation was performed at 4 to 6 weeks following the second dose. Maintenance therapy was then given at 15-20 mg/m^2 every 4 to 6 weeks if disease regression or stability was observed.

If the WBC was less than 3000 or the platelets were less than 75,000 immediately prior to the next dose, treatment was withheld until weekly counts demonstrated recovery. Table I shows the adjustments made for bone marrow suppression.

TABLE I. Dose Alteration (Mitomycin C)

WBC	Platelets	Dose
>5000	>150,000	100%
4000-5000	100-150	75%
3000-4000	75-100	50%
<3000	<75	Hold

All patients required a pathologic diagnosis of epidermoid cancer of the lung. Patients had either recurrent or inoperable disease. To be eligible for evaluation *two* courses of drug had to be given with a minimum survival of at least 8 weeks. All patients considered to be responders had to have at least a 50% reduction in measurable disease. This was calculated as the difference in size of the sums of the products of the largest perpendicular diameters of the lesions. The duration of response was determined from the time of onset of the response until relapse, and survival was measured from the onset of therapy until death. The quality of survival was evaluated using the performance status criteria of the Eastern Cooperative Oncology Group and is shown in Table II.

There were 17 patients who had received no prior therapy of any kind. Eight patients received prior radiation therapy to the primary lesion. Only four patients had received and failed to respond to prior chemotherapy. Surgery had been performed on two patients.

TABLE II. Performance Status

0	Fully active—asymptomatic
1	Ambulatory—symptomatic
2	Resting in chair or bed <50% time
3	Resting in chair or bed >50% time
4	Completely bedridden

III. RESULTS

Fifteen patients had a performance status (PS) of 1 while an additional 11 patients were PS 2. Only 2 patients were PS 3, and there were no patients in either the PS 0 or 4 category.

There was a total of 57 doses of mitomycin C given ranging from 20 mg to 40 mg per injection. Seventeen patients received more than two courses of treatment. Only four patients received five or more doses. Gastrointestinal disturbances were not frequent, and only an occasional patient suffered significant alopecia. There was no renal or hepatic toxicity seen.

Hematologic toxicity was encountered in all three cell lines and is presented in Table III. WBC depression was mild and seen in about 50% of the patients. No instances of infection secondary to severe neutropenia were encountered. The range varied from 2300 to 24,800 WBC during the study. There was a gradual decrease in the percentage of hematocrit with each cycle of treatment. Hematocrits of 30% or lower were observed in approximately 1/3 patients after two courses of therapy.

TABLE III. Blood Counts

	Start of therapy	Prior to 2nd dose	Prior to 3rd dose	Prior to 4th dose	Prior to 5th dose	Prior to 6th dose
WBC (mean x $10^3/mm^3$)	11.8	7.9	7.3	7.8	5.6	6.8
HCT (mean %)	38	36	34	32	31	29
Platelets (mean x $10^3/mm^3$)	413	309	206	134	103	93
Number of pts.		28	22	15	11	7

Subsequent dose reduction appeared to decrease further hematocrit depression. Transfusions of packed RBCs were used for symptomatic anemia with good palliative results. Platelet counts dropped by 50% after the first two doses. By the start of the fourth dose 80% of the patients had platelet counts below normal. Recovery was usually seen in 4 weeks but some patients required prolonged periods (> 8 weeks). Counts rarely fell below 40,000 and platelet transfusions were not required. No instances of severe bleeding could be attributed to decreased platelets. When midcycle counts were measured there was some partial reversibility seen after the first dose in all cell lines, but thereafter a gradual cumulative depressive effect was observed.

There were 10 objective partial responses seen in 28 patients. All responses occurred within 8 weeks, and no further responses were seen after more than two doses in previously stable patients. Antitumor activity was observed in most patients (9/10) within 4 weeks, and the criteria for partial response was met in 6 patients at 4 weeks and in the additional 4 patients at 8 weeks (Table IV).

Improvement in performance status (PS) was seen in 4 patients with stability observed in another 4 patients. A decrease in PS was seen in only 2 patients. The improvement was observed within the first 2 weeks of starting treatment (Table IV). The duration of responding patients was approximately 3.5 months (Table IV). Overall survival for responders was 4.9+ months and 4.4+ months for nonre-

TABLE IV. Mitomycin C in Epidermoid
Lung Cancer: Response Characteristics

Response rate:	10PR/28 pts.[a]
Onset of response:	6PR/after 1st dose
	4PR/after 2nd dose
Duration of response:	3.4+ months
Performance status:	Improvement 4 pts.
	Stable 4 pts.
	Decrease 2 pts.

[a] PR: partial response.

sponders. It must be emphasized that all patients had to survive at least 8 weeks before inclusion into the study for evaluation purposes.

There were 5 patients who relapsed in the area of previous radiation therapy for their primary lung cancer. None of these 5 patients had additional evidence of distant metastases. There were no antitumor responses seen in this group. However, this group had a mean survival of 6.6 months compared to 3.5+ months for the other nonresponders. When the survival data is adjusted to omit this group of patients, a trend toward increased survival in the responding group becomes evident (4.9 months versus 3.5+ months). Furthermore, the adjusted response rate also increases to 10/23 as compared to 10/28.

IV. DISCUSSION

Neyazaki *et al.* (1975) has shown antitumor activity in epidermoid cancer of the lung when bronchial artery infusion of mitomycin C is employed. Furthermore, Godfrey and Wilbur (1972) and Kenis and Stryckmans (1972) have shown the feasibility of giving mitomycin C in large intermittent bolus doses. Previous reviews (Crooke and Bradner, 1976; Whittington and Close, 1970) have disclosed very little activity of mitomycin C against epidermoid cancer of the lung. The results reported were obtained using low daily, or frequent intermittent, schedules for mitomycin C. Because large bolus doses may produce the pharmacologic effects seen with intraarterial infusion, this study was undertaken. Indeed, there was clear cut antitumor activity obtained in 10 of 28 patients. Furthermore, there was an improvement in quality of survival with no serious toxicities. Survival figures are inconclusive, but in certain circumstances they indicate a positive trend.

In patients who relapse only in the site of previously irradiated disease, there appears to be no benefit from mitomycin C therapy. This group survives longer than patients with distant metastases and obscures any survival benefit comparison that may accrue to responding patients. This group is still too small to result in clinically significant results; however, further patient accrual will ultimately decide this issue.

REFERENCES

Crooke, S. T., and Bradner, W. T. (1976). *Cancer Treat. Rev. 3,* 121-139.
Godfrey, T. E., and Wilbur, D. W. (1972). *Cancer 29,* 1647-1652.
Kenis, Y., and Stryckmans, P. (1972). *Cancer Chemother. Rep. 56,* (part 1), 151.
Neyazaki, T. Ikeda, M., Seki, Y., Egawa, N., and Suzuki, C. (1969). *Cancer 24,* 912-922.
Neyazaki, T., Kimura, S., and Suzuki, C. (1975). *Panminerva Medica 17,* 290-293.
Selawry, O. S. (1973). *Cancer Chemother. Rep. 4,* (part 3), 177-188.
Whittington, R. M. and Close, H. P. (1970). *Cancer Chemother. Rep. 54,* (part 4), 195-198.

Chapter 22

MITOMYCIN C BLADDER INSTILLATION THERAPY FOR BLADDER TUMORS

Teruo Mishina
Hiroki Watanabe

I. INTRODUCTION

Topical therapy for bladder tumors was first described by Semple in 1948, who used podophyllin on four patients with bladder papillomas. The effectiveness of thio-TEPA as topical therapy for superficial bladder tumors was reported by Jones and Swinney (1961), Oravisto (1965), Esquivel et al. (1965), Abbassian et al. (1966), Veenema et al. (1969), and Saito et al. (1977).

The use of mitomycin C for bladder instillation therapy and satisfactory results were described by Shida et al. (1967), Nishiura et al. (1968), Sai and Hayakawa (1968), Ogawa (1969), Oomaru et al. (1973), and Saito et al. (1977).

In our clinic, topical bladder instillation therapy with mitomycin C has been used since 1967 in the treatment of bladder tumors. Some results have already been reported (Mishina et al. 1975). In Japan, 5-fluorouracil, ftorafur, adriamycin, bleomycin, neocarzinostatin, and carboquone are now used for bladder instillation therapy as well as mitomycin C, thio-TEPA. In our clinic, we have used mitomycin C, thio-TEPA, 5-fluorouracil, ftorafur, adriamycin, neocarzinostatin, bleomycin, and carboquone for the treatment of bladder tumors; and mitomycin C is thought to be the best of these for topical therapy.

In the examination of B strains of *Escherichia coli,* mitomycin C was proved to inhibit selectively deoxyribonucleic acid novo synthesis in a low concentration (0.1 μg/ml), in which ribonucleic acid and protein synthesis cannot be influenced (Shiba *et al.,* 1959). This action is believed to contribute to the inhibition of tumor growth.

Ogawa (1969) discovered that mitomycin C histologically has direct and indirect actions on bladder tumors in bladder instillation therapy. It directly causes degenerative changes in the cell plasma, and indirectly causes secondary necrosis of the cells, because of ischemia from the fibrinoid degeneration of the interstitial tissue and the necrotic degeneration of vessels. These degenerative changes are thought to be caused by the thickening and hyalinization of the media of the arterioles. Fifty cases of mitomycin C bladder instillation therapy are described herein.

II. MATERIALS AND METHODS

A. Mitomycin C Bladder Instillation Therapy

The 50 patients who underwent topical therapy for bladder tumors were requested to reduce fluid intake for about 12 hr to maintain adequate drug concentration within the bladder. The patients were asked to lie on the examination table after they had voided, and 20 mg mitomycin C in 20 ml sterilized distilled water (1000 μg/ml) was instilled into the bladder through a catheter. The drug was held in the bladder for as long as possible, on the average for 3 hr.

The concentration of mitomycin C acting on the surface of the tumors is 1000 μg/ ml immediately after bladder instillation and 167 μg/ml 3 hr later. Meanwhile, about 100 ml urine may be excreted and, therefore, the volume will become 120 ml 3 hr after instillation. This concentration of mitomycin C is much higher than the level required for inhibiting the development of tumor cells. The procedure was performed 3 times weekly, and 1 course of therapy consisted of 20 such procedures. Cystoscopic examination was performed before, during, and after therapy. Hematocrit, white blood cells, and platelets were examined every 10 days to check general side effects.

TABLE I. Tumor Size and Effect

Tumor size	No. pts.	Complete disappearance	Partial disappearance	No effect	Effective rate (%)
3mm	7	7	0	0	100
5mm	19	6	9	4	79
10mm	12	7	4	1	92
15mm	3	1	1	1	67
Pigeon's egg	3	1	1	1	67
Walnut	4	0	1	3	25
Hen's egg	2	0	0	2	0
Totals	50	22	16	12	

B. Mitomycin C Absorption Through the Bladder Epithelium

We measured the serum level of mitomycin C by bioassay in five patients with clinically evident bladder tumor 1 hr after 20 mg mitomycin C bladder instillation and in three normal adult rabbits 1 hr after bladder instillation of 1 mg mitomycin C per 1 kg of body weight.

III. RESULTS

A. Mitomycin C Bladder Installation Therapy

The tumors disappeared completely in 22 of the 50 patients studied (44%), partially disappeared in 16 patients (32%), and were not affected in 12 patients (24%). The total effective rate was 76%. The results are discussed from the standpoint of size, number, form, stage, and grade of tumors.

Size

As shown in Table I, the 3 mm tumors in all 7 patients completely disappeared, an effective rate of 100%. The 5 mm tumors in 19 patients completely disappeared in 6 cases, partially disappeared in 9 cases, and were not affected in 4 cases. Thus, an effective rate of 79% was observed. The 10 mm tumors in 12 patients completely disappeared in 7 cases, partially disappeared in 4 cases, and in 1 case there was no effect; thus, an effective rate of 92%. The 15 mm tumors in 3 patients completely disappeared in 1 case, partially disappeared in 1 case, and in the remaining case there was no effect; thus, an effective rate of 67%. Effective rates for pigeon's egg size, walnut size, and hen's egg size tumors were 67, 25, and 0%, respectively.

Number

In patients with 1, 3, and more than 6 tumors, the effective rates were 67, 60, and 73%, respectively. In patients with 2, 4, and 5 tumors, the effective rates were 100% in all (see Table II). No correlation between the number of tumors and the effect was detected.

TABLE II. Tumor Number and Effect

No. tumors	No. pts.	Complete disappearance	Partial disappearance	No effect	Effective rate (%)
1	21	10	4	7	67
2	9	5	4	0	100
3	5	1	2	2	60
4	1	1	0	0	100
5	3	1	2	0	100
More than 6	11	4	4	3	73
Totals	50	22	16	12	

TABLE III. Tumor Form and Effect

Tumors	No. pts.	Complete disappearance	Partial disappearance	No effect	Effective rate (%)
Papillary, pedunculated	23	14	7	2	91
Papillary, sessile	22	8	7	7	68
Non-papillary, sessile	5	0	2	3	40
Totals	50	22	16	12	

Form

As shown in Table III, in 23 cases of papillary and pedunculated tumors, results were complete disappearance in 14, partial disappearance in 7, and no effect in 2, for an effective rate of 91%. In 22 cases of papillary and sessile tumors, results were complete disappearnace in 8, partial disappearance in 7, and no effect in 7, for an effective rate of 68%. In 5 cases of nonpapillary and sessile tumors, results were partial disappearance in 2 and no effect in 3 for an effective rate of 40%.

Stage

Stages of bladder tumors are shown in Fig. 1. The numbers 1, 2, 3, 4, and 5 represent mucosa, submucosa, muscle, fat, and lymph nodes, respectively.

Stage 0 means that the growth is limited to the mucosa; stage A, to mucosa and submucosa. Stage B indicates muscle invasion; stage B_1, invasion to the superficial muscular layer, stage B_2, invasion to the deep muscular layer. Stage C indicates tumor invading the perivesical fat, and stage D those that have metastasized. In 44 cases of low-stage tumors (A and B_1) results were the complete disappearance of

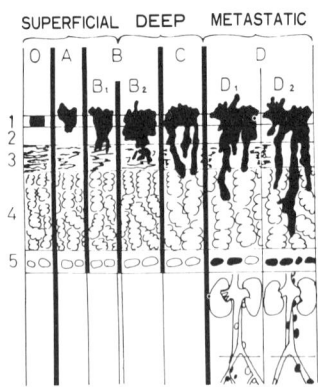

Fig. 1.   Stages of bladder tumors.

TABLE IV. Stage and Effect

Stage	No. pts.	Complete disappearance	Partial disappearance	No effect	Effective rate (%)	
A	33	20	9	4	88	84
B_1	11	2	6	3	73	
B_2	0	0	0	0	0	
C	3	0	0	3	0	17
D	3	0	1	2	33	
Totals	50	22	16	12		

the tumor in 22, partial disappearance in 15, and no effect in 7 for an effective rate of 84%.

In 6 cases of high stage tumors (B_2, C, and D) results were partial disappearance in 1 and no effect in 5 for an effective rate of 17% (see Table IV).

Grade

In 18 cases of low grade tumors (I and II), results were the complete disappearance of the tumor in 10, partial disappearance in 6 and no effect in 2, for an effective rate of 89%. In 11 cases of high grade tumors (III and IV) results were the complete disappearance of the tumor in 1, partial disappearance in 3, and no effect in 7, for an effective rate of 36% (see Table V).

Side Effects

Local side effects of frequent and painful urination were observed in 3 patients. The topical therapy could, however, be completed in each case.

For 2 patients, interruption of the therapy was not necessary and for the remaining patient, interruption was required only for a week. Neither bone marrow dysfunction (leukopenia, thrombocytopenia, and anemia) nor other general side effects were observed.

Case Report

One case of successful treatment with mitomycin C instillation therapy will be demonstrated here. Figure 2 shows cytoscopic findings of a 65-year-old male, who

TABLE V. Grade and Effect in 29 Patients Who Underwent Transurethral Biopsies

Grade	No. pts.	Complete disappearance	Partial disappearance	No effect	Effective rate (%)	
I	0	0	0	0	0	89
II	18	10	6	2	89	
III	9	1	3	5	44	36
IV	2	0	0	2	0	
Totals	29	11	9	9		

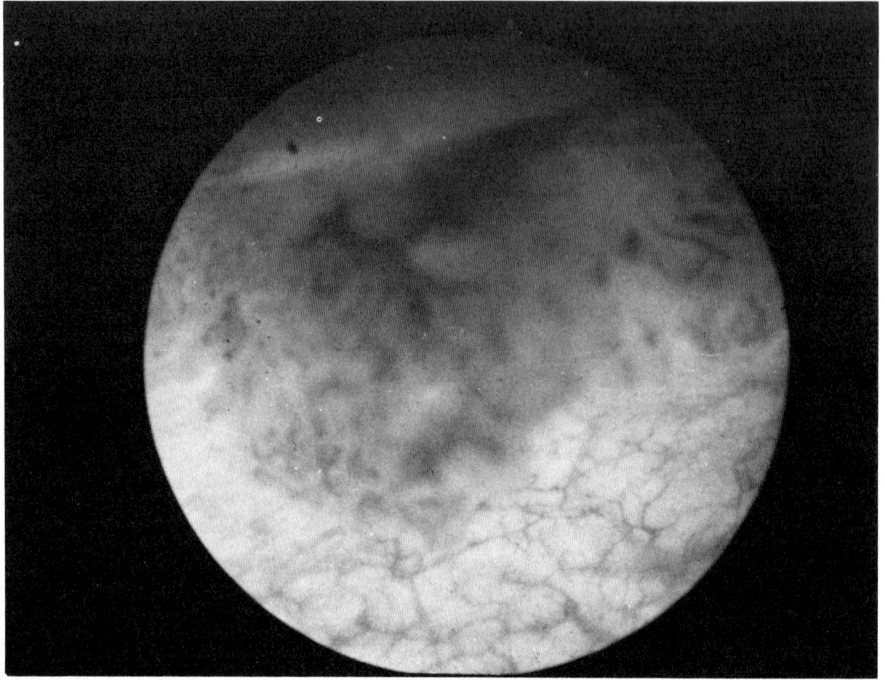

Fig. 2. Cystoscopic findings of a 65-year-old male with a bladder tumor before the MMC bladder instillation therapy.

underwent partial cystectomy in May 1971, and who revisited the clinic in October suffering from macrohematuria. On cystoscopic examination, a small finger-tip-sized, papillary and sessile tumor located at the neck of the bladder was observed. Transurethral biopsy of the tumor revealed that the tumor was transitional cell carcinoma, stage A, grade II. Mitomycin C instillation therapy was begun immediately.

Figure 3 shows the tumor partially disappearing after bladder instillation of 20 mg mitomycin C 10 times. The tumor disappeared completely after bladder instillation of 20 mg mitomycin C 20 times (Fig. 4). No tumor cells were detected by transurethral biopsy. This patient did not complain of any local or general side effects during the treatment.

B. Mitomycin C Absorption Through the Bladder Epithelium

The mean serum level of mitomycin C in rabbits was 0.003 $\mu g/ml$, whereas only trace levels were detected in the serum of patients with bladder tumor 1 hr after bladder instillation of mitomycin C (see Fig. 5).

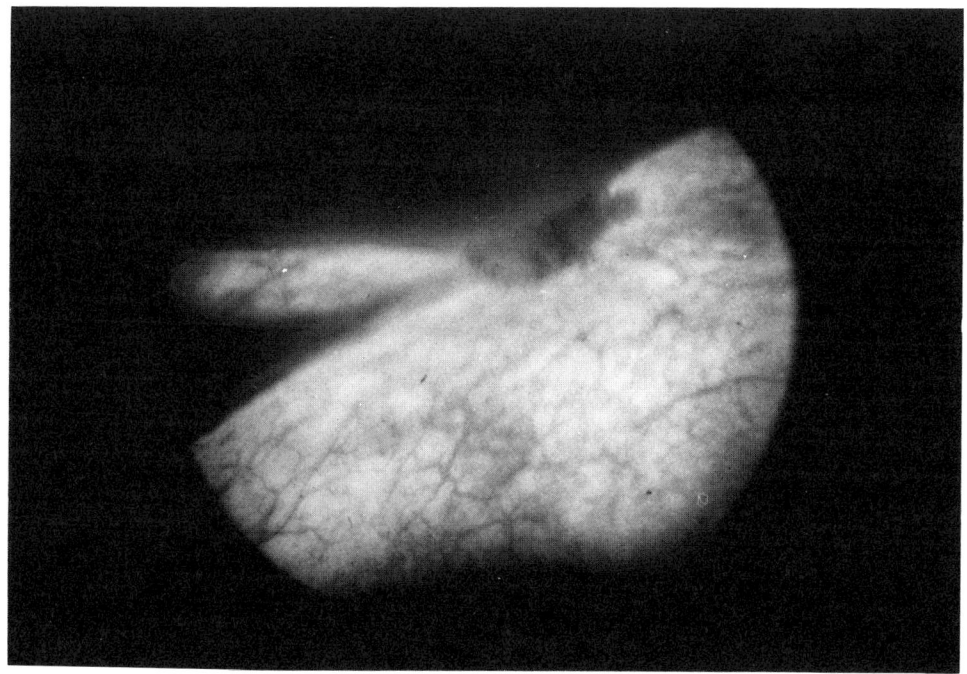

Fig. 3. Cystoscopic findings of the patient during therapy.

IV. DISCUSSION

It is generally stated that the following four points must be satisfied for anti-cancer drugs to be suitable for topical therapy for bladder tumors: (*a*) effectiveness on transitional cell carcinoma; (*b*) ability to kill tumor cells on contact with them for a short duration; (*c*) little local irritation on the normal bladder epithelium; and (*d*) little transfer into the blood.

In 1977, Kato showed that half the number of T-24 cells which were successfully isolated from human bladder transitional cell carcinoma by Bubenick *et al.* (1973) were killed after contact for 2 hr with a special culture fluid containing 0.02-0.1 μg/ml mitomycin C (see Fig. 6).

Shimoyama and Kimura (1973) examined the number of living cells of the L-1210 cell line after several sessions of contact with mitomycin C in various concentrations. They found that all the cells were killed after contact with 10 μg/ml mitomycin C for 30 min, and presumed that the action of mitomycin C was cytocidal depending on its concentration (see Fig. 7). Concerning the local irritability of mitomycin C on the normal bladder epithelium, Shida *et al.* (1967) observed that severe bladder irritation occurred in 44% and slight bladder irritation in 32% of 45 patients with bladder tumors after daily bladder instillation of mitomycin C.

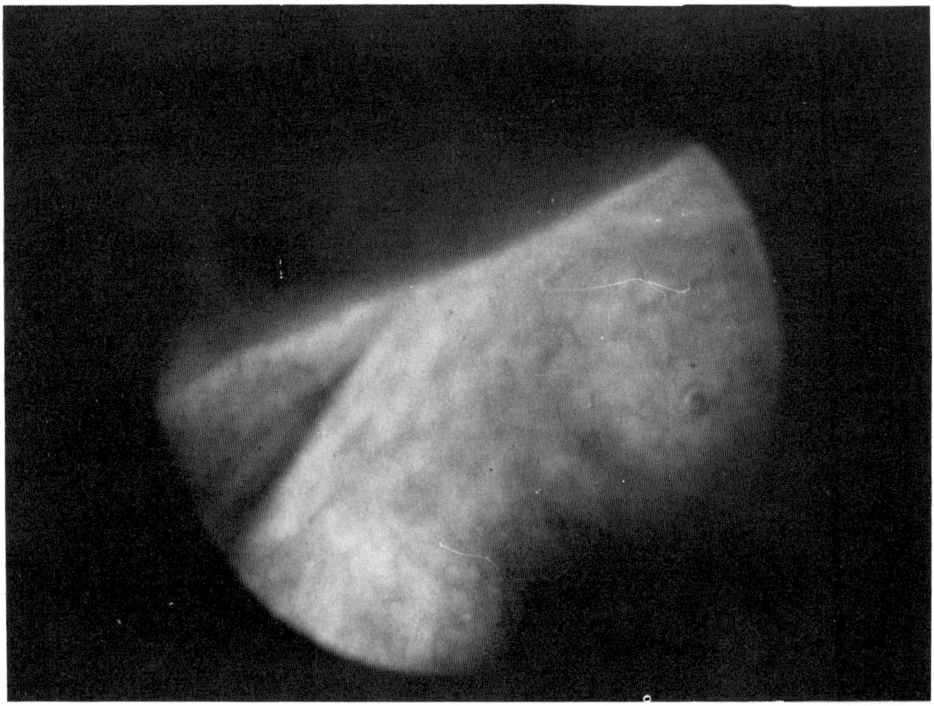

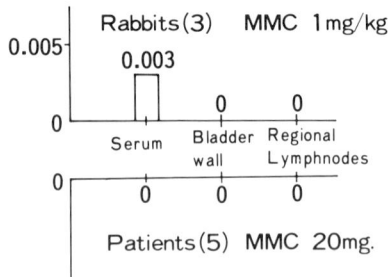

Fig. 4.   Cystoscopic findings of the patient after therapy.

The irritation, however, disappeared spontaneously without special treatment. This was also confirmed in our series. Imamura *et al.* (1976) found that the local irritability from mitomycin C instillation was reduced with the simultaneous administration of dexamethasone into the bladder.

Although Ogawa (1969) reported to the contrary, we observed that mitomycin C could be absorbed slightly from the rabbit bladder epithelium. No absorption occurred, however, from the normal or cancerous human bladder epithelium.

Rabbits(3)   MMC 1mg/kg

0.005

0.003

0

Serum   Bladder   Regional
              wall   Lymphnodes

0

0   0   0

Patients(5) MMC 20mg.

Fig. 5.   MMC absorption through the bladder epithelium.

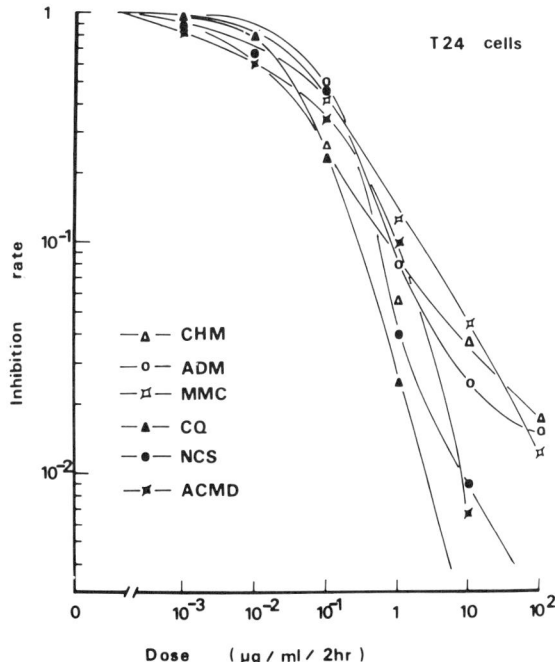

Fig. 6. Cytotoxic effect of 6 anticancer drugs measured by ^{14}C-leucine incorportation (Kato, 1977).

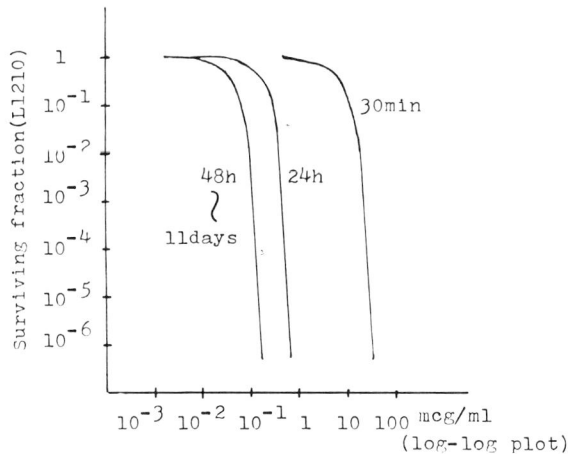

Fig. 7. Cytocidal action of MMC (Shimoyama and Kimura, 1973).

In our series, neither evidence of bone marrow dysfunction nor other general side effects were noticed.

From these points of view, mitomycin C is thought to be the most suitable anti-cancer drug for topical therapy of bladder tumors. We used mitomycin C bladder instillation therapy on 50 cases of bladder tumors and obtained a total effective rate of 76%.

It is presumed from our results that mitomycin C bladder instillation might be effective in tumors of (a) papillary form; (b) less than 10 mm in diameter; (c) low stage; and (d) low grade. No relation was recognized between the effectiveness and the number of tumors (Mishina *et al.*, 1975).

The results of mitomycin C bladder instillation therapy for low-stage and small tumors reported in Japan are shown in Table VI. The total effective rate was 80%, and no severe general side effects were reported.

From these clinical trials in Japan, it is advised that 20 mg mitomycin C in 20 ml sterilized distilled water might be instilled into the bladder three times weekly, and one course of the therapy might consist of 10 instillations. For the past 3 years, we have used this course of therapy routinely for most suitable patients visiting our clinic and have obtained good results.

Although these are not confirmed, the following advantages of mitomycin C bladder instillation therapy might be considered:

1. Carcinoma *in situ* or precancerous changes can not be determined by cystoscopy, and these changes will be missed at surgery. The preoperative bladder instillation of mitomycin C may help to destroy these changes.
2. In cases of diffuse papillomatosis, the number of patients needing to undergo total cystectomy can be minimized if some partial regression takes place by the bladder instillation of mitomycin C.
3. Mitomycin C topical therapy may reduce the dissemination of tumor cells into the operative field by destroying superficial tumor cells.

TABLE VI.   Mitomycin C Bladder Instillation Therapy Reported in Japan

	No. of cases	Complete disappearance	Partial disappearance	No effect
Shida *et al.* (1967)	35	16	14	5
Nishiura *et al.* (1968)	9	1	6	2
Ogawa (1969)	18	15	3	0
Oomaru *et al.* (1973)	23	6	9	8
Mishina *et al.* (1975)	44	22	15	7
Saito *et al.* (1977)	40	16	13	11
Totals	169	76 (45%)	60 (35%)	33

REFERENCES

Abbassian, A., and Wallace, D. M. (1966). *J. Urol. 96,* 461-465.

Bubenik, J., Baresova, M., Viklicky, V., Jakoubkova, J., Sainerova, H., and Donner, J. (1973). *Int. J. Cancer 11,* 765-773.

Esquivel, E. L., Jr., Mackenzie, A. R., and Whitmore, W. F., Jr. (1965). *Invest. Urol. 2,* 381-386.

Imamura, K., Yoshida, H., Maruyama, K., Ikeuchi, T., Yjima, N., Koshino, Y., and Saito, T. (1976). *Jap. J. Clin. Urol. 30,* 241-245.

Jones, H. C., and Swinney, J. (1961). *Lancet 2,* 615-618.

Kato, T. (1977). *In* "Abstracts of the 42nd Annual Meeting of the Eastern Section of the Japanese Urological Association," p. 21. Jap. Urol. Assoc. Press, Tokyo, Japan.

Mishina, T., Oda, K., Murata, S., Ooe, H., Mori, Y., and Takahashi, T. (1975). *J. Urol. 114,* 217-219.

Nishiura, T., Kumamoto, E., Nishimaru, Y., Tahara, M., Mizutani, H., Kawata, Y., Shimano, E., Miyamura, R., and Takasaki, E. (1968). *Igaku no Ayumi 65,* 637-643.

Ogawa, H. (1969). *Jap. J. Urol. 60,* 717-723.

Oomaru, K., Hidaka, M., and Fujii, K. (1973). *Nishinihon J. Urol. 35,* 510-514.

Oravisto, K. J. (1965). *Urol. Int. 20,* 23-28.

Sai, E., and Hayakawa, T. (1968). *Med. Consult. and New Remedies 5,* 1933-1935.

Saito, S., Takahashi, Y., Ohshima, H., and Matsuda, G. (1977). *Jap. J. Clin. Med. 35,* 1983-1987.

Semple, J. E. (1948). *Brit. Med. J. 1,* 1235-1237.

Shiba, S., Terawaki, A., Takagi, T., and Kawata, J. (1959). *Nature 183,* 1056-1057.

Shida, K., Douguchi, T., Sasazaki, T., Sato, H., Takahashi, U., Tatani, M., Kato, N., Urano, E., Oogoshi, M., Tazaki, H., Ozeki, Z., Matsunaga, S., Yajima, H., Nakagami, Y., and Nakamura, Y. (1967). *Jap. J. Clin. Urol. 21,* 1057-1059.

Shimoyama, M., and Kimura, (1973). *The Saishin-Igaku 28,* 1024-1040.

Veenema, R. J., Dean, A. L., Jr., Roberts, M., Fingerhut, B., Chowhury, B. K., and Tarassoly, H. (1962). *J. Urol. 88,* 60-63.

Chapter 23

TREATMENT OF MULTIPLE SUPERFICIAL TUMORS OF THE URINARY BLADDER WITH INTRAVESICAL MITOMYCIN C

R. Bruce Bracken

Douglas Johnson

I. INTRODUCTION

Superficial transitional cell carcinomas arising from the urinary bladder mucosa pose complex therapeutic problems due to their multifocal origin and their tendency to recur in over 60% of patients. Frequently, "subcystoscopic" areas of dysplasia and carcinoma *in situ* are interspersed between visible tumors (Melicow and Hollowell, 1952; Eisenberg *et al.*, 1960; Schade and Swinney, 1968, Cooper *et al.*, 1955; Koss *et al.*, 1974), making a technique that bathes the entire bladder mucosa with antitumor medication more desirable than transurethral resection or local excision of visible tumors. In the past, other treatment modalities such as external (Miller and Johnson, 1973) and intracavitary irradiation (Werf-Messing, 1971; Wallace, 1971), mucosal denudation (Harada and Kusunoki, 1968), local heat (Hall *et al.*, 1974), and pressure techniques (Helmstein, 1972) have proved disappointing in the management of these cases. Consequently, when conservative measures have failed to control the disease, radical cystectomy and urinary diversion have usually been required.

Topical therapy with triethylene thiophosphoramide (Thio-TEPA) was developed independently by Jones and Swinney (1961) and Veenema *et al.* (1965) in the early 1960s, and for years has been the only agent routinely employed for intravesical therapy of superficial bladder tumors (Table I). Its lack of effectiveness in patients with large tumor burdens and its potential myelosuppressive toxicity (14%) with an occasional reported death (Abbassian and Wallace, 1966; Bruce and Edcomb, 1967) has prompted investigators to search for more effective drugs with less severe potential side effects. Previous use of other agents such as podophyllin, phenol and glycerin, 5-fluorouracil, and formalin has proved either less effective or too toxic for clinical use (Abbassian and Wallace, 1966; Semple, 1948; Bunge, 1952; Veenema, 1968). Recent reports using butoxytolune (Barsel *et al.*, 1977), carboquone (Washida *et al.*, 1977), adriamycin (Banks *et al.*, 1976; Uyama and Kagawa, 1977; Ozaki, 1977), *cis*-platinum (Yagoda, personal communication), bleomycin (Bracken *et al.*, 1977), cytosine arabinoside (Yoshida *et al.*, 1977), and epodyl (Robinson *et al.*, 1977) as intravesical agents have suggested that they may be superior to Thio-TEPA in this disease (Table II).

Mitomycin C, an alkylating agent isolated from *streptomyces caepitosus*, is clearly active against bladder carcinoma when used systemically or regionally (Wakaki *et al.*, 1958; Eonly *et al.*, 1975; Ogata *et al.*, 1973). Mishina and colleagues from Japan (Mishina *et al.*, 1975) also demonstrated its topical activity when they reported a 44% complete and a 32% partial response rate for patients treated with 20 mg of intravesical mitomycin C three times a week for a total of 20 treatments. Treatment was effective when tumor size was less that 10 mm, regardless of the number of tumors. Systemic toxicity was absent. In view of these encouraging but preliminary results, we undertook a study to determine (*a*) the clinical efficacy (measured objectively by tumor regressions) of intravesical mitomycin C therapy; (*b*) the optimum induction dose and frequency of administration; (*c*) the amount of local absorption of the drug from the urinary bladder into the systemic circulation; and (*d*) the incidence, nature, and severity of side effects accompanying its use.

II. MATERIALS AND METHODS

Enrolled in this study were 32 informed and consenting patients with recent biopsy-proven transitional cell carcinoma of the urinary bladder, clinically staged as O or A (TIS or T1), in whom endoscopic excision was impossible due to multiplicity of tumors, increasing frequency of recurrences, tumor location, or health factors. Patients were excluded from investigation if (*a*) the neoplasm extended into or beyond the muscular layer of the bladder; (*b*) the white blood cell count was less than 3500 mm^3 or the platelet count was less than 150,000 mm^3, (*c*) serum creatinine was greater than 2.0 mg%; or (*d*) if other antineoplastic (systemic or local) agents were to be given during the duration of the study.

A complete history and physical examination, bimanual examination, and accurate endoscopic documentation of all measurable intraluminal disease were re-

TABLE I. Effects of Thio-TEPA on Bladder Tumors[a]

Author	No. of patients	Dose schedule	Response		
			Complete	Partial	None
Jones and Swinney (1961)	13	30-120 mg/50 ml every 2-3 days x 4 doses	4	7	2
Esquivel et al. (1965)	10	60 mg/week 4-12 weeks	3	4	3
Abbassian and Wallace (1966)	13	90 mg/50 cc H_2O every 4 days x 4	3	5	5
Veenema et al. (1965, 1969)	46	60 mg/week/1-2 weeks repeated at intervals	17	16	13
Edsmyer and Boman (1971)	29	50 mg/alt. day x 6	12	12	5
Nieh et al. (1978)	27	30-60 mg/weekly/8 weeks	15	NS	NS

[a] Modified from Williams (1975).
*NS: not stated.

TABLE II. Response Rates For Various Drug Programs

Author	Drug	Dose schedule	No. of patients	Response		
				Overall (%)	Complete	Partial
Barsel et al. (1977)	Butyloxytoluene	10% solution/12-55 instillations	66	86	NS*	NS*
Uyama and Kagawa (1977)	Adriamycin	30-60 mg/30 ml saline 3-21 treatments	49	45	5/49	17/49
Ozaki (1977)	Adriamycin	20-60 mg/20-30 ml saline 3 days/week for 1-2 weeks	80	71	22/80	35/80
Washida et al. (1977)	Carboquone	10 mg/50 ml water twice weekly for 5 weeks	7	71	2/7	3/7
Yoshida et al. (1977)	Cytosine arabinoside	400 mg/20 treatments	6	33	NS*	NS*
Robinson et al. (1977)	Epodyl	100 mg infusion as a 1% saline solution/week x 12	48	94	16/35	17/35
Bracken et al. (1977)	Bleomycin	30-120 units/30-60 ml H_2O weekly x 8	26	38	7/26	3/26

*NS: not stated.

quired for all patients within 21 days prior to institution of therapy. The extent of disease remaining following transurethral biopsy and/or resection and prior to intravesical therapy was categorized as follows: minimal (1+)—one or two well-defined small papillary tumors; limited (2+)—less than 25% of the vesical mucosa involved by apparent neoplasia; moderate (3+)—neoplastic involvement ranging from 25-50% of the bladder mucosa; and severe (4+)—tumor involvement exceeding 50% of the vesical mucosa. In addition, a complete blood count, platelet count, chest x ray, excretory urogram, serum multiple analysis (SMA), urinalysis, and urine culture and sensitivity were obtained in all patients. In an effort to minimize the risk of the drug absorption, therapy was not begun until 3 weeks after transurethral resection.

Patients were urged to withhold fluid intake for 12 hr prior to treatment, thereby permitting maximum retention and concentration of the drug within the bladder during treatment. A urethral catheter was inserted aceptically into the bladder and all urine was removed. Mitomycin C, dissolved in sterile water, was placed in the bladder, the catheter was removed, and the drug was retained intravesically for 2 hr, after which the patient was asked to void. Blood was routinely drawn for serum determinations of mitomycin C levels before, and at 60, 120, and 150 minutes after drug instillation recorded from the time of the first instillation. The volume of urine voided at the termination of the vesical instillation was recorded and a 20 ml aliquot obtained. The collected serum and urine samples were frozen and forwarded to Bristol Laboratories for bioassay of mitomycin C levels.

Although the same concentration of drug (1 mg/ml) was used, four different drug regimens were studied. Initially, 20 mg of mitomycin C were dissolved in 20 cc of sterile water (10 patients). Later the amount of drug was increased to 25 mg in 25 cc of sterile water (11 patients), 30 mg in 30 cc sterile water (6 patients), and more recently 40 mg in 40 cc of sterile water (5 patients). Cystoscopy, usually under local anesthesia, was repeated immediately prior to the eighth treatment. One month elapsed without treatment, and during the eleventh week endoscopy under anesthesia was performed at which time response to the treatment was evaluated.

At the eleventh-week cystoscopy, response was recorded according to the following criteria: complete remission—disappearance of all evidence of vesical malignant disease; partial remission—a decrease of the total cross-section areas of tumor by 50% or greater with no new lesions developing; improvement—regression of every evidence of disease by less than 50% but without evidence of progression; and progression—any measurable increase in tumor cross-section area or evidence of a new lesion.

III. RESULTS

Patient response to mitomycin C is given in Table III. The overall response rate in this series was 81% with complete responses noted in 50% of the patients, partial responses in 25%, and improvement in 6%. Progressive disease was recorded in only 19% of the patients. Although complete and partial responses were obtained with

TABLE III. Treatment Results According to Dose of Intravesical Mitomycin C

	Milligrams of mitomycin C dissolved in milliliters of water			
Results	20/20	25/25	30/30	40/40
Complete response	4	7	3	2
Partial response	2	1	2	3
Improvement	–	1	1	–
Progression	4	2	–	–
Total	10	11	6	5

all four drug regimens, two-thirds of the tumor progressions occurred at the 20 mg level, but none was seen when doses exceeded 25 mg.

Results of intravesical therapy evaluated according to the degree of tumor burden present at the initiation of treatment is given in Table IV. Although too few patients have been evaluated for the results to be statistically significant, they do suggest that reduced dosage rather than the extensiveness of disease is related to treatment failure.

Absorption of mitomycin C was not detected in any patient. The mean percentage of administered drug recovered in the urine was 51% for the 20 mg dose, 46% at 25 mg, 61% at 30 mg, and 73% at 40 mg. Since serum determinations showed no detectable mitomycin C levels, we assume that the failure to account for all the drug was a result of incomplete bladder emptying due either to anatomic or to functional abnormalities or to the circumstances of the test situation. Furthermore, no clinical evidence of drug toxicity was noted in any patient. White blood cell counts, platelet counts, liver profile studies (alkaline phosphatase, SGOT, serum bilirubin), and renal function tests (blood urea nitrogen and serum creatinine) remained unchanged during therapy.

IV. DISCUSSION

The concentration of mitomycin C acting directly on the vesical mucosa and surface of the tumor has been estimated by Mishina *et al.* (1975) to be 1000 μg/ml

TABLE IV. Results of Intravesical Chemotherapy Related to Tumor Burden

	Milligrams of mitomycin C dissolved in milliliters of water				
Tumor burden	20/20	25/25	30/30	40/40	Total
Minimal (1+)	–	NR	3CR, PR	–	5
Limited (2+)	2CR, 3NR	5CR, PR, I NR	PR, I	CR, PR	17
Moderate (3+)	CR, 2PR, NR	2CR	–	PR	7
Extensive (4+)	CR	–	–	CR, PR	7
Totals	10	11	6	5	32

immediately after instillation and 167 μg/ml at 3 hr. Similar results were obtained in the current study, with drug concentrations ranging from 83 μg/ml to 220 μg/ml 2 hr after the drug had been instilled into the bladder. The reduced concentration of mitomycin C at 2 hr was a result of dilution due to the continuous efflux of urine into the bladder in spite of restricted fluid intake. In no case was absorption of the drug detected in the serum. The concentration within the bladder is reportedly much higher than the level required for inhibiting tumor growth (Mishina *et al.,* 1975).

Normal bladder epithelium appears resistant to mitomycin C, while neoplastic cells have greater susceptibility. Although the action of mitomycin C on bladder carcinoma is incompletely understood, the drug has been said to have both a direct and indirect action (Mishina *et al.,* 1975). It may have an oncolytic effect by causing degenerative changes within the cell as well as an indirect action by producing thickening and hyalinization of the walls of arterioles resulting in secondary necrosis of cells due to ischemia.

Side effects from the topical vesical applications in this series have been minimal. Systemic toxicity is unlikely; and no patient experienced systemic toxicities since little, if any, of the drug is absorbed from the normal bladder. Local side effects have likewise been rare, consisting only of lower urinary tract irritative symptoms in a few patients. However, mitomycin C is a carcinogen and the potential for carcinogenesis remains a major concern. The frequent findings of diffuse mucosal field changes ranging from hyperplasia to dysplasia to carcinoma *in situ* in patients with bladder cancer have been well documented. Whether a potential carcinogen like mitomycin C, applied to carcinogen-sensitive tissue, will have long-term adverse effects remains to be determined. However, provisions have been made for long-term follow-up of our patients, paying careful attention to the rate of progression to more malignant neoplasms.

Our results would suggest that 30 mg in 30 ml sterile water is the minimum induction dose that can routinely be effective using a weekly instillation regimen, and perhaps higher drug concentrations may prove more beneficial. The need for maintenance therapy can only be ascertained if tumors recur in patients who achieve a complete response. Should the need for long-term treatment arise, additional factors requiring consideration would include patient selection, drug dose, frequency and duration of administration as well as criteria for treatment evaluation. Although the size (volume) of individual tumors may adversely affect the response rate, no correlation has been noted with regard to the number of tumors. The overall effective rate of 76 to 81% for mitomycin C suggests that it is the preferred drug available today for vesical chemotherapy.

REFERENCES

Abbassian, A., and Wallace, D. M. (1966). *J. Urol. 96,* 461.

Banks, M. D., Pontes, J. E., Izbicki, R. M., and Pierce, J. M., Jr. (1976). *J. Urol. 118,* 757.

Barsel, V. A., Dulkin, L. M. and Demidov, A. T. (1977). *Vopr. Onkol. 23,* 50.

Bracken, R. B., Johnson, D. E., Rodriguez, L. H., Samuels, M. L. and Ayala, A. (1977). *Urology* *9*, 161.

Bruce, D. W., and Edgcomb, J. H. (1967). *J. Urol. 97*, 482.

Bunge, R. G. (1952). *J. Urol. 68*, 475.

Cooper, P. H., Waisman, J., Johnson, W. H., and Skinner, D. G. (1955). *Cancer 31*, 1055.

Edsmyer, F., and Boman, J. (1971). *Acta. Radio. 9*, 395.

Eisenberg, R. B., Roth, R. B., and Schweinsbert, M. H. (1960). *J. Urol. 84*, 544.

Eonly, K., Elias, E. G., Mittleman, A., Albert, P., and Murphy, G. P. (1973). *Cancer 31*, 1150.

Esquivel, E. L., Jr., Mackenzie, A. R., and Whitmore, W. F., Jr. (1965). *Invest. Urol. 2*, 381-386.

Hall, R. R., Schade, R. O. K., and Swinney, J. (1974). *Brit. Med. J. 2*, 593.

Harada, N., and Kusunoki, T. (1968). *J. Urol. 99*, 725.

Helmstein, K. (1972). *Brit. J. Urol. 44*, 434.

Jones, H. C. and Swinney, J. (1961). *Lancet 2*, 615.

Koss, L. G., Tiamson, E. P., and Robbins, M. A. (1974). *JAMA 225*, 281.

Melicow, M. M., and Hollowell, J. W. (1952). *J. Urol. 68*, 763.

Miller, L. S. and Johnson, D. E. (1973). "Seventh National Cancer Congress," pp. 771-782. J. B. Lippincott Co., Philadelphia, Pa.

Mishina, T., Oda, K., Murata, S., Ooe, H., Mori, Y., and Takahashi, T. (1975). *Urol. 114*, 217.

Nieh, P. T., Daly, J. J., Heaney, J. A., Heney, N. M., and Prout, G. R. (1978). *J. Urol. 119*, 59.

Ogata, J., Migita, N., and Nakamura, T. (1973). *J. Urol. 110*, 667.

Ozaki, Y. (1977). *Jap. J. Urol. 68*, 934.

Robinson, M. R., Shelley, M. B., Richards, B., Bostable, J., Blashan, R. W., and Smith, P. H. (1977). *J. Urol. 118*, 972.

Schade, R. O. K., and Swinney, J. (1968). *Lancet 2*, 943.

Semple, J. R. (1948). *Brit. Med. J. 1*, 1235.

Uyama, T., and Kagawa, S. (1977). *Nishinihan J. Urol. 39*, 916.

Veenema, R. J. (1968). *JAMA 206*, 2725.

Veenema, R. J., Dean, A. L., Jr., Roberts, M., Fingerhut, B., Choevhury, B. K., and Tarassaly, H., (1965). *Urol. 2*, 381.

Veenema, R. J., Dean, A. L., Jr., Uson, A. C., Roberts, M., and Longo, F. (1969). *J. Urol. 101*, 711.

Wakaki, S., Muramo, H., Tamora, K., Shipmpizu, G., Kato, E. Kamada, H., Kudo, S., and Fujimoto, Y. (1958). *Antibiot. Chemother. 8*, 228.

Wallace, D. M. (1971). *Brit. J. Urol. 43*, 177.

Washida, H., Ueda, K., Watanabe, H., and Watari, N. (1977). *Acta. Urol. Jap. 23*, 567.

Werf-Messing, V. D. (1971). *Clin. Radiol. 22*, 101.

Williams, R. E. (1975). In "The Biology and Clinical Management of Bladder Cancer" (E. H. Cooper and R. E. Williams, eds.), p. 182. Blackwell Scientific Publications, London.

Yoshida, H., Saito, T., Ikeuchi, T., Maruyama, K., and Imamuka, K. (1977). *Acta. Urol. Jap. 23*, 51.

Chapter 24

MITOMYCIN C IN CHILDHOOD CANCER: A REVIEW

Manuel L. Gutierrez

I. INTRODUCTION

Mitomycin C was first introduced for clinical trials in the United States in 1958, and initial studies showed demonstrable chemotherapeutic activity but a discouragingly high level of toxicity (Jones, 1959; Evans, 1961). Subsequent refinements in the dose scheduling have resulted in the reduction of myelosuppression associated with mitomycin C.

As a single agent, mitomycin C has shown activity in breast, stomach, colorectal, pancreatic, and head and neck carcinomas (Manheimer and Vital, 1966; Wise et al., 1976; Moore et al., 1968; Crooke and Bradner, 1976). It is also possibly active in adenocarcinoma of the lung, ovary, biliary tree, and cervix (Manheimer and Vital, 1966; Moore et al., 1968; Crooke and Bradner, 1976). In combination with other agents, mitomycin C has demonstrated significant antitumor activity against several diseases such as adenocarcinoma of the stomach (Ota et al., 1972) and squamous cell carcinoma of the cervix (Baker et al., 1974).

Although it has a wide range of antineoplastic activity in adults, mitomycin C has demonstrated relatively limited activity in the treatment of childhood malignancies (Evans, 1961; Baker et al., 1974; Sutow et al., 1971; Evans et al., 1969; Jaffe et al., 1971). The fact that only very limited clinical trials have been performed is probably due to the impact of the disappointing results obtained by early workers. A review of the limited studies on mitomycin C in childhood cancer is the basis of this report.

II. DOSAGE SCHEDULES

Evans (1961) reported the first clinical trial of mitomycin C in children. In the first few patients entered in the study, varying dose schedules were used. The highest dose was 2.5 mg/kg given over 15 weeks. Subsequent doses varied from 0.4 mg/kg to 1.0 mg/kg given over 2-10 days. Doses higher than 0.6 mg/kg were associated with severe toxicity. Doses between 0.4 and 0.6 mg/kg given as a 0.1 or 0.2 mg/kg per day injection were suggested as the most satisfactory in avoiding significant toxicity (Evans *et al.*, 1969).

Sutow *et al.* (1971) of the Southwest Oncology Group initiated in 1970 a phase I trial utilizing several dose schedules. The number of patients included in each regimen, however, was too small for proper evaluation of its efficacy. Table II presents information on the various dosage schedules of mitomycin C used in children.

In combination with vincristine and phenylalanine mustard Jaffe *et al.* (1971) used mitomycin C at a dose of 0.1 mg/kg. The three drugs were administered intravenously at weekly intervals. Sinniah *et al.* (1974) adopted a combination of mitomycin C and vincristine in treating patients with hepatoblastoma. Mitomycin C was given at a dose of 0.04-0.09 mg/kg or 2 mg/m^2 IV weekly from 1 to 4 doses before surgery.

A. Antitumor Activity

1. As a Single Agent

Forty-two children with leukemia and various types of solid tumors were included in the initial study by Evans (1961). Significant tumor regression occurred

TABLE I. Objective Responses to Mitomycin C as a Single Agent in Childhood Cancer

Tumor types	Evans (1961)	Evans *et al.* (1969)	Sutow *et al.* (1971)
	References		
	(Responders/evaluable cases)		
Osteosarcoma	3/14	0/13	0/5
Rhabdomyosarcoma		2/7	1/4
Hodgkin's disease	1/3		
Neuroblastoma		0/2	0/1
Ewing's sarcoma		0/3	0/2
Neurofibrosarcoma			1/1
Unclassified sarcoma			1/5
Acute leukemia	0/3		
Chronic leukemia			1/1
Miscellaneous		0/9	0/3

TABLE II. Mitomycin Dosage Schedules in Childhood Cancer

References	Dosage schedules	No. of patients treated	No. of courses or pulses
Evans, (1961)	0.4-1.0 mg/kg given in 2-10 days	62	
Evans et al. (1969)	0.2 mg/kg or 6 mg/m^2 q 14 days for 5 doses in 10 weeks	16	
Sutow et al. (1971)	0.1 mg/kg/day x 4		1
	0.1 mg/kg/day x 5		8
	0.15 mg/kg/day x 4		2
	0.15 mg/kg/day x 5	21	10
	0.4 mg/kg x 1		7
	0.6 mg/kg x 1		2
	1.0 mg/kg x 1		1

in 3/17 patients with metastatic osteogenic sarcoma. Two of the 7 patients with rhabdomyosarcoma, 1/3 with Hodgkin's disease and 1/1 with chronic granulocytic leukemia also showed objective responses. In this particular study, the overall response rate to mitomycin C was approximately 16%. This regimen was associated with severe myelosuppression observed in over 50% of the patients. A follow-up study was undertaken by the same group utilizing an intermediate dose schedule to lessen toxicity (Evans et al., 1969). Thirteen patients with metastatic osteogenic sarcoma received mitomycin C at a dose of 0.2 mg/kg or 6 mg/m^2 every 14 days for 5 doses in 10 weeks. Toxicity varied from none to severe myelosuppression. However, no response was obtained. Using multiple dose schedules as outlined in Table II, Sutow et al. (1971) of the Southwest Oncology Group treated 21 patients with various types of solid tumors. Three responses were reported, one each in unclassified sarcoma, neurofibrosarcoma, and rhabdomyosarcoma.

2. In Combination with Other Antineoplastic Agents

Due to the poor objective tumor responses and the severe toxicities encountered in the early studies, clinical trials using mitomycin C in combination with other chemotherapeutic agents are very few.

Jaffe et al. (1971) reported the effect of a combination of mitomycin C, phenylalanine mustard, and vincristine against metastatic osteogenic sarcoma. Ten patients were treated with the combination regimen. Although dose limiting toxicity was not encountered, only one transient partial response was obtained.

In a review of 20 patients with primary hepatic cancer in Kuala Lumpur, Malaysia, Sinniah et al. (1974) reported an increase in the duration of survival of patients if chemotherapy was employed before or after surgery. Mitomycin C and vincristine appeared to be the most effective combination. Six patients ranging in age from 1 to 2½ months were given vincristine and mitomycin C prior to surgery. Postoperatively, 5/6 patients received a single dose of the same combination. One pa-

TABLE III. Mitomycin C in Combination Regimens in Childhood Cancer

References	Combination regimens	Diagnosis	No. of patients treated	No. of responders
Jaffe et al. (1971)	MMC: 0.1 mg/kg/week PAM: 0.2 mg/kg/week VCR: 0.025 mg/kg/week	Metastatic osteogenic sarcoma	10	1
Sinniah et al. (1974)	MMC: 0.04-0.09 mg/kg or 2 mg/m^2/week x 1-6 doses VCR: 2 mg/m^2/week x 1	Hepatoblastoma	6	3

tient received 8 weekly doses after surgery. Three of the 6 patients were alive and well from 36-54 months after surgery at the time of the report.

III. TOXICITY

Myelosuppression affecting particularly the leukocytes and platelets was the most prominent toxicity encountered in adults. The hematologic toxicity was dose related and was usually delayed. Other less common side effects included gastrointestinal disturbances, alopecia, stomatitis, severe cellulitis at the injection site if extravasation occurred and, rarely, skin rash.

In children, the toxic effects of mitomycin C were similar to those in adults. Over 50% of those patients who received a total dose of 0.5 mg/kg or more in the study by Evans (1961) developed severe toxicity. Each subsequent course of therapy was usually associated with more prolonged depression of the bone marrow. In the clinical trials conducted by Sutow et al. (1971), all the dose regimens used were frequently associated with moderate to severe leukopenia and thrombocytopenia. The single large infrequent intravenous doses were better tolerated, however. The nadir of the thrombocytopenia usually occurred in the latter part of the third to the sixth week of treatment. The nadir of leukopenia usually coincided with the lowest platelet count. Bone marrow recovery to its pretreatment value was achieved approximately 2 weeks after the last dose of mitomycin C in most patients.

IV. DISCUSSION

Mitomycin C was studied initially in children with cancer several years ago but failed to be of significant value. The disappointing results obtained by early workers probably accounted for the subsequent limited studies utilizing this drug in childhood neoplasms.

Recently developed single large infrequent dosage regimens have resulted in improved clinical utility in adults (Wise et al., 1976; Godfrey and Wilbur, 1972; Baker et al., 1976). The use of such dosage regimens has never been extensively studied in pediatric tumors. Thus it may be of value to study the effects of mitomycin C administered on the high dose infrequent schedule in children with cancer.

REFERENCES

Baker, L. H., Caoli, F. M., Izbicki, R. M., Opipari, M. I., and Vaitkevicius, V. K. (1974). *Proc. Am. Assoc. Cancer Res. 15,* 182.

Baker, L. H., Izbicki, R. M., and Vaitkevicius, V. K. (1976). *Med. Rediatr. Onco. 2,* 207-213.

Crooke, S. T., and Bradner, W. T. (1976). *Cancer Treat. Rev. 3,* 121-139.

Evans, A. E. (1961). *Cancer Chemother. Rep. 14,* 1-9.

Evans, A. E., Heyn, R., Nesbit, M., and Hartmann, J. R. (1969). *Cancer Chemother. Rep. 53,* 297-298.

Godfrey, T., and Wilbur, D. (1972). *Cancer 29,* 1647-1652.

Jaffee, N., Traggis, D., and Enriquez, C. (1971). *Cancer Chemother. Rep. 55,* 189-191.

Jones, R., Jr. (1959). *Cancer Chemother. Rep. 3,* 3-7.

Manheimer, L., and Vital, J. (1966). *Cancer 19,* 207-212.

Moore, G. E., Bross, I. D., Ausman, R., Nadler, S., Jones, R., Slack, N., and Rimm, A. (1968). *Cancer Chemother. Rep. 52,* 675-684.

Ota, K., Kurita, S., Nishimura, M., Ogawa, M., Kamei, Y., Kunyuki, I., Murahami, M., Oyama, A., Hoshero, A., Amo, H., and Kato, T. (1972). *Cancer Chemother. Rep. 56,* 373-385.

Sinniah, D., Campbell, P. E., and Colebatch, J. H. (1974). *Prog. Pediatr. Surg. 7,* 141-170.

Sutow, W. W., Wilbur, J. R., Vietti, T. H., Vuthibhagdee, P., and Fujimoto, T. (1971). *Cancer Chemother. Rep. 55,* 285-289.

Wise, G. R., Kuhn, I. N., and Godfrey, R. E. (1976). *Med. Pediatr, Oncol. 2,* 55-60.

Chapter 25

CLINICAL AND PATHOLOGIC STUDY OF MITOMYCIN C NEPHROTOXICITY

Voravit Ratanatharathorn
Laurence H. Baker
Pravit Cadnapaphornchai
Barbara F. Rosenberg
Vainutis K. Vaitkevicius

I. INTRODUCTION

Since mitomycin C was introduced into clinical practice over a decade ago, much has been learned regarding optimal dose schedule and antitumor activity. Despite extensive phase I and II studies, little had been mentioned regarding its potential nephrotoxicity until it was reported by Liu *et al.* (1971). In this review, we will attempt to analyze the previous reports of nephrotoxicity caused by administration of mitomycin C and the data that we have accumulated at our institution and at the Southwest Oncology Group over the past 4 years.

Mitomycin C is an antibiotic that was isolated from *Streptomyces caespitosus.* Animal and human pharmacology has been extensively studied both in this country and Japan over the last two decades (Jones, 1959; Philips *et al.,* 1960; Schwartz *et al.,* 1961; Schwartz *et al.,* 1963; Fujita *et al.,* 1971). In the experimental animals, two types of pathologic changes in the urinary system were described. A papillomatous proliferation of the epithelium at the uretero-pelvic junction was seen following prolonged intraperitoneal injections of subtoxic doses, leading to ureteral obstruction (Matsuyama *et al.,* 1964). A similar lesion has not been reported in man. Secondly, when Philips *et al.* (1960) administered 2 mg/kg of mitomycin C intravenously to two rhesus monkeys, both developed severe watery diarrhea. The histopathologic picture of tubular necrosis was noted. These histologic changes could also be due to volume depletion and shock secondary to severe diarrhea. A single dose of mitomycin C equivalent to that given to the rhesus monkeys has not been used in man.

In the review of 14 series of clinical trials of mitomycin C in the English literature published from 1959 to 1977, only 8 out of 1245 patients treated with various dose schedules were reported to have developed nephrotoxicity (Table I). Of the eight cases, only the three reported by Liu *et al.* (1971) contained detailed clinical information. Kidney biopsy of Liu's cases showed characteristic changes of the glomerular tufts, especially on the nuclei. The true incidence of mitomycin C nephrotoxicity cannot be estimated accurately from the literature reviewed because of short follow-up in those phase I-II studies, lack of clinical detail to exclude other causes, and, most frequently, lack of serial renal function studies.

Questions still remain: Is mitomycin C nephrotoxic? If so, is there any dose relationship to this toxicity? Finally, are there any characteristic histopathologic changes in the kidney?

Although nephrotoxicity related to mitomycin C has been reported in several previous studies, true incidence remains unknown. Difficulties in establishing the clinical nephrotoxicity of mitomycin C are due to several factors:

1.   The diversity of known nephrotoxic agents that patients may be receiving concomitantly with mitomycin C at the time renal failure is recognized. The most common drugs frequently implicated as a cause of renal failure are the antibiotics, especially the aminoglycoside group (Appel and Neu, 1977). In addition, combinations of antitumor agents are also frequently employed, and some of these agents are known to be nephrotoxic, for example, *cis*-platinum (Talley *et al.*, 1973), streptozotocin (Broder and Carter, 1973), mithramycin (Kennedy, 1970), methotrexate (Pitman *et al.*, 1975), and cytoxan (Lopes, 1967).

2.   Complexity of the clinical course associated with advanced carcinoma:
     a. Dehydration due to poor fluid intake or diuretic administration.
     b. Effusion in the thoracic and peritoneal cavities which often necessitates drainage of symptomatic relief.
     c. Cardiocirculatory failure due to underlying arteriosclerotic heart disease, anthracycline-induced cardiomyopathy, sepsis.
     d. Obstructive uropathy along the course of the ureter, which is most common in pelvic tumors. Occasionally, obstruction can occur in the tubular level by tumor metabolities such as myeloma protein (Martinez-Maldonado *et al.*, 1971) or uric acid crystal. Rarely, renal parenchymal invasion by the tumor itself leads to renal failure.
     e. Miscellaneous metabolic disturbance, for example, hypercalcemia: hypokalemia if prolonged can eventually lead to renal failure (Epstein, 1971).
     Only when all these clinical factors are dissected in each patient with renal

TABLE I. Review of Clinical Trial of Mitomycin C in Adults

Report	No. of patients treated[a]	Dose schedule	Total dose (mg)	Total dose (mg/kg)	Nephrotoxicity
Jones et al. (1959)	120	0.1-25 mg/kg IV daily	–	0.3-1.0	Not mentioned.
Miller et al. (1962)	33	10-30 mg daily continuous IV infusion	60-80	1.1-21	One patient who developed uremia died 14 days after initiation of treatment. Another patient developed azotemia but recovered uneventfully.
Manheimer and Vital (1966)	46	IV daily, weekly and twice weekly	12-147	0.2-2.0	One patient developed azotemia.
Moertel et al. (1968)	95	0.15 mg/kg daily x 5 0.15 mg/kg daily x 6	24-60	–	Not mentioned.
Horton et al. (1968)	75	0.075 mg/kg weekly	–	–	Not mentioned.
Moore et al. (1968)	346	0.05 mg/kg daily x 6 then Q. O. D.	12-50	–	Not mentioned.
Mansfield (1969)	23	0.05 mg/kg daily x 6 then Q. O. D.	17.7-155.5	–	Not mentioned.
Whittington and Close (1970)	257	0.05 mg/kg IV daily x 10	–	–	One patient developed uremia.
Liu et al. (1971)	32	0.5-1.0 mg/kg IV every 4-8 weeks	–	–	Three patients developed nephrotoxicity. Total doses were given 105, 230, and 245 mg.
Godfrey and Wilbur (1972)	106	20-30 mg IV every 3-4 days	18-168	0.27-3.0	No nephrotoxicity observed.
Van Dyke et al. (1972)	45	10 mg IV twice weekly x 5 doses	50	–	No nephrotoxicity observed.
Early et al. (1973)	21	0.25-1.0 mg/kg biweekly	–	–	One patient died from nephrotoxicity. Total dose received was not mentioned.
Baker (1976)	32	22.5 mg/m² every 8 weeks	–	–	No nephrotoxicity observed.
Buroker et al. (1977)	14	15 mg/m² every 8 weeks	–	–	No nephrotoxicity observed.

[a] Total number of patients treated: 1245.   [b] Number of patients with nephrotoxicity reported: 8.

function abnormalties and no other causes found can mitomycin C be implicated as a potential nephrotoxic agent.

3. When clinical nephrotoxicity due to mitomycin C is suspected, it is often difficult to justify a kidney biopsy in the presence of progressive primary disease. Only 3 case reports on histopathology of the kidney associated with mitomycin C have been published.

4. Previous reports suggest that mitomycin C nephrotoxicity is most likely dose related. To reach a critical cumulative dose, the follow-up period at the dose schedule commonly employed would have to exceed 24 weeks. The majority of the patients who were treated with mitomycin C will usually not survive long enough to develop this complication; therefore, large numbers of patients will be required to determine the incidence of nephrotoxicity.

II. MATERIALS AND METHODS

We originally studied 68 patients treated at the Department of Oncology, Wayne State University from 1972 to 1974. Complete clinical data were available on all patients. All patients but one have died; at the time of this writing one patient (J. F.) remains alive and well, off therapy for the past 92 weeks. Forty-seven patients underwent autopsy, and three were excluded because of poor tissue preservation of autopsy materials. Tumor types and patient stratification according to total dose administered are shown in Table II. All these patients had received similar dose schedules of mitomycin C given by bolus injection of 15-20 mg/m^2 intravenously

TABLE II. Patient Characteristics

	Group I	Group II	Group III
Cumulative dose (mg)	≤49	50-99	>100
Total No. of patients	19	20	29
Age:			
Range	36-77	43-75	29-70
Mean	59	58	56
Sex:			
Male	13	13	17
Female	6	7	12
Tumor Type:			
CA cervix	2	2	0
CA stomach	3	5	11
CA rectum	4	4	10
CA pancreas	3	3	4
CA esophagus	0	3	0
Hepatoma	2	0	2
CA gallbladder	1	0	1
Renal cell CA	1	1	0
Miscellaneous	3	2	1
Total No. with autopsy	18	17	12
No. with evaluable autopsy material	17	16	11
No. without autopsy	1	3	17

every 6 to 8 weeks. Abnormal renal functions were defined as BUN of above 20 mg/dl and/or creatinine above 2 mg/dl. Renal failure was considered present if creatinine was consistently elevated above 2 mg/dl. Renal histology obtained at autopsy was reviewed by the pathologist who participated in this study with no knowledge of the clinical data. Statistical analysis was performed using Student's T test and chi-square test where applicable.

Mean BUN and serum creatinine values for the three groups were 22.2 mg/dl (range 7-65 mg/dl) and 1.2 mg/dl(range 0.3-1.9 mg/dl) for group I; 24 mg/dl (range 9-65 mg/dl) and 1.3 mg/dl (range 0.8-18 mg/dl) for group II; and 21.6 mg/dl (range 7-65 mg/dl) and 1.4 mg/dl (range 0.5-2.8 mg/dl) for group III. There were no statistical differences among the groups.

III. RESULTS

Although the ranges of the BUN serum creatinine values varied, only 10 patients had BUN higher than 30 mg/dl and/or serum creatinine higher than 2 mg/dl; for these 10 patients the clinical data were analyzed in detail (Table III). In nine patients, renal histology was available for evaluation. Of these, four had normal findings and five were abnormal; three had fibrin thrombi in the glomeruli, one had renal cortical necrosis, and the remaining patient had pyknotic glomerular nuclei with segmental collapse and bizarre giant cells. Three patients were hypotensive 24 hr before death; one patient was in congestive heart failure and had received large doses of furosemide. Three patients had received concomitant administration of gentamicin.

Four of the 68 patients developed renal failure: one in group II and three in group III; the frequency of renal failure had no correlation with the total dose received ($p = 0.32$).

The last patient in group III (J. F.) showed persistent elevation of the BUN (37 mg/dl) and serum creatinine (2.8 mg/dl) 92 weeks after the last dose of mitomycin C. She also had recurrent urinary tract infection (*E. Coli*) and had been treated with several courses of oral cephalosporin. Intravenous pyelography was not done because of previous anaphylatic reaction to the contrast medium. Renal scan and renogram subsequently showed no evidence of obstruction. Chronic pyelonephritis was suggested to be the cause of renal failure in this patient.

Histologic findings of the kidneys in the autopsied group were summarized in Table IV. Changes consistent with acute tubular necrosis were seen in three patients: one in group I and two in group III. Two patients had sepsis and hypotension. All three patients had received gentamicin. Although none of these patients had BUN and serum creatinine values above 30 mg/dl and 2 mg/dl respectively, this could be related to the rapid clinical course of the disease.

Pyknotic glomerular nuclei with segmental collapse and bizarre giant cells were seen in five patients. Two of the five patients had hypotension, and one of these had also received gentamicin. Hypotension was secondary to pulmonary embolism

TABLE III. Clinical and Histologic Findings of Patients with Abnormal Renal Functions
(BUN 30 mg/dl and/or Creatinine 2 mg/dl)

Group	Name	BUN	Creat.	Hypo-tension	Dehy-dration	CHF	Urinary Obs.	Infection UTI	Infection Sepsis	Infection Others	Other Nephro-toxic agents	Histologic findings of the kidneys
I	O.P.	65	1.8	none	none	none	Rt. ureter	none	none	none	none	Fibrin thrombi in the glomeruli
	H.A.	52	1.6	none	none	none	none	Gram. neg. org.	E. coli	none	none	Fibrin thrombi in the glomeruli
	G.G.	32	1.6	present	present	none	none	none	none	none	none	Renal cortical necrosis
II	A.O.	31	1.7	none	present	present	none	none	none	none	none	Normal
	E.H.	31	1.7	none	none	none	none	none	none	none	none	Normal
	J.V.[a]	65	1.8	present	present	none	none	none	none	none	Genta	Pyknotic glomerular nuclei with seg. collapse & bizarre giant cells
	E.C.[b]	43	2.8	present	present	none	none	none	none	none	Genta	Fibrin thrombi in the glomeruli
III	J.E.	65	2.6	none	none	none	Bilat.	none	Pseudomonas	Pneumonia Klebsiella	none	Normal
	F.P.	24	2.1	none	present	none	none	none	none	Broncho-pneumonia	Genta	Normal
	J.F.[c]	37	2.8	none	none	none	none	E. Coli	none	none	none	Not available

[a] J. V. also had massive pulmonary embolism on autopsy.
[b] Four patients were considered to have renal failure (E. C., J. E., F. P., J. F.) where creatinine was elevated above 2 mg/dl.
[c] This patient is still alive; BUN and creatinine values were obtained 23 months following the last dose of MMC. She also has recurrent UTI and has been treated with several courses of oral cephalosporin antibiotic.

TABLE IV. Cross Tabulation of Dose Range and Histologic Findings[a]

Dose range	No. of patients	Normal	Consistent with acute tubular necrosis	Pyknotic glom. nuclei & segmental collapse & bizarre giant cells	Fibrin thrombi in the glom.	Subcapsular scarring & chronic interstitial nephritis	Others
49	17	10	1	1	2	1	2[b]
50-99	16	11	0	1	1	2	1[c]
100	11	5	2	3[d]	1	0	0
Total	44	26	3	5	4	3	3

[a]Chi-square value 10.236 and p value of 0.4201.
[b]One had renal cortical necrosis, the other had nephrosclerosis.
[c]Findings consistent with diabetic glomerulopathy.
[d]These 3 patients also had fibrin thrombi in the glomeruli.

in one patient, and the other had staphylococcal aureus sepsis. In the latter, multiple staphylococcal microabscesses were found in the kidneys at autopsy. The third patient had bacterial meningitis which caused rapid death. The remaining two patients died from far-advanced carcinoma, one of whom was also found to have pneumonitis at autopsy. Only one of the five patients (J.V.) had abnormal renal function with BUN OF 65 mg/dl and creatinine of 1.8 mg/dl. These findings could be explained by the presence of hypotension and gentamicin administration.

Fibrin thrombi in the glomeruli were noted in seven patients. None of these patients was suspected of having disseminated intravascular coagulation prior to death. Three of the four patients in group III who had these findings also had pyknotic glomerular nuclei with segmental collapse. Three patients in this group had abnormal renal functions (Table III). Only one patient had a serum creatinine above 2 mg/dl; this patient had also received concomitant gentamicin.

Subcapsular scarring and findings consistent with chronic interstitial nephritis were seen in three patients. Unilateral ureteral obstruction associated with infections were present in two patients. None of these patients had significant renal function impairment.

Miscellaneous histologic findings consisted of one case each of diabetic glomerulopathy, nephrosclerosis, and renal cortical necrosis. These lesions were related to the patient's preexisting diabetes, hypertension, and volume depletion.

From this study several conclusions can be drawn. In the relatively small group of patients treated, we cannot demonstrate any conclusive evidence of mitomycin C nephrotoxicity. Although the incidence of renal failure (creatinine > 2mg/dl) is higher in the group who had received more than 100 mg total dose, this is not statistically significant. There were other factors that could have explained their renal function abnormalities: Of the four patients with renal failure (1 in group II, 3 in group III), two patients had been receiving gentamicin, one patient had bilateral ureteral obstruction, and one had recurrent urinary tract infection.

Histopathologic findings as described by Liu *et al.* (1971) in their three patients who developed nephrotoxicity were also noted in 5 of 44 autopsied patients in one series. These five patients were distributed among three groups who received various cumulative dosages. There is no statistical difference in the distribution of the pathologic findings among these three groups. Clinical evidence of nephrotoxicity was also lacking. Pyknotic glomerular nuclei with segmental collapse and the presence of giant cells appears to be a nonspecific pathologic change and bears no relationship to the cumulative dose of mitomycin C received. Various histopathologic findings in the kidneys of severely ill patients also had been noted by other investigators, but these were without apparent effect on renal function.

A. Southwest Oncology Group Study

Because of the inconclusive evidence of mitomycin C nephrotoxicity in the Wayne State University study, we felt that a larger number of patients would be required to answer this important question. In 1974, SWOG had activated a phase

III randomized trial of 5-FU infusion and mitomycin C versus 5-FU infusion and methyl-CCNU. Since neither 5-FU nor methyl-CCNU has been reported to produce nephrotoxicity, the incidence of renal insufficiency developed in each group allows an estimation of nephrotoxicity and dose response relationships to mitomycin C.

Of the 150 evaluable patients with various gastrointestinal carcinomas treated in the SWOG study from 1974 to 1977, 272 patients were randomized to receive 4-day infusion of 5-FU at the dose of 100 mg/m^2/day every 4 weeks and mitomycin C at 15-20 mg/m^2 every 8 weeks. The remaining 238 patients received similar dose schedules of 5-FU and methyl-CCNU at 175 mg/m^2 orally every 8 weeks. All patients had normal renal functions prior to initiation of treatment and had to have at least one set of renal function tests available 4 weeks after the first course of treatment. Only the last or highest values of BUN creatinine were used in the statistical analysis.

B. Results

To ensure comparability of renal function follow-up of the 510 patients randomized to both treatment arms, the durations from the time that chemotherapy started to the last available renal function tests were determined. The median duration of follow-up (17 weeks) was similar in both groups. Results of renal function studies are summarized in Table V. The mean BUN and creatinine values were higher in the group who received 5-FU + mitomycin C compared to the group who received 5-FU + methyl-CCNU (18.85 mg/dl and 1.35 mg/dl versus 16.79 mg/dl and 1.09 mg/dl, respectively). However, the difference only reached a statistically significant level with creatinine values ($p = 0.01$). Of the 510 patients in this study, only 326 patients had serial determination of creatinine: 171 in the 5-FU + mitomycin C group and 155 in the 5-FU + methyl-CCNU group. When the criteria for renal failure (creatinine > 2 mg/dl) were applied to determine the incidence of renal failure in the two groups, 17 of 171 in the 5-FU + mitomycin C group and 5 of 155 in the 5-FU + methyl-CCNU group developed renal failure following initiation of chemotherapy; this difference is statistically significant ($p = 0.01$). Higher incidence of renal failure in the 5-FU + mitomycin C group, therefore, explained the overall higher creatinine values in the group receiving 5-FU + mitomycin C. Correlation was found between the incidence of renal failure and total dose of mitomycin C administered (Table VI).

TABLE V.   Renal Function Studies: 5-FU + Mitomycin C versus
5-FU + Methyl-CCNU

	No.	5-FU + MMC	5-FU + MeCCNU
Mean BUN (mg/dl)	476	18.85 (3-88)	16.79 $p = 0.064$ (6-101)
Mean Creatinine (mg/dl)	326	1.35 (0.6-9.3)	1.09 $p = 0.01$ (0.6-5.3)
Freuency of Renal		17/77	5/155 $p = 0.01$

TABLE VI. Frequency of Renal Failure in Patients Who Received
5-FU + Mitomycin C

Total dose of mitomycin C (mg)	≤49	50-99	≥100
No. of patients	45	85	41[a]
No. with renal failue	5	4	8

The conclusions from the SWOG study can be summarized as follows:

1. Incidence of renal failure is higher in the group that received 5-FU + mito-mycin C compared to the group that received 5-FU + methyl-CCNU. Although other causes of renal failure could not be identified from this large cooperative group study because of unavailability of detailed clinical information, these varia-bles should be negated in this large randomized study. The only difference between the treatment arms was the inclusion of either mitomycin C or methyl-CCNU. We therefore concluded that mitomycin C is probably nephrotoxic.

2. Nephrotoxicity of mitomycin C appears to be dose related.

IV. DISCUSSION

It took several years of wide use of the drug before we recognized the possible nephrotoxic effect of mitomycin C. Despite extensive analysis of our clinical and pathologic data, several controversies remain. Our data suggest nephrotoxic poten-tial, but the true incidence and histopathologic characterisitics still have to be verified. The answers to these questions can only be arrived at by a large prospec-tive study in a single institution with careful serial monitoring of renal functions, and with all clinical details available for final analysis. Until such information be-comes available, physicians should be aware of the nephrotoxic potential of mito-mycin C. Meticulous review of the patient's clinical course will usually help to determine the cause of nephrotoxicity.

REFERENCES

Ansfield, F. J. (1969). *Cancer Chemother. Rep. 53*, 287-289.

Appel, G. B., and Neu, H. C. (1977). *N. Engl. J. Med. 296*, 663-670. 722-728, 784-787.

Baker, L. H., Izbicki, R. M., and Vaitkevicius, V. K. (1976). *Med. Pediatr. Oncol. 2*, 207-213.

Broder, L. G., and Carter, S. K. (1973). *Ann. Int. Med. 79*, 108-118.

Buroker, T. R., Baker, L. H., Correa, J., Schwartz, L. S., and Vaitkevicius, V. K. (1977). *Cancer Treat. Rep. 61*, 463-467.

Early, K., Elias, E. G., Albert, D., and Murphy, G. P. (1973). *Cancer 31*, 1150-1153.

Epstein, F (1971). *In* "Diseases of the Kidney" (M. B. Straus and L. G. Welt, eds.), pp. 903-931. Little, Brown, Boston, Mass.

Fujita, H. (1971). *Jap. J. Clin. Oncol. 12*, 151-162.

Godfrey, T. E., and Wilbur, D. W. (1972). *Cancer 29*, 1647-1652.

Horton, J., Olson, K. B., Cunningham, T. and Sullivan, J. (1968). *Cancer Chemother. Rep. 52*, 597-600.

Jones, R., Jr. (1959). *Cancer Chemother. Rep. 2,* 3-7.

Kennedy, B. J. (1970). *Am. J. Med. 49,* 494.

Liu, K., Mittelman, A., Sproal, E. E., and Elias, E. G. (1971). *Cancer 28,* 1314-1320.

Lopes, V. M. (1967). *Lancet 1,* 1060.

Manheimer, L. H., and Vital, J. (1966). *Cancer 19,* 207-212.

Martinez-Maldonado, M., Yium, J., Suki, W. N., and Eknoyan, G. (1971). *J. Chron. Dis. 24,* 221-237.

Matsuyama, M., Suzumori, K., and Nakamura, T. (1964). *Nature 202,* 99-100.

Miller, E., Sullivan, R. D., and Schryssochoos, T. (1972). *Cancer Chemother. Rep. 21,* 129-135.

Moertel, C. E., Reitmeier, R. J., and Hahn, R. G. (1968). *JAMA 204,* 1045-1048.

Moore, G. E., Bross, I. D. J., Ansman, R., Nadler, S., Jones, R., Slack, N., and Rimm, A. A. (1968). *Cancer Chemother. Rep. 52,* 675-684.

Philips, F. S., Schwartz, H. S., and Sternberg, S. S. (1960). *Cancer Res. 20,* 1345-1361.

Pitman, S. W., Parker, L. M., Tattersall, M. H. N., Jaffe, N., and Frei, E. III. (1975). *Cancer Chemother. Rep. 6,* 43-49.

Schwartz, H. S. and Philips, F. S. (1961). *J. Pharm. Exp. Ther. 33,* 335-342.

Schwartz, H. S., Sternberg, S. S., and Philips, F. S. (1963). *Cancer Res. 23,* 1125-1136.

Talley, R. W., O'Bryan, R. M., Gutterman, J. U., Brownlee, R. W., and McCredie, K. B. (1973). *Cancer Chemother. Rep. 57,* 465-471.

Van Dyke, J. J., Falkson, G., and Falkson, H. C. (1972). *S. Afr. Med. J. 46,* 1921-1926.

Whittington, R. M., Close, H. P. (1970). *Cancer Chemother. Rep. 54,* 195-198.

Chapter 26

PULMONARY TOXICITY OF MITOMYCIN

Silvana Martino
Laurence H. Baker
Richard J. Pollard
Juan J. Correa
Michael D. DeMattia

I. INTRODUCTION

The most common toxicities of mitomycin C have been well described. The most significant toxicity in man is myelosuppression. Leukopenia, thrombocytopenia, and to a lesser extent anemia commonly occur (Baker *et al.,* 1974; Moore *et al.,* 1968). Other toxicities that have been reported are severe local cellulitis if extravasation of the drug occurs (Moore *et al.,* 1968; Buzdar *et al.,* 1978), and gastrointestinal symptoms such as anorexia, nausea, vomiting, and diarrhea. Fever, alopecia, stomatitis, and skin rashes have been observed (Bristol, 1977). Other side effects whose causal relationship to mitomycin is less clear have also been described: headaches, blurring of vision, confusion, drowsiness, syncope, fatigue, edema, thrombophlebitis, and hematemesis (Bristol, 1977). An unusual toxicity described with mitomycin use is renal failure (Liu *et al.,* 1971; Ratanatharathorn *et al.,* 1977). Changes in hepatic function concomitant with mitomycin administration have been described (Robert *et al.,* 1968). An uncommon, and only recently described, toxicity of mitomycin is a histologic picture of interstitial pneumonitis and pulmonary fibrosis. We have observed a number of patients who have

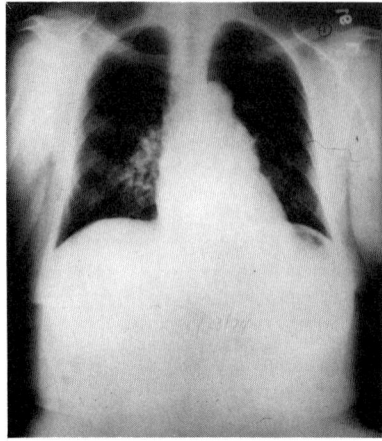

Fig. 1a.   Bilateral pulmonary infiltrate following six doses of mitomycin C.

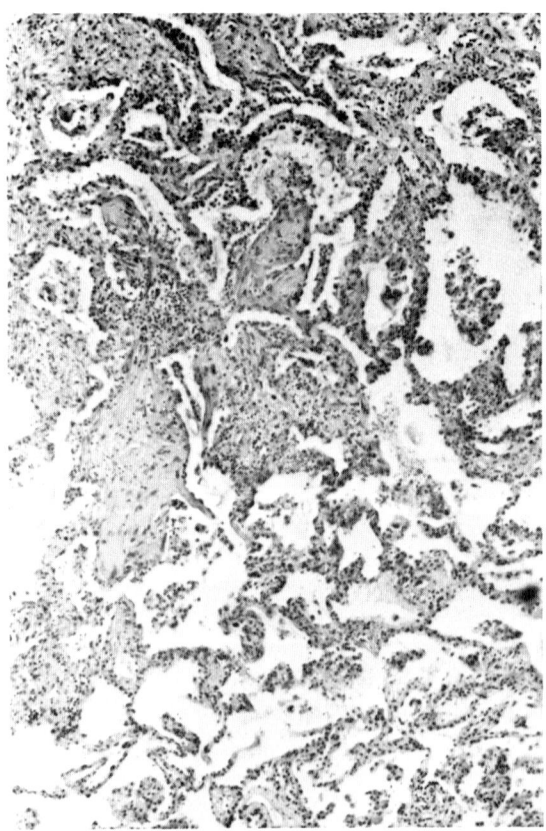

Fig. 1b.   Interstitial fibrosis (x 19.5).

developed pulmonary infiltrates during mitomycin therapy, with failure to ascribe these findings to any other cause. Five such patients are described.

II. PATIENTS AND METHODS

Case 1

A 58-year-old black woman was diagnosed as having adenocarcinoma of the stomach. She underwent gastrojejunostomy and choledocojejunostomy. In February 1973, combination chemotherapy with 5-fluorouracil 1100 mg/m² x 5 days given every 4 weeks and mitomycin 20 mg/m² IV bolus given every 8 weeks was started. A total of 6 doses of mitomycin and 14 doses of 5-FU were given until May 1974, when the patient developed shortness of breath and nonproductive cough without fever. She was hospitalized, and an extensive evaluation that included sputum for gram stain and routine bacterial cultures, AFB stains and cultures, fungal stains and cultures, viral studies for adenovirus, influenza A and B, respirating syncytial virus, parainfluenza 1, 2, 3, and pneumocystis carinii failed to reach a specific etiology for the pulmonary infiltrate (Fig. 1a). On May 15, 1974, she underwent thoracotomy, when pleural and multiple lung biopsies were taken. Histologic section demonstrated focal areas of fibrosis of the pleura and alveolar septa, with infiltration of numerous lymphocytes, plasma cells, and mononuclear cells and a few eosinophils. The alveolar septa in these areas were moderately thickened, and there was hyperplasia of the alveolar lining cells. Some of the alveoli contained macrophages and desquamated granular pneumocytes with PAS positive material in the cytoplasm. No vasculitis was present. No evidence of fungi or pneumocystis carinii was found. These findings were felt to be a chronic interstitial pneumonitis (Figs. 1b, 1c).

Case 2

A 68-year-old caucasian man underwent right hemicolectomy for Duke's C adenocarcinoma of the ascending colon. In August of 1974, the patient developed local recurrence, and was started on chemotherapy consisting of 5-fluorouracil infusion of 1100 mg/m² x 5 days repeated every 4 weeks and mitomycin C 20 mg/m² IV bolus to be given every 8 weeks. After 2 complete courses of this treatment, the patient developed increasing dyspnea, weakness, and nonproductive cough without fever. The arterial blood gases demonstrated severe hypoxia with PO_2 ranging between 35-40. Chest x ray showed bilateral pulmonary infiltrates (Fig. 2a). Evaluations for infectious causes were negative. A lung biopsy demonstrated interstitial pulmonary fibrosis. Corticosteroids were started, and the patient demonstrated both symptomatic improvement and decreased infiltrates on chest x ray. Chemotherapy with the same two agents was resumed with only one more course of mitomycin being given. The patient's respiratory symptoms recurred in October of 1975. A new extensive noninvasive workup failed to reveal the etiology of the pul-

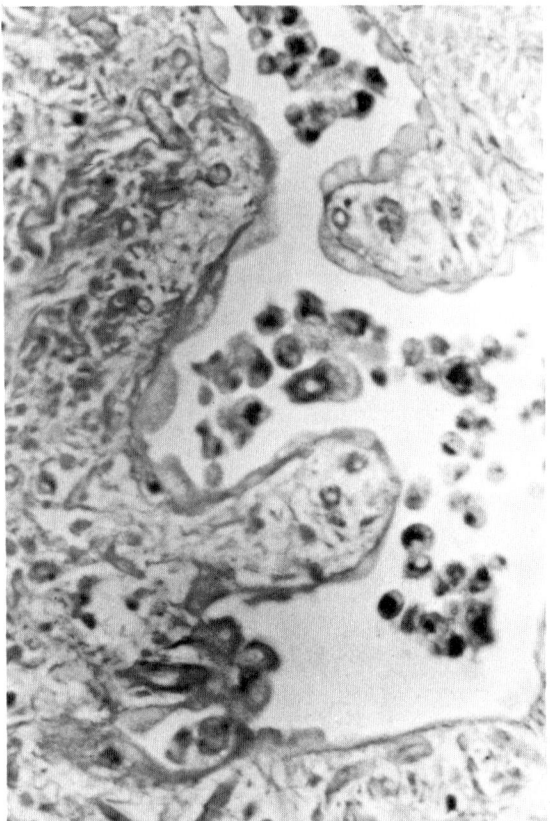

Fig. 1c.   Chronic interstitial pneumonia with desquamated cells into alveoli (x 98.15).

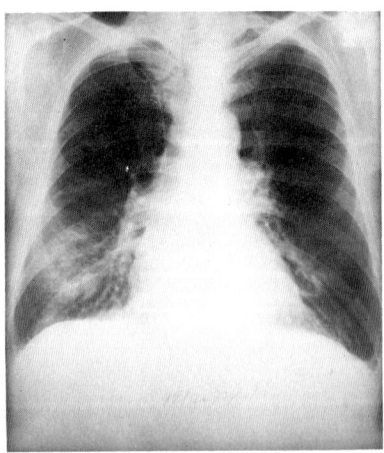

Fig. 2a.   Bilateral pulmonary infiltrates after two courses of mitomycin.

monary infiltrates. A second lung biopsy was done and interstitial pulmonary fibrosis was again demonstrated (Fig. 2b). The alveolar septa were thickened by a relatively acellular fibrous connective tissue. There was hyperplasia of the alveolar lining cells with exfoliation of some of the cells into the lumina of the alveoli. The small arteries exhibited slight fibrous thickening of the intima. The PAS stain was negative for fungi. Steroid therapy was restarted, but the patient failed to improve.

Case 3

A 68-year-old white male was diagnosed in June of 1973 as having adenocarcinoma of the rectum with metastases to lymph nodes, omentum, and liver. One month after hemicolectomy he was started on monthly 5-day continuous infusion of 1100 mg/m^2 of 5-fluorouracil and mitomycin C 20 mg/m^2 IV bolus at 8-week intervals. A partial response of greater than 50% was observed with this chemotherapy. After the second course of mitomycin, he developed symptoms of dyspnea, a cough productive of small amounts of white sputum, but no fever.

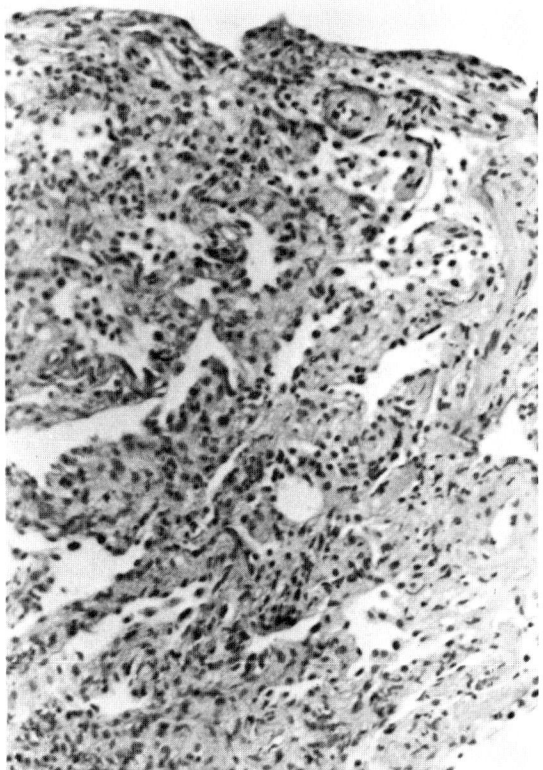

Fig. 2b.   Pulmonary interstitial fibrosis (x 48.75).

Chest x ray demonstrated bilateral interstitial infiltrates (Fig. 3a). Initial treatment was with digitalis and diuretics, to which minimal symptomatic improvement occurred. Following an additional course of mitomycin, the patient's x ray demonstrated increasing infiltrates. No further mitomycin was given but 5-FU was continued, and the partial remission of his tumor was maintained. Bronchoscopy with AFB, fungal, and routine cultures of bronchial washings, and silver stains for pneumocystis carinii demonstrated no evidence of an infectious etiology. Titers for cytomegalovirus and toxoplasma were within normal limits.

Open lung biopsy performed on December 19, 1973 demonstrated focal fibrosis of the parenchyma associated with hyperplasia of pneumocytes. Occasional hyaline membranes showed fibrous organization. Acute and chronic interstitial inflammatory infiltrates of moderate degree was present. There was thickening and tortuosity of arterioles (Fig. 3b). The pattern suggested diffuse alveolar damage that had progressed to fibrosis (Fig. 3c).

Treatment with digitalis, diuretics, and steroids resulted in no improvement. The patient died of respiratory failure on December 19, 1973. Postmortem examination demonstrated interstitial pulmonary fibrosis without evidence of bacterial, fungal, protozoan, or tuberculous disease.

Case 4

A 60-year-old caucasian male underwent a right hemicolectomy for adenocarcinoma in November of 1974. Local recurrence was found in November 1975, and 2 months later a right malignant pleural effusion developed. Systemic chemotherapy was begun in January 1976 with monthly 4-day continuous infusion of 5-fluorouracil and mitomycin C 15 mg/m^2 given every 8 weeks. Radiation therapy to a painful

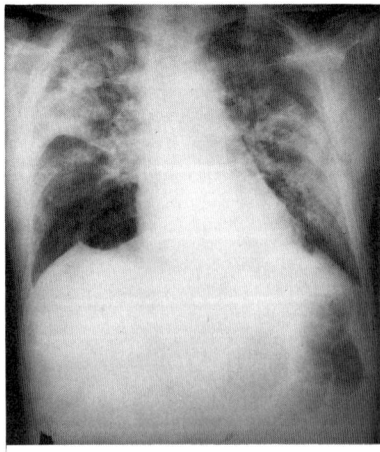

Fig. 3a.   Bilateral pulmonary infiltrates.

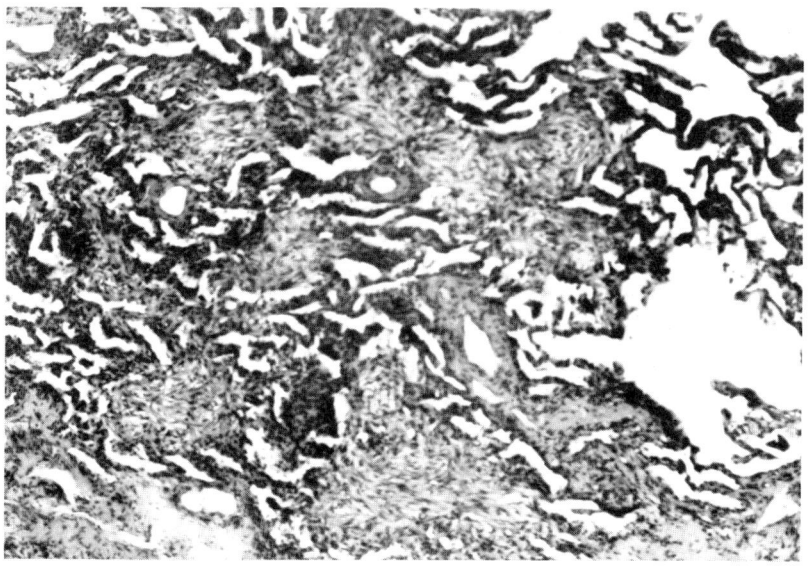

Fig. 3c. Pulmonary interstitial fibrosis (x 19.5).

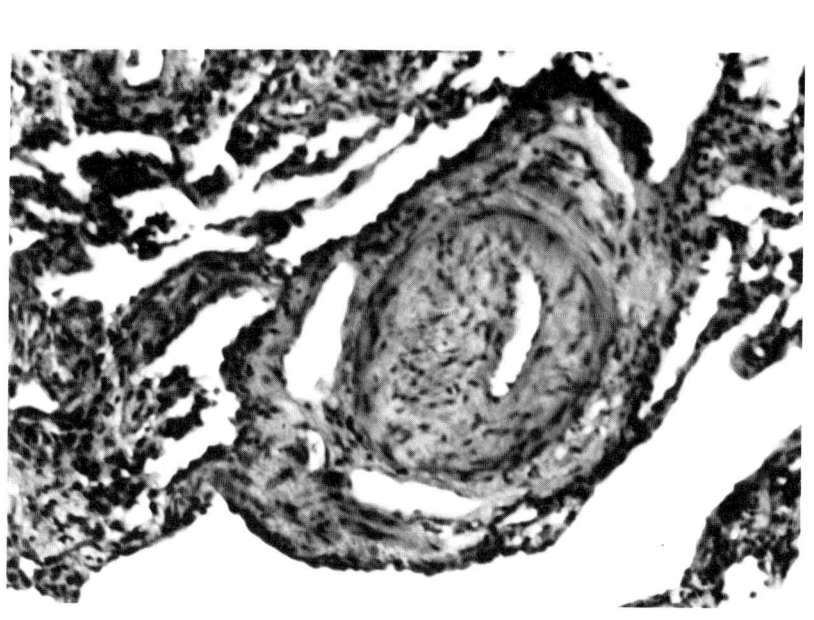

Fig. 3b. Pulmonary interstitial fibrosis with marked sclerosis of blood vessel (x 48.75).

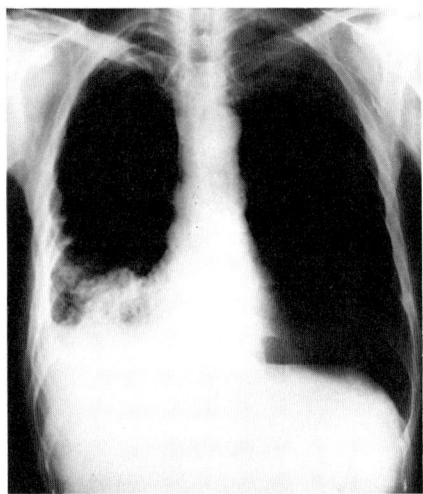

Fig. 4.   Localized pulmonary infiltrate of right lower lobe.

mass in the right lower quadrant of the abdomen was also given. The painful mass disappeared and the pleural effusion did not recur. Evaluation of the patient in April 1976 demonstrated no tumor.

In May of 1976 the patient developed exertional cough and dyspnea, with chest x ray showing a right lower lobe infiltrate (Fig. 4). An extensive work-up including studies for cytology, AFB, fungi, and pneumocystis carinii was done, and demonstrated no specific etiology for the infiltrate. Bronchography and bronchoscopy with bronchial washings and biopsy also failed to define a cause for the infiltrate. A chest x ray 3 weeks after initial evaluation showed the infiltrate to be decreasing in size. Since the patient had only minimal symptoms, no open lung biopsy was done. Therapy was continued with 5-FU alone. The pulmonary infiltrate remained unchanged.

Case 5

A 55-year-old caucasian female was diagnosed as having ascending colon carcinoma with pelvic metastasis in January 1973. She was known to have tricuspid incompetence and a patent foramen ovale. In July 1973 after palliative hemicolectomy she was started on 5-FU and mitomycin. She had evidence of improvement on this chemotherapy by disappearance of a mass that was pressing on the right ureter. In September of 1973, after the second course of mitomycin, the patient began to demonstrate marked lethargy and shortness of breath, with increased pulmonary wedge pressure which was thought to be a result of the cardiac anomaly. Treatment with diuretics, digitalis, and steroids resulted in clinical improvement. No further mitomycin was given; 5-FU was continued. The patient began to show

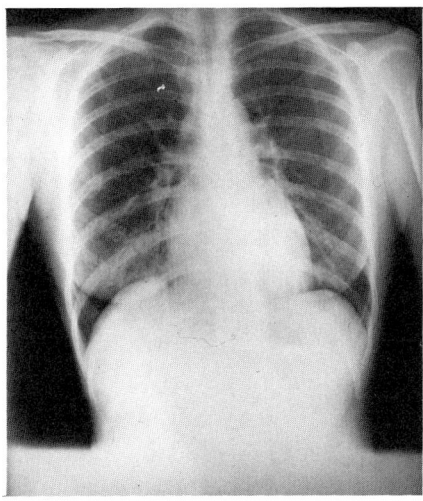

Fig. 5a.   Bilateral interstitial infiltrates following two courses of mitomycin.

evidence of continued pulmonary interstitial x ray findings (Fig. 5a) and worsening respiratory status. She became unresponsive to steroids, diuretics, and digitalis. Pulmonary function showed marked decrease in oxygen saturation. Bronchoscopy was performed, and biopsy demonstrated interstitial fibrosis. The patient continued worsening and expired on December 19, 1976. Postmortem examination confirmed interstitial fibrosis. Extensive alveolar macrophage proliferation with desquamation into the lumina was present. The alveolar walls appeared thickened and focally fibrotic, with an infiltrate of plasma cells, lymphocytes, and neutrophils. The arterioles demonstrated medial hypertrophy and narrowed lumina. Strands of fibrin in the alveolar spaces demonstrated focal early organization. A recticulum stain showed increased recticulum and thickening of alveolar walls. The trichrome stain also demonstrated focal fibrous thickening of alveolar walls (Fig. 5b).

III. RESULTS

That mitomycin C is an agent that causes pulmonary toxicity was suggested by Samson *et al.* (1978). In a group of 35 evaluable patients with primary lung carcinoma being treated with mitomycin C 20 mg/m^2 at a 6-week interval, one patient was found to develop pulmonary fibrosis for which no other etiology was found at postmortem. Orwoll *et al.* (1978) described three patients receiving mitomycin 20 mg/m^2 at 4-6 week intervals who developed respiratory symptoms and an interstitial infiltrate on chest x ray. The histology of lung biopsy was similar to ours but differed in that interstitial fibrosis was not prominent.

Histologic confirmation of pulmonary fibrosis was not obtained in our fourth

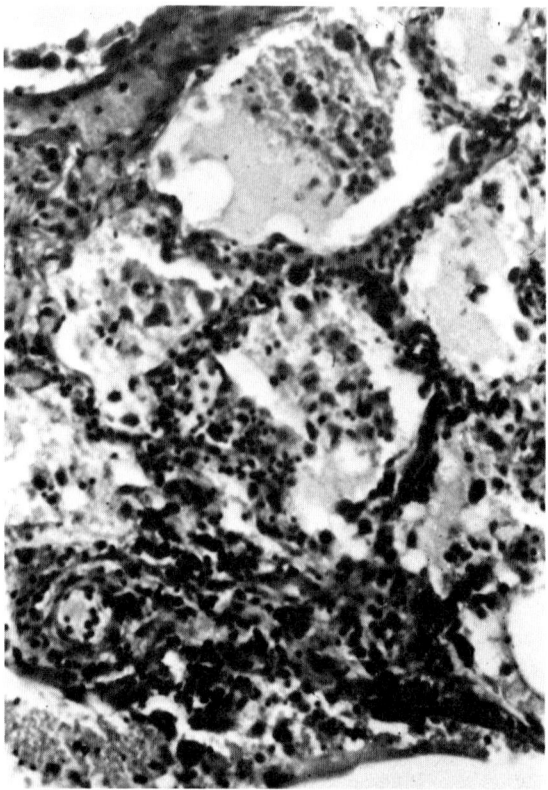

Fig. 5b.   Pulmonary interstitial fibrosis and pneumonitis.

case. Tissue from our other four cases demonstrated a similar picture. Focal fibrosis of alveolar septa was observed in all specimens. Two cases demonstrated visceral pleural fibrosis, and in one case there was thickening of the basement membrane. Capillaries and small arteries demonstrated thickening of their walls with luminal compression and narrowing. Some vessels contained thrombi. The alveolar pattern was distorted with hyperplasia of the alveolar lining cells and with exfoliation of these cells into the alveoli. One sample demonstrated a scant mononuclear infiltrate, and two others had an infiltrate of neutrophils, lymphocytes, and histiocytes. Vasculitis, necrosis, granuloma, and tumor were absent in all specimens. The clinical presentation of all five patients was similar; dyspnea, nonproductive cough, and hypoxia without fever. Case 3 and case 5 were treated with diuretics and digitalis. Some improvement was observed only in case 5, who had a history of underlying tricuspid insufficiency and a patent foramen ovale. However, this patient was also treated with steroids, and perhaps clinical improvement was on that basis and not due to diuretics and digitalis. Case 3 was also placed on steroids but only shortly prior to his death.

Case 2 was initially treated with steroids only, and demonstrated both clinical improvement and decreased infiltrate on chest x ray. Steroids were then stopped and one more course of chemotherapy was given. His symptoms increased, and steroids were resumed but resulted in no clinical improvement the second time. Cases 1 and 4 received no steroids or other specific treatment.

In four of the five patients, clinical symptoms occurred following the second course of mitomycin C (and fourth course of 5-FU). Two of these patients were then given one more course of both mitomycin and 5-FU; all four continued to deteriorate. Case 1 demonstrated symptoms after 6 doses of mitomycin C and 14 courses of 5-FU. In all five patients, studies for routine bacteria, AFB, fungi, and pneumocystis carinii were all negative. None of our patients had received radiation to thoracic structures or previous chemotherapy. Neither tumor, granuloma, nor infectious agents could be identified in pulmonary tissues obtained at biopsy or postmortem evaluation. All 5 patients were being treated for carcinomas of the gastrointestinal tract with 5-fluorouracil and mitomycin C. We suspected that our patients were experiencing pulmonary toxicity from chemotherapy. Since 5-fluorouracil has had wide clinical use and no pulmonary toxicity has been described with it, it seems most likely that mitomycin C is the toxic agent.

IV. DISCUSSION

Within the group of drugs that have thus far been described in the literature as causing pulmonary toxicity leading to fibrosis, drugs that appear to function at least in part as alkylating agents predominate, for example, busulfan (Schein et al., 1975; Rosenow, 1972; Sostman et al., 1977; Hankins et al., 1978; Stott et al., 1976) cyclophosphamide (Rosenow, 1972; Sostman et al., 1977; Stott et al., 1976; Scully et al., 1978; Mark et al., 1978; Patel et al., 1976), BCNU (Bailey et al., 1978; Crittenden et al., 1977), chlorambucil (Cole et al., 1978), and uracil mustard (Hankins et al., 1978). That their toxicity is directly related to their alkylating mechanism seems quite possible. It would therefore not be unlikely that other alkylating drugs such as mitomycin C result in similar pulmonary toxicity.

That the toxicity seen in our patients was dose related seems unlikely as four patients had received only two doses of mitomycin when symptoms began. The value of steroids once symptoms and x ray changes are present cannot be evaluated from our few patients. Nor is it entirely certain at present whether the toxicity is due to the combination of 5-FU and mitomycin rather than mitomycin alone.

Since mitomycin C is a commonly used antineoplastic drug, and since, similar to several other alkylating agents, it may produce pulmonary toxicity in the form of interstitial pneumonitis and fibrosis, we wish to alert physicians that in a patient who has a pulmonary infiltrate for which no other cause can be identified, mitomycin induced pulmonary toxicity may be the cause. In such situations no specific treatment can be advised from our limited experience, but a course of steroids and cessation of mitomycin C therapy would seem prudent.

REFERENCES

Bailey, C. C., Marsden, H. B., and Jones, P. H. M. (1978). *Cancer 42*, 74-76.

Baker, L. H., Caoli, F. M., Izbicki, R. M., Opipari, M. I., and Vaitkevicius, V. M. (1974). *Proc. Am. Assoc. Cancer Res. 15*, 182 (Abst.).

Bhat, K. S. S., Anderson, K. R., and Stewart, R. D. H. (1974). *Aust. N.Z. J. Med. 4*, 277-280.

Bristol Laboratories (1977). "Mutamycin in Selected Bibliography and Abstracts," pp. 84-86.

Brown, W. G., Hasan, F. M., and Barbee, R. A. (1978). *JAMA 239*, 2012-2015.

Buzdar, A. U., Tashima, C. K., Blumenschein, G. R., Hortobagyi, G. N., Yap, H. Y., Krutchik, A. N., Bodey, G. P., and Livingston, R. B. (1978). *Cancer 41*, 392-395.

Codling, B. W., and Chakera, T. M. H. (1972). *J. Clin. Pathol. 25*, 668-673.

Cole, S. R., Myers, R. J., and Klatsky, A. U. (1978). *Cancer 41*, 455-459.

Crittenden, D., Tranum, B. L., and Haut, A. (1977). *Chest 72*, 372-373.

Daskal, Y., Gyorkey, F., Gyorkey, P., and Busch, H. (1976). *Cancer Res. 36*, 1267-1272.

Einhorn, L., Krause, M., Hornback, N., and Furnas, B. (1976). *Cancer 37*, 2414-2416.

Elion, G. B. (1967). *Fed. Proc. 26*, 898-904.

Gutin, P. H., Green, M. R., Bleyer, W. A., Bauer, V. L., Wiernik, P. H., and Walker, M. D. (1976). *Cancer 38*, 1529-1534.

Hankins, D. G., Sanders, S., MacDonald, F. M., and Drage, C. W. (1978). *Chest 73*, 415-416.

Iacovino, J. R., Leitner, J., Abbas, A. K., Lokich, J. J., and Snider, G. L. (1976). *JAMA 235*, 1253-1255.

Jones, S. E., Moore, M., Blank, N., and Castellino, A. (1972). *Cancer 29*, 498-500.

Lascari, A. D., Strano, A. J., Johnson, W. W., and Collins, J. G. P. (1977). *Cancer 40*, 1393-1397.

Liu, K., Mittelman, A., Sproul, E. E., and Elias, E. G. (1971). *Cancer 28*, 1314-1320.

Mark, G. J., Lehimgar-Zadeh, A., and Ragsdale, B. D. (1978). *Thorax 33*, 89-93.

Moore, G. E., Bross, I. D. J., Ausman, R., Nadler, S., Jones, R., Jr., Slack, N., and Rimm, A. A. (1968). *Cancer Chemother. 52*, 675-684.

Nesbit, M., Krivit, W., Heyn, R., and Sharp, H. (1976). *Cancer 37*, 1048-1054.

Orwoll, E. S., Kiessling, P. J.,and Patterson, J. R. (1978). *Ann. Intern Med. 89*, 352-355.

Patel, A. R., Shah, P. C., Rhee, H. L., Sasson, H., and Rao, K. P. (1976). *Cancer 38*, 1542-1549.

Ratanatharathorn, V., Cadnapaphornchai, P., Rosenberg, B., Baker, L. H., Taher, S., Ruffner, B. W., McDonald, F. D., and Vaitkevicius, V. K. (1977). *Proc. Am. Soc. Clin. Oncol. 18*, 293 (Abst.).

Robert, J., Barbier, P., Manaster, J., and Jacobs, E. (1968). *Digestion 1*, 229-232.

Rosenow, E. C. III (1972). *Ann. Inter. Med. 77*, 977-991.

Rubin, G., Baume, P., Vandenberg, R. (1972). *Aust. N. Z. J. Med. 3*, 272-274.

Samson, M. K., Comis, R. L., Baker, L. H., Ginsberg, S., Fraile, R. J., and Crooke, S. T. (1978). *Cancer Treat. Rep. 62*, 163-165.

Samuels, M. L., Johnson, D. E., Holoye, P. Y., and Lanzotti, V. J. (1976). *JAMA 235*, 1117-1120.

Schein, P. S., and Winokur, S. H. (1975). *Ann. Intern. Med. 82*, 84-95.

Scully, R. E., Galdabini, J. J., and McNeely, B. U. (1978). *Case Records of the Mass. General Hospital 298*, 729-736.

Sostman, H. D., Matthay, R. A., and Putnam, C. E. (1977). *Am. J. Med. 62*, 608-615.

Stott, H., Stephens, R., Fox, W., Simon, G., and Roy, D. C. (1976). *Thorax 31*, 265-270.

Chapter 27

CLINICAL PHARMACOLOGY OF MITOMYCIN C

Steven D. Reich

I. INTRODUCTION

Mitomycin C has been in clinical use for about 20 years. Yet a paucity of information relating to the clinical pharmacology of the drug is available. The lack of a convenient, sensitive, specific assay for mitomycin C probably has been the factor that limited the number of studies on the clinical pharmacology of the drug.

II. RESULTS

A. Assay Methodology

The method of measurement that appears to be most widely used is a microbiological assay using growth inhibitory zones on agar plates as the parameter proportional to concentration (Schwartz and Philips, 1961; Fujita, 1971). The limit of sensitivity appears to be 0.1 $\mu g/ml$ with this method except when a particularly sensitive microorganism is available. The minimum assayable concentration of mitomycin C when this organism was employed was 0.002 $\mu g/ml$ (Fujita, 1971). A spectrophotometric procedure is available but is suitable for *in vitro* experiments only since the absorption maximum used is at a wave length at which plasma constituents would interfere (Schwartz and Philips, 1961). This method is probably not as sensitive as the microbiological assay. A high-pressure liquid chromatography method for assaying bulk samples of mitomycin C has been described (Sanhueza and Vulcano, unpublished report) using a μ Bondapak C_{18} column with detection at 254 nm, but this method is not sensitive enough for biological samples. Mass spectroscopy has been tried to both detect and quantitate drug and metabolites, but to date there have been no published reports of clinical studies using this method. Although the methodology available for mitomycin C assay is limited, the studies done thus far do give some information on the clinical pharmacology of the drug.

B. Absorption

Absorption from the gastrointestinal tract occurs in man and animals. Tests in rats innoculated with intramuscular Walker 256 tumor cells demonstrated a therapeutic ratio similar to intraperitoneal dosing, but 8 times as much drug was required with the oral route (Bradner, 1968). Other animal studies again showed similar toxic effects with oral and intraperitoneal routes, but the oral route required up to 12 times the comparable intraperitoneal dose (Philips et al., 1960). On the basis of these animal experiments and reports from Japan of oral activity in patients with cancer (Hibino, 1964), a phase I study of oral mitomycin was performed in the United States (Crooke et al., 1976). Of the 24 patients who were evaluable for response in this study of 31 patients with various advanced malignancies, no complete or partial responses were noted. However, of the 27 patients who were evaluable for toxicity, 6 experienced significant myelosuppression as shown in Table I. In general, toxic effects were observed in patients treated at the higher dose levels, and patients with peak serum concentrations of 0.4 μg/ml appeared uniformly to develop toxicity. Peak serum concentrations did not appear to correlate with dose, and the time to reach this peak was variable from patient to patient. The study concluded that the oral absorption of mitomycin C was erratic and that toxicity did not correlate with dose; the drug, therefore, could not be recommended for oral use.

Since encouraging results have been reported for intravesical treatment of bladder papillomas (Crooke et al., 1978), it should be noted that little absorption of active drug into the systemic circulation occurs when mitomycin C is directly in-

TABLE I. Myelosuppression after One Dose of Mitomycin C

Dose (mg/m^2)	Nadir ($\times 10^3$)	Time to nadir (days)	Peak serum concentration (μg/ml)	Previous chemotherapy
		Leukopenia (WBCs $<4000/mm^3$)		
30	2.6	51	0.4	5-FU, CTX
45	3.5	20	Unevaluable	None
45	3.7	16	0.4	None
		Thrombocytopenia (platelets $<100,000/mm^3$)		
22.5	54	12	0.4	Cooper, ADR
45	27	16	0.4	None
45	72	33	Unevaluable	None

stilled into the bladder. A report from Japan where a dose of 20 mg twice daily for more than 20 days was used demonstrated peak blood levels in the range of 0.002 to 0.0025 µg/ml (Imamura *et al.,* 1974). This range is below that detectable by assays available in the United States. The phase I-II trial of intravesical mitomycin C in the United States resulted in serum concentrations below 0.1 µg/ml and no serious systemic toxicity when 40 mg was instilled as a single dose (Crooke *et al.,* 1978).

C. Distribution

The distribution of mitomycin C was determined at 5 min in Guinea pigs given a dose of 5 mg/kg using a sensitive microbial assay (Fujita, 1971). The highest tissue concentration was obtained in the kidney and was about 7% of the serum concentration of 3.35 µg/ml. Urine and bile concentrations were about 25 µg/ml at this time. Muscle, heart, eye, tongue, and lung had concentrations above 0.1 µg/g of tissue. Liver, spleen, and brain had undetectable concentrations.

Different routes of administration can alter distribution as reflected in maximum blood concentrations. Perfusion can achieve a concentration of mitomycin C about five times as high as that of intravenous injection (Fujita, 1971). Arterial infusion can also give local concentrations about three times as high as those reached by the intravenous route. The concentrations for these various routes were reported in the Japanese literature, and details concerning the method of administration with respect to species and timing are lacking. A study done in the United States demonstrated that concentrations in the range of 2-15 µg/ml could be obtained in patients with pelvic perfusions (Mori *et al.,* 1962). However, severe toxicity to skin of the pelvic area was reported, especially in previously irradiated areas, and systemic toxicity was encountered when leakage occurred during the perfusion.

D. Metabolism

Metabolism of mitomycin C readily occurs in the presence of reducing agents. Mitomycin C can be reduced chemically by sodium hydrosulfite or biochemically by an NADPH-dependent system (Crooke and Bradner, 1976). The liver is thought to be the major organ of biotransformation, but most tissues have the capability of metabolizing the drug (Fujita, 1971). Homogenates of liver, spleen, kidney, brain, heart, lung, and testis have high capacities for metabolizing mitomycin C. The process may be enzyme mediated since the microsomal enzyme fraction has the greatest ability to metabolize the drug. Heating the homogenates for 5 min at 100°C completely inhibits the reaction. Dialysis of homogenates against water also inhibits the reaction, which suggests that low molecular weight cofactors are necessary for the reaction (Fujita, 1971). The presence of oxygen markedly decreases the rate of metabolism of mitomycin C (Schwartz and Philips, 1961).

The metabolism of mitomycin C appears to be related to that of other quinone-containing anticancer drugs such as doxorubicin (adriamycin) and lapachol (Bachur *et al.*, 1978). These agents interact with mammalian microsomes and function as free radical carriers. A free radical intermediate has been confirmed by electron paramagnetic resonance spectroscopy (EPR). Quinone drugs appear to augment the flow of electrons from NADPH to molecular oxygen. Flavoproteins may be intermediates in the transfer of electrons. The EPR signal suggests that the free radical intermediate has an extremely short half-life.

Metabolism of mitomycin C and the mechanism of action of the drug are closely related. Metabolism leads to unstable, reactive species with alkylating potential. Once these moieties react, they cannot react further. If the mitomycin C molecule is in the vicinity of a biologically important molecule such as DNA, irreversible damage may occur with metabolism. Otherwide, damage would be minimal, and the drug will be inactivated.

E. Excretion

Metabolism appears to be the major route of elimination of mitomycin C, but urinary excretion does play a role, especially at higher drug dosages. The urinary clearance of active mitomycin C in dogs approximates that of creatinine (Schwartz and Philips, 1961). The drug does not appear to be tightly bound to plasma proteins. These findings are compatible with glomerular filtration as the main route of kidney elimination.

Recovery of mitomycin C in urine is dependent on the dose of mitomycin C, as shown in Table II. The percentage of drug excreted by rats during a 24-hr period was increased with increasing dose (Schwartz and Philips, 1961). However, at lower dose levels, the degree of renal function did not play a major role in determining plasma concentrations, as shown in Fig. 1. At a dose (2 mg/kg) at which 18% of the drug would be expected to be excreted in urine during the first 24 hr, only minor changes in the plasma disappearance curve were noted. The β phase half-life increased from about 17 min in a normal rat to about 26 min in a nephrectomized rat. The significance of this increase is not known since no data was supplied on the variance associated with the assay procedure or on interanimal variability.

F. Pharmacokinetics

Unfortunately, studies of mitomycin C pharmacokinetics in man are rare. An early study done in Japan reported blood concentration data for 4 dose levels of

TABLE II. Recovery of Mitomycin C from Urine of Rats

Dose (mg/kg)	Recovery (%)
1.0	13
2.0	18
4.0	24
8.0	35

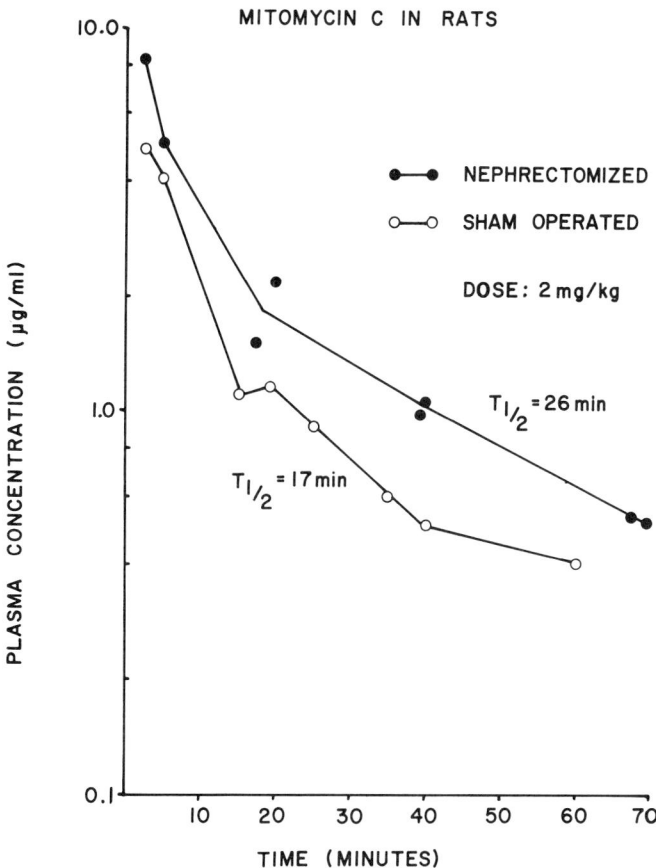

Fig. 1. Plasma disappearance of mitomycin C in rats after nephrectomy (●-●) or sham operation (0-0). Half-lives ($T_{1/2}$) are approximate (redrawn from Schwartz and Philips, 1961).

mitomycin C (Fujita, 1971). No detailed information on the assay or patient characteristics was given. The information supplied is in the form of a concentration versus time curve drawn on a linear scale. Redrawing the curve on a semilogarithmic scale gives more information. The redrawn curves are shown in Fig. 2. From the curves, distribution (alpha) and elimination (beta) phases can be identified. The possibility that another phase exists beyond the 120-min time point cannot be excluded. The beta phase half-lives determined from the redrawn figure are shown in Table III. These half-lives are different from those calculated by the authors of the Japanese paper who reported shorter values, as shown in Table III.

Too few points are available to determine the distribution phase half-lives. Extrapolation of the concentration curve to 0 min gives estimates of the initial volume of distribution from 4 to 15 L with an average of 9 L which suggests that mitomycin C is initially distributed in extracellular fluid.

Metabolism and excretion appear to be dose-dependent. Longer serum half-lives

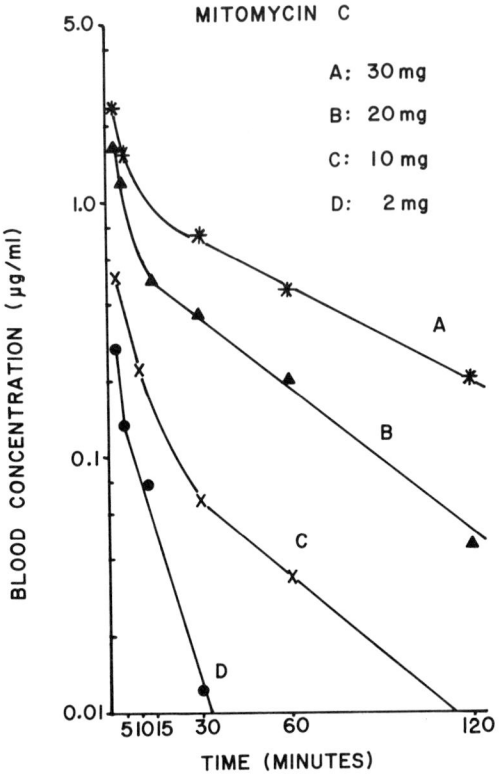

Fig. 2. Plasma disappearance curves of mitomycin C in man (redrawn from Fujita, 1971).

were found at the higher dose levels, and at least in animal studies a greater percentage of drug is excreted in urine during the first day at the higher dose levels. These findings are consistent with nonlinear kinetics, perhaps of the Michaelis-Menten type, due to saturation the enzymatic systems necessary for metabolism. Saturation of these mechanisms lead to prolonged levels in plasma, and therefore more is excreted by the kidneys. Renal function might therefore be a determinant of toxicity at higher dose levels since severe dysfunction might lead to elevated and markedly prolonged plasma levels. Liver function is probably important as well since mitomycin C is metabolized in this organ and is excreted into bile (Fujita,

TABLE III. Terminal Half-Lives of Mitomycin C Curves

Curve	Dose (mg)	$T\frac{1}{2}\beta$ (min) Original	Redrawn
A	30	17	49
B	20	10	33
C	10	9	30
D	2	6	7.5

1971). The studies needed to document increased plasma concentrations with associated increased toxicity in the presence of renal or liver dysfunction have not been performed.

G. Scheduling

The value of clinical pharmacological studies is that they can often help determine proper schedules of drug administration. Although it was found empirically that a high-dose intermittent schedule was efficacious with less toxicity than a low dose continuous schedule, the pharmacokinetics of mitomycin C are consistent with this observation. Since the cytotoxic effects of mitomycin C are not phase specific, the activity of the drug (both beneficial and adverse) should be related to drug exposure (Jusko, 1971). Drug exposure is defined as the area under the plasma concentration versus time curve. Because of the dose-dependent characteristics of this curve, large doses would give greater drug exposure than if the same total dose were given as multiple small doses. Although damage to normal tissues would also be greater with large doses, toxicity could be kept minimal if a sufficient length of time were allowed between courses. This argument is complicated by the report that doses of mitomycin C between 1.1 and 2.1 mg/kg administered by continuous intravenous infusion over 24 hr given in periods ranging from 3 to 12 days gave an incidence of hematopoietic toxicity comparable to a dose range of 0.9 to 1.2 mg/kg by single, daily injection over the same period (Sullivan, 1964). Of 30 patients treated with the infusion, no cases of stomatitis, nausea, or vomiting were noted, but eight objective and subjective responses were seen. These findings may be related to not only the clinical pharmacology of the drug, but also to the cytokinetics of normal and tumor cells.

H. Alteration of Pharmacokinetics

The clinical pharmacokinetics of mitomycin C can be manipulated in a variety of ways in an attempt to improve the therapeutic index of the drug. Different schedules can be employed, but it is often difficult to predict the resultant effects since cytokinetics may play a role in determining cytotoxicity. Since the drug is metabolized by microsomal enzymes, changing the metabolic profile of the liver may change the pharmacokinetics of the drug. Microsomal enzyme inducers such as phenobarbital or liver enzyme inhibitors such as *C. parvum* or cyclophosphamide may alter the toxicity to host or tumor. Timed-release agarose bead conjugates of mitomycin C can change both drug exposure and tissue distribution. Although these agarose bead conjugates have been prepared and shown to release active drug *in vivo* (Hashida *et al.*, 1977), their antitumor effect has not been reported on. The incorporation of mitomycin C into emulsions can also change the clinical pharmacokinetics of the drug with enhancement of the lymphatic transport of mitomycin C (Nakamoto *et al.*, 1975). High concentrations of drug within the lymphatic system might prove to be useful in the treatment or prevention of metastases.

III. DISCUSSION

A more complete knowledge of the clinical pharmacology of mitomycin C would be helpful in determining the factors that affect tumor response and toxicity to the host. Until a specific, sensitive, and reliable assay suitable for routine use is devised, the clinical pharmacologic studies of mitomycin C will be limited. Hopefully, now that there has been renewed interest in this active antineoplastic agent, more effort will be directed to the development of such an assay.

REFERENCES

Bachur, N. R., Gordon, S. L., and Gee, M. V. (1978). *Cancer Res. 38,* 1745-1750.

Bradner, W. T. (1968). *Cancer Chemother. Rep. 52,* 389-391.

Crooke, S. T., and Bradner, W. T. (1976). *Cancer Treat. Rev. 3,* 121-139.

Crooke, S. T., Henderson, M., Samson, M., and Baker, L. H. (1976). *Cancer Treat. Rep. 60,* 1633-1636.

Crooke, S. T., Johnson, D. E., and Bracken, R. B. (1978). *Proc. Amer. Soc. Clin. Oncol. 19,* 321.

Fujita, H. (1971). *Jap. J. Clin. Oncol. 12,* 151-162.

Hashida, M., Kojima, T., Takahasi, Y., Muranishi, S., and Sezaki, H. (1977). *Chem. Pharm. Bull. 25,* 2456-2458.

Hibino, S. (1964). *Acta. Un. Int. Cancer 20,* 267-270.

Imamura, K., Yoshida, H., Nakano, H., Ikeuchi, T., Yajima, N., and Shibaki, K. (1974). *Acta. Urol. Jap. 20,* 33-38.

Jusko, W. J. (1971). *J. Pharmacol. Sci. 60,* 892-895.

Mori, S., Clarkson, B., O'Connor, A., and Lawrence, W., Jr., (1962). *Clin. Pharmacol. Therap. 3,* 447-463.

Nakamoto, Y., Fujiwara, M., Noguchi, T., Kimura, T., Muranishi, S., and Sezaki, H. (1975). *Chem. Pharm. Bull. 23,* 2232-2238.

Philips, F. S., Schwartz, H. S., and Sternberg, S. S. (1960). *Cancer Res. 20,* 1354-1361.

Schwartz, H. S., and Philips, F. S. (1961). *J. Pharmacol. Exptl. Therap. 133,* 335-342.

Sullivan, R. D. (1964). *Antimicrob. Agents Chemother. 51,* 540-544.

Chapter 28

REFLECTIONS AND PROSPECTS

Stephen K. Carter

An old drug can always have a new lease on life. Mitomycin C proves the truth of that statement as well as any in the annals of modern chemotherapy. Discovered in Japan, initial clinicals trials of the drug in the United States date back nearly 20 years. The clinical trials in the United States validated that mitomycin C was an active drug especially in gastrointestinal cancer. Along with that activity was seen severe marrow toxicity, and the drug was considered to have a slim therapeutic index. This slim therapeutic index, on the schedules used, put the drug into a semi-limbo state where it was available only for investigational studies, which were not extensive. The reawakening of interest in mitomycin C came about with the uncovering of the high single-dose approach at a reasonable dose level. The high-dose intermittent schedule had been reported by the Japanese many years ago. An old study of the Eastern Cooperative Oncology Group at doses of 1-2 mg/kg had proven so toxic that it was discontinued. Years later when the 20 mg/m^2 dose level was used, activity was seen with a reasonable therapeutic index. The improved therapeutic index has made combination studies also more feasible, and several active regimens have been developed which were reported at this symposium.

Gastrointestinal cancer has always been one of the major indications for mitomycin C. The Japanese clinical data emphasized the activity in gastric cancer, which is the most common oncologic problem in that country. The initial studies in the United States emphasized colorectal cancer, reflecting its prominence in this country. In the early 1960s there was an assumption that all gastrointestinal adenocarcinomas were similar in terms of drug responsiveness. Therefore poor activity in colorectal cancer would be predictive for a similar fate in gastric and pancreatic lesions. The data of recent years has revealed that gastric cancer is more responsive to drugs than is large bowel cancer. Adriamycin is totally inactive in the low-lying adenocarcinomas but has significant activity in gastric cancer. Mitomycin C, while slightly active in colon and rectal tumors, demonstrated higher activity in stomach malignancies. The new emphasis on specific protocols for gastric cancer has exploited this activity of mitomycin C and brought it to renewed prominence and study.

Gastric cancer appears to be most sensitive, large bowel the least sensitive, and pancreas possibly intermediate. The data of Schein *et al.* (this volume), comparing the FAM regimen in all three sites is a good example. It is clear that adriamycin is an active drug in stomach cancer and an inactive drug in bowel cancer. While mitomycin C appears to have activity to some degree in all sites, there does appear to be a higher activity in gastric cancer, especially within the framework of combination studies.

Breast cancer is a tumor in which mitomycin C should have a greater role to play in future studies. Crooke, in his review, reports a cumulative response rate of 34.7% with 26 responses in 75 patients. The largest series is that of Moore, where 15/42 responses were reported. These 75 total cases are restricted to studies that clearly defined an objective response as a 50% decrease in the multiple of the two longest dimensions of a measurable mass. For a long time this activity has not been exploited in combination approaches, the probable reason being the perception of a slim therapeutic index for the drug that would make combination with other cytotoxic drugs difficult. The demonstration of the effectiveness of combining mitomycin with adriamycin and 5-FU in other solid tumors has opened up the possibility of these combinations being effective in breast cancer. The Northern California Oncology Group data on FOAM presented by Friedman (this volume) indicate that mitomycin C may have something meaningful to offer in breast cancer combination treatment.

Analog development in the mitomycin C area has received emphasis both in the United States and Japan but predominately in the latter country. In the United States porfiromycin received extensive clinical trial. Porfiromycin is N-methyl mitomycin C and was developed by the Upjohn Company with clinical trials sponsored by the National Cancer Institute. Porfiromycin showed no advantage over mitomycin C in either efficacy or toxicity. Baker *et al.* reported on a randomized prospective study of the two drugs. Thirty-two patients received mitomycin C 22.5 mg/m^2 Q 6-8 weeks and 31 received porfiromycin on an identical schedule (75 mg/m^2). Eleven patients (32%) who received mitomycin C achieved remission as compared tp 10 of 31 (32%) with porfiromycin. Both drugs produced significant myelosuppression; however, the porfiromycin toxicity appeared more cumulative.

In Japan several analogs have been clinically tested. The most prominent of which is carbazilquinone. This drug has shown an activity spectrum similar to that of mitomycin C but has also shown significant marrow toxicity. Trials in the United States are not currently contemplated.

Analogs are developed with the hope of improving the therapeutic index of active drugs. This includes increasing the response rate and/or diminishing the toxicity. A major limitation for mitomycin C is its bone marrow toxicity. An analog compound having a gentler marrow toxicity would have two major advantages: (*a*) to increase the potency of the active moeity in the mitomycin C so as to increase the overall response rate achievable; (b) to enable combination studies with other drugs at closer to full therapeutic doses for each component drug. One approach to analog development would be to select all compounds with comparable or superior experimental tumor activity as compared to mitomycin C and study these for experimental marrow toxicity. Those with the least marrow toxic potential could then be considered for clinical evaluation.

An important development in analog evaluation is the screening for toxicologic effects as well as for antitumor effect. With mitomycins this has involved screening for marrow toxicity and renal toxicity. Bradner (this volume) has described a prescreen of P-388 leukemia and toxicity in mice. The toxicity evaluation has included blood count depression in the mouse with a 35% decrease in WBC considered meaningful myelosuppression. This prescreen approach offers a matrix of 16 possible results on which to base decisions (Table I). Seven would be negative and indicate no further study, 5 would be positive, and 4 would indicate further study is possibly warranted.

The clinical study of a new mitomycin C analog will pose some specific problems. If the analog is predicted to be less myelosuppressive, the phase I study is to establish the highest dose of a drug that can be given safely to a patient. This is predicated on the cell-kill hypothesis that has governed so much of the chemotherapy clinical surgery study. We can expect that severe toxicity will be dose limiting for a mitomycin C analog. If it is not marrow, it might well be kidney, an organ damaged by mitomycins in large animal studies. If it is not renal, it will be hepatic, neurologic, or some other organ toxicity which will ultimately limit the dose. It must be hoped that if an analog is not myelosuppressive, its limiting toxicity will not be so severe or unpredictable as to prejudice future use of the compound.

If the compound is myelosuppressive in phase I, it could be hoped that the toxicity would not be as severe or cumulative as with mitomycin C. This could be manifested as a shallower dose response curve or as an increase in the quantity of drug administered.

Phase II would have to involve studies in mitomycin-responsive tumors such as gastrointestinal adenocarcinoma, breast cancer, and uterine cervix cancer. The end point would be a level of activity indicating some hope that the analog would be superior to mitomycin C. If more acceptable toxicity were the end point, then comparable activity to mitomycin C would be acceptable. Phase II studies in previously untreated large bowel and pancreas cancers would be easy to obtain as would trials in previously untreated non-oat-cell lung. In breast cancer, trials in patients failing primary combinations not utilizing mitomycin would also be easy to perform.

TABLE I. Marrow Toxicity

P-388 Activ.	None	<MMC	= MMC	>MMC
None	Neg.	Neg.	Neg.	Neg.
<MMC	?	?	Neg.	Neg.
= MMC	Pos.	Pos.	?	Neg.
>MMC	Pos.	Pos.	Pos.	?

Gastric cancer and uterine cervix would cause some difficulties since mitomycin C is used in the first-line effective combinations, but these also could be overcome.

The end result for phase III study of an analog is to clearly establish whether the analog is superior to mitomycin C or not. The perfect trial involves a prospective controlled comparison of the analog as a single agent versus mitomycin C as single agent. These trials are no longer common or popular in cancer chemotherapy. If a drug is active in phase II, it becomes quickly integrated into combinations. The new combination goes through a pilot study process that encompasses phase I and phase II and then, if positive, moves in phase III study. The problem of combination study is that it is often difficult to dissect out the absolute value of a single drug component. Thus, the oncology literature is full of data on drugs in combination whose true value and status in comparison with other analogs has still not been established. The nitrosoureas are examples that quickly come to mind.

Mitomycin C was first studied clinically in the United States in 1958. Twenty years later the drug is experiencing a renaissance of interest and clinical study. It is active in solid tumors with a broad spectrum and offers exciting potentials for combination study. Analog development is receiving renewed interest and, hopefully, we can look forward to even better effects in the future.